ETHICAL DIMENSIONS
in the Health Professions

FIFTH EDITION

RUTH B. PURTILO, PHD, FAPTA
Professor Emerita of Ethics
MGH Institute of Health Professions
Boston, Massachusetts;
John Marsh Visiting Professor
University of Vermont
Burlington, Vermont

REGINA F. DOHERTY, OTD, MS, OTR/L
Lecturer
Tufts University
Department of Occupational Therapy
Medford, Massachusetts;
Senior Occupational Therapist
Massachusetts General Hospital
Boston, Massachusetts

ELSEVIER
SAUNDERS

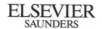

ELSEVIER
SAUNDERS

3251 Riverport Lane
St. Louis, Missouri 63043

ETHICAL DIMENSIONS IN THE HEALTH PROFESSIONS,
FIFTH EDITION   ISBN: 978-1-4377-0896-7

Notices

Knowledge and best practice in this field are constantly changing. As new research and experience
broaden our understanding, changes in research methods, professional practices, or medical
treatment may become necessary.

   Practitioners and researchers must always rely on their own experience and knowledge in evaluating and using any information, methods, compounds, or experiments described herein. In using
such information or methods they should be mindful of their own safety and the safety of others,
including parties for whom they have a professional responsibility.

   With respect to any drug or pharmaceutical products identified, readers are advised to check
the most current information provided (i) on procedures featured or (ii) by the manufacturer of
each product to be administered, to verify the recommended dose or formula, the method and
duration of administration, and contraindications. It is the responsibility of practitioners, relying
on their own experience and knowledge of their patients, to make diagnoses, to determine dosages
and the best treatment for each individual patient, and to take all appropriate safety precautions.

   To the fullest extent of the law, neither the Publisher nor the authors, contributors, or editors,
assume any liability for any injury and/or damage to persons or property as a matter of products
liability, negligence or otherwise, or from any use or operation of any methods, products,
instructions, or ideas contained in the material herein.

Library of Congress Cataloging-in-Publication Data

Purtilo, Ruth B.
   Ethical dimensions in the health professions / Ruth B. Purtilo, Regina F. Doherty. — 5th ed.
   p. ; cm.
   Includes bibliographical references and index.
   ISBN 978-1-4377-0896-7 (pbk. : alk. paper) 1. Medical ethics. I. Doherty, Regina F. II. Title.
   [DNLM: 1. Ethics, Professional. 2. Patient Rights—ethics. W 50]
   R724.P82 2011
   174'.2—dc22

                                                                                    2010038396

Executive Editor: Kathy Falk
Associate Developmental Editor: Lindsay Westbrook
Publishing Services Manager: Catherine Jackson
Senior Project Manager: Mary Pohlman
Senior Book Designer: Paula Catalano

Printed in the United States of America

Last digit is the print number: 9   8   7   6   5   4   3   2   1

Working together to grow
libraries in developing countries

www.elsevier.com | www.bookaid.org | www.sabre.org

ELSEVIER   BOOK AID   Sabre Foundation
            International

With gratitude to
the patients, professional colleagues, and students
whose experiences have taught us
volumes about the value and meaning of care.

Foreword

As a nurse ethicist in a tertiary care institution, I observe, hear about, and become involved in many of the complex cases that challenge interdisciplinary health professionals, patients, and surrogates on a daily basis. Health professionals are immersed in day-to-day clinical decisions that are increasingly complex and often require more from them than their requisite professional specialty training can offer. Today's health professional must have the language, forums, interdisciplinary collaboration, and support to effectively acknowledge and process these complex situations. Ruth Purtilo and Regina Doherty provide a readily accessible and clinically relevant format in the fifth edition of *Ethical Dimensions in the Health Professions* to support interdisciplinary health professionals in this quest. Dr. Purtilo has long been a leader in the concept and practice of interdisciplinary ethics and my opportunity to work with Dr. Doherty in her position as Co-Chair of the Massachusetts General Hospital Ethics in Clinical Practice Committee successfully demonstrated her skill in highlighting the benefits of interdisciplinary collaboration in ethically challenging cases.

This book makes ethical theory applicable for the practicing clinician by placing its use within the Six-Step process of analysis and highlighting the ethical decision-making process utilizing a wide variety of case studies. The Six-Step model assists health professional students and practicing clinicians in approaching the often overwhelming nature of a clinical ethics situation that can be replete with high emotion, a multitude of facts, and lack of clarity. For many years now, I have used the Six-Step process in teaching students and practicing professionals. It is highly accessible to both. Its common sense problem-solving approach allows a weaving in of ethical theory in context that otherwise can become overly theoretical and difficult for the student or professional to embrace in the absence of the model. The fifth edition of *Ethical Dimensions in the Health Professions* continues to make this contribution to both the student and the lifelong learner at a time when ethical complexities are on the rise. The addition of new Chapter 2, "The Ethical Goal of Professional Practice: A Caring Response" and Chapter 11, "Communication and Information Sharing" represents topics that are current and needed for ethical analysis and decision making. The "caring response" as articulated in the text draws attention to behaviors that help to accomplish this essential goal, beautifully expressed in a way that is understandable and tangible. Never in the history of the professions is the recognition of "empathic communication" more needed in both education and practice. The authors urge readers to embrace reflection on the impact of their roles as they practice. Through doing so the reader is better prepared to provide ethically sensitive care.

As a consummate supporter of interdisciplinary collaboration in the clinical setting, I am excited about the fifth edition of *Ethical Dimensions in the Health Professions*. In my role as Co-Chair of the MGH Optimum Care Committee, I have consistently observed that patients and their surrogates benefit most when health professionals of all disciplines involved in their care come together to share their expertise, challenge assumptions, and, in the end, arrive at creative alternatives that could not possibly be derived through the eyes of a single discipline. I am certain you will find that use of this book will bring clinical ethics alive for you as a student and practicing health professional.

Ellen M. Robinson, RN, PhD
Nurse Ethicist, Institute for Patient Care
Co-Chair, MGH Optimum Care Committee
Massachusetts General Hospital
Boston, Massachusetts

Preface

Every day health professionals confront ethical issues in their practice. This text gives readers the basic tools to use for recognizing ethical issues, building understanding, and working toward the resolution of ethical problems. The goal is to improve the lives of patients, the community, and themselves. Practitioners in the health professions are members of society who are transformed from simply caring to learn to also learning to care. The tone of this book is practical throughout, designed for people on the front lines of health care decision making. Society expects its health professionals to be informed about current ethical issues and to be moral agents in helping to address them.

This fifth edition of *Ethical Dimensions in the Health Professions* reflects the authors increased awareness that ethics has to be taught, and taught well, so that students will be well prepared for their role. Today's health professional must not only have knowledge and skills, but effectively balance these with sound judgment and responsibility for action. Effective ethical decision making in clinical practice demands that the professional use clinical reasoning—a complex thought process that entails thinking, analyzing, decision making, acting, and reflecting upon professional practice. Ethical reasoning is not used in isolation, but rather in concert with other types of clinical reasoning. Administrators and teachers in professional education continue to work toward offering more and better professional ethics courses, seminars, and continuing education opportunities that emphasize this shift. Furthermore, in many educational programs, educators skillfully have woven ethics theory and practice into the very fabric of the student's learning experiences in the clinic as well as the classroom. Our goal in preparing this updated and expanded edition has been to reflect these positive changes.

What's New in this Edition

At the outset you will notice the addition of Regina Doherty, a respected occupational therapy clinician and educator as a co-author. Whose training, professional experience, and expertise in ethical reasoning enhance the pages of this text. Our collaborative work in interdisciplinary classroom teaching, the development of curricular materials, and leadership in the development of an international consortium on ethics education, were prompts to enrich this book through a co-authored effort. The text remains deeply interdisciplinary and clinically oriented. Readers of previous editions will notice signature features carried through into this edition, among them the overarching goal of professional practice, a caring response; the three prototypes of ethical problems; the six-step process of ethical decision making; narrative accounts to illustrate relevant ethics themes in everyday practice; built- in reflective exercises; summary statements; and questions for thought and discussion at the end of each chapter. Cases and federal statutes and regulations that have ethical bearing in practice have been updated.

In Section One the reader is introduced to the idea of morality and ethical study, which includes an expanded section on law and ethics. A new chapter is now devoted entirely to care. This includes the concept of care and characteristics of a caring response in the health professions. A new section on modes of clinical reasoning helps the reader to set the context for more critical reflection on the various ethical dimension of practice. Section Three has been reorganized to reflect updated national standards and challenges. The most recognizable change is the addition of a new chapter on communication, a foundational aspect of therapeutic relationships. Given the heightened reliance on new mechanisms of communicating in health care, this chapter focuses directly on the ethical dimensions of information sharing. It provides insights to help students examine communication through the lens of ethical decision making. Given the increased awareness on health disparities, Section Five includes an expanded emphasis on social justice. As in previous editions, our intent is to help readers prepare for their role as moral agents and enhance their ability to effectively confront ambiguities in practice. The final chapter highlights moral agency and responsibility in its expanded forms. Here opportunities present in societal spheres where the roles of the health professional and citizen meld.

The fifth edition stands on the shoulders of the previous four, grounded securely in theory and those enduring concerns that have supported the need for professional ethics and ethical professionals since the beginnings of health care. It also builds on our abiding conviction that health professionals can and should assume a strategic position to help shape the contours of today's health care environment so that it embraces and protects cherished social values. We hope that *Ethical Dimensions in the Health Professions* will serve as a guide and welcome companion on your journey in professional ethics. This journey is, we believe, a key to finding self-fulfillment in professional life.

Ruth B. Purtilo
Regina F. Doherty

Acknowledgments

Edition Five

The first edition of this book was co-authored by Ruth Purtilo and Dr. Christine Cassel. Readers familiar with Dr. Cassel's outstanding contributions to health care and health policy will recognize her ideas and insights still woven into the very warp and woof of the text.

We owe a debt of gratitude to the health professions students and colleagues we have had the opportunity to teach and learn from at our respective current places of employment, including the MGH Institute of Health Professions, The University of Vermont at Burlington, Tufts University, and the Massachusetts General Hospital. We have led and served on several ethics committees throughout our careers, and these interdisciplinary discussions have expanded our understanding of how ethical issues impact the lives of patients, their families, health professionals, and institutions. Our mentors and supporters along the way are too numerous to mention here. We have benefitted greatly from their generosity and care.

Lastly, a heartfelt thanks to our husbands, Vard Johnson and Dan Doherty, whose deep support and respect for our professional endeavors nourish our work and lives; and to Regina's young daughter, Olivia Grace, and Ruth's goddaughter, Allison Cole, whose inquisitive spirits and open hearts are sources of great motivation and joy.

Ruth B. Purtilo
Regina F. Doherty

Notes to Instructors on Using This Edition

The core purpose of this book is to provide the tools for addressing common, everyday ethical issues in the health professions. Our hope is that both you and your students will find it user-friendly! The goal of a caring response (Chapter 2), and the concept of moral agency (Chapter 3) provide a framework throughout the text for ethical analysis and action.

Instructional Tools

A Six-Step Process of Ethical Decision Making

The Six Steps	Building Blocks
Step 1: Gather relevant information	One must pay critical attention to the details of a situation. This means learning to distinguish clinical, legal, and ethical content.
Step 2: Identify the type of ethical problem	The three prototypes of ethical problems introduced in Chapter 3 help to organize the details of a narrative into the appropriate category (or categories) for ethical analysis.
Step 3: Analyze the problem using ethics theories or approaches	In Chapter 4 the skills of ethical reasoning are put into play. The foundational theories, approaches, and methods of ethics (i.e., moral virtues, rights, duties, and principles) are introduced here as tools for analysis.
Steps 4: Explore the practical alternatives	This step focuses on the realistic options for carrying through with ethically appropriate action. Openness and creativity are essential.
Step 5: Act	In this step, action is required. The resolve and courage to proceed are needed.
Step 6: Evaluate the process and outcome	In this final step, the professional/s reflect on the ethical decision, action, and outcomes. Attention is paid to what can be learned for future situations.

Each chapter contains:
- *A Narrative* to illustrate key themes in that chapter
- Educational *Objectives* for the chapter
- *New Terms* introduced in the chapter
- A list of *Key Concepts* used in the chapter and where each first appeared in the book
- *Reflection* exercises throughout the text encourage students to pause for their own response during their study when a key concept or point has been made.
- *Numerous Summary Statements* within each chapter and at the end of each chapter help guide the reader along.
- *Questions for Thought and Discussion* are included at the end of each chapter for group discussion or individual reflection. This includes additional cases along with other exercises reinforcing the main points of the chapter.
- *References* are provided for those interested in learning more about a particular topic.

Objectives

Through studying this book and discussing the *Questions for Thought and Discussion,* students will be able to:
1. Increase their knowledge and understanding of the ethical dimensions of professional practice.
2. Identify how the goal of finding a caring response factors into a wide range of ethical issues in professional practice.
3. Recognize the nature and scope of their moral agency as a health professional.
4. Competently apply ethical reasoning with the help of a straightforward problem-solving method designed for ethical situations.
5. Become competent in utilizing basic ethics theories, approaches, and concepts widely used today to address ethical challenges in professional practice.
6. Recognize current and longstanding themes in professional ethics and cite examples of concrete ethical situations reflecting them.
7. Gain insight into ethical situations and problems that are unique to their own profession, in contrast to those shared by a wide range of health professionals.
8. Recognize the ethical issues that present in the societal context of health care.
9. Find resources that are useful for more in-depth study of professional ethics.

Contents

Guide to Stories in Text

Introduction to Ethical Dimensions in the Health Professions

1

Morality and Ethics: What Are They and Why Do They Matter?

Objectives

The reader should be able to:
- Define morality and ethics and distinguish between the two.
- Describe the differences among and relationship of personal, group, and societal moralities that health professionals must integrate into their own moral life.
- Describe the function of a health professions code of ethics in terms of professional morality.
- List three ways in which ethics is useful in everyday professional practice.
- Compare the basic function of law and ethics in professional practice.
- Identify some laws and policies that protect the personal moral convictions of health professionals while upholding ethical standards of the profession.
- Delineate a basic distinction between theories of action and virtue and between approaches that emphasize individuals or communities as the primary moral concern of ethics.

New terms and ideas you will encounter in this chapter

plateau	integrity	ethics committees
morality	societal morality	Constitutional law
moral judgment	group morality	statutory law
values	professional morality	administrative law
moral value	code of ethics	common law
moral duty	Hippocratic Oath	state interests
moral character/virtue	ethics	licensing laws
personal morality	ethicists	moral repugnance

Introduction

Your adventure into the world of health care ethics begins with a story. Throughout this textbook you will meet patients, health professionals, families, and others who face challenges posed by their situations and the health care environment. Their stories illustrate the types of ethical issues you yourself may face as a caregiver, a patient, or a family member. The underlying ethical themes in the stories are woven into the very fabric of health care. This book attempts to pull out the threads, examine them for their unique or interesting characteristics, and assess the role each plays in the overall scheme of good professional practice.

The following story concerns the Harvey family and the health care system into which they are catapulted after the tragic events of a beautiful late spring day.

🦋 The Story of the Harvey Family and the Health Care Team

Drew Harvey was undoubtedly one of the most popular students at Mountmore College. Now in his senior year, he was captain of the college basketball team, which had had its best season ever, going to regional competition, and he had his own band that played every Saturday night at the most popular local pub, the Mole Hole. He had played more than studied during his first 2 years of college, never having to "crack the books" in high school. But after his sophomore year, he worked as an assistant in a local law firm. When he returned in his junior year, he announced that he was going to become a lawyer. He buckled down, gaining an almost straight "A" record, without having to give up basketball or the band.

May 20

The violent incident that occurred the weekend before commencement rocked the entire community. Drew's band was playing at the Mole Hole at an event reserved for the college seniors and their friends. At the end of the first set, just as Drew was acknowledging the band members to the applause and howls of the audience, he suddenly staggered backward; blood appeared on his forehead as he fell forward off the platform. After a moment of stunned silence, someone screamed, "He's been shot!" Pandemonium broke out. Someone called 911. Drew mumbled, a confused and frightened look on his face, "What's going on?" Then he lost consciousness. He was taken to the emergency department of a hospital, where a bullet was determined to have lodged in his skull, penetrating it above his left temple.

The physician assistant and nurses on duty administered first aid trauma measures. By now his parents had arrived. The physician on call asked

Drew's mother, Alice, to sign informed consent, insurance, and other forms and began to prepare Drew for immediate surgery to remove the bullet and for subsequent admission to the hospital.

Mrs. Harvey wept. When a nurse put an arm across Alice's shoulder and said, "I'm sorry," Alice began to cry inconsolably. Alfonso Harvey, Drew's father, stood off to one side, staring straight ahead as if in shock. The nurse offered to get Alice a drink of water and guided them to a private waiting room while explaining what would happen next. Police were everywhere.

June 11

After 2 weeks in the intensive care unit, Drew regained consciousness. The shunt that had been placed in his skull to relieve the swelling of his brain was working well. He was beginning to focus his gaze, and the nurses believed he was trying to say something, although no one else saw this gesture yet. On the 18th day, the physician reported that Drew would be transferred to the medical unit. This morning, 22 days after the shooting, the physician told Alice that Drew's condition was stabilized and he would be going home soon. "Home!" Alice gasped. "How can we possibly manage at home? He can barely talk, can't walk, can't go to the bathroom alone!" The social worker who was standing at the foot of the bed explained that the Harveys would be visited by a home care nurse and for some time (depending on his progress) by an occupational therapist, physical therapist, speech therapist, and others. The physician reminded the Harveys that Drew's progress exceeded their expectations, likely a reflection of the excellent physical shape he was in before his trauma. The social worker added that a home health aide also would visit periodically. The physician did caution that although Drew's condition was improving, how much it would finally improve was impossible to predict. However, she said the entire team was hopeful.

July 11

At home, Drew's right arm and hand regained function so that he could almost dress himself. He could not walk because of spasticity of the right leg, although the spasticity seemed at times to be subsiding. He suffered from a limited vocabulary but increasingly caught himself when he used a wrong word. Because of this progress, the case manager authorized another 6 weeks of physical therapy, speech therapy, and occupational therapy.

Mr. and Mrs. Harvey were understandably anxious but very supportive throughout the entire ordeal, encouraging their son toward as much independence as possible and offering support when needed. Drew's older brother made some adjustments in the Harveys' home to accommodate Drew's impaired functional status.

Today (August 1)

The several health professionals working with Drew have grown attached to him and his family. They have rejoiced with every sign of progress and have struggled with him through the frustration and depression that accompany such a catastrophe. But the health professionals are now faced with a difficult situation. Another treatment review is due. Understandably, when no further progress can be shown, authorization for his treatments (and therefore, the reimbursements for them) will be discontinued. At the moment, his progress seems to have stopped.

Anyone who works with patients who experience brain trauma knows that the team faces a critical and delicate situation. The rate of "progress" is not always constant. It may be marked by periods of rapid improvement interspersed with other periods of almost no perceptible change (*plateaus*). If the patient ceases to receive maintenance treatments during these plateau periods, a dramatic loss in functioning may occur. Yet many insurance plans or other reimbursement mechanisms make little or no allowance for these plateau periods, and treatment usually is discontinued. A patient must have a symptom that becomes acute again before treatment can be reinstituted. In summary, although progress eventually does end, the failure to allow for a plateau period often results in the patient's premature discontinuation from treatment altogether. This is precisely the ambiguity facing the health professionals who have been treating Drew Harvey.

The Story of the Harvey Family (continued)

Drew's speech and progress in performing activities of daily living have reached a plateau. Yet the health professionals have not reached an agreement regarding whether more improvement may be on the way if his condition is not allowed to slip back. Maybe he will be able to avoid lifelong use of a wheelchair if his treatment is not discontinued at this critical juncture. But his university's health plan insurers use success ("outcomes") measures that make it unlikely he will continue to be reimbursed for therapy costs. The health professionals know that continued payments for treatment depend on their report of his progress. What should they do?

• Should they "bend the truth a little," reporting that Drew continues to make daily progress, so that he is less likely to lose an opportunity for possible further progress?

• Should they tell the truth, knowing that Drew will be discontinued from treatment at this time?

- What other alternatives to an either/or solution to this perplexing problem should they pursue?
- Should they get involved in trying to change the insurance company policies that put them in this difficult situation in the first place?

 Reflection

Suppose you are treating Drew and believe you are the one who has to be an advocate for him and his family. What, if anything, should you do to figure out some way to report on his condition that gives him a chance at a few more treatment sessions? Questions with a broader outlook might occur as well. For instance, is it fair to continue treating him if you are not prepared to make a similar defense for all patients in a comparable situation? Or an even broader scope may be encompassed: Are you as a health professional responsible for trying to change the insurance system or hospital policies so that such situations do not occur and you can more easily give patients what you think they need?

Take a minute to jot down what you think are the most important challenges facing health professionals involved with Drew Harvey's situation, regardless of whether they are suggested in the text:

1. _____

2. _____

3. _____

4. _____

Responses to these challenges are not found in the textbooks that deal with the technical skills of your chosen field. You are beginning to use your understanding of morality and how ethics figures into your professional life if you are concerned with what would be right or wrong conduct for you in this situation and why; what your duties are to everyone involved and what your (and everyone else's) rights are; also if you are thinking about the type of character traits you want to preserve; or what constitutes fairness for all patients in similar situations. In a word, what is involved in showing Drew and his family that you care?

 SUMMARY

Facing difficult human questions about right and wrong conduct, duties, rights, character traits, and fair treatment is part and parcel of your professional ethical life.

These considerations may even make you think about what type of society you want to help build in your professional career. In all of these areas of your professional life, you are dealing with morality and moral values.

Morality and Moral Values

When *morality* is mentioned, you might think of what you were told to do or not to do as a child. You are right. That is a part of morality. But morality is a much richer set of ideas than that. From the earliest societies onward, people have established guidelines designed to preserve the very fabric of their society. The guidelines become a natural language and behavior that describe the way things ought to be and what types of things we should value. Most members of society accept these guidelines, allowing the assumptions on which morality is based to prescribe decisions about many aspects of daily life.

Morality is not simply an intellectual exercise. Individuals and groups feel strongly about what is right and wrong, good or bad. A part of moral development is to instill these assumptions into children at a deep emotional level so that acting on the guidelines is not only habitual but makes them feel as if the right decision was taken. Viewed collectively, these guidelines constitute a society's morality.

First and foremost, morality is relational. It is concerned with relationships between people and how, ultimately, they can best live in peace and harmony. The goal of morality is to protect a high quality of life for an individual or for the community as a whole. Ethicists Tom Beauchamp and James Childress summarize it this way: "certain things ought or ought not to be done because of their deep social importance in the ways they affect the interests of other people."[1] It follows that morality is context dependent. A *moral judgment* is needed when the particulars of a specific situation arise. When you are faced with being an advocate for Drew, you are forced into thinking of him in very specific terms as a human in relationship to his family, to the health professionals, and to society.

Values is the language that has evolved to identify intrinsic things a person, group, or society holds dear. Not all values are *moral values* of course. For instance, some things are cherished for their beauty, novelty, or efficiency they bring to our lives. Things that uphold our ideas of what is needed for morality to survive and thrive are viewed as moral values. Many moral values describe qualities that support individuals in their desire to live full lives, allowing them to pursue their own basic interests and providing help for others to do so. We ascribe moral value to character traits of persons or societies, too, making a moral judgment of their being praiseworthy or blameworthy traits. A compassionate person is judged as praiseworthy and a cruel one as blameworthy; a just society is praiseworthy and one that holds its citizens in a grip of terror is blameworthy.

Moral duty and *moral character* also are associated with morality. Duty is a language that has evolved to describe actions in response to claims placed on a person or society. Not all duty is moral duty, just as not all we value is of moral value. Moral duty describes certain actions required of you if you are to play your part in preventing harm and building a society in which individuals can thrive. Specific duties and the ethical theories based on this aspect of morality are described in Chapter 4. Moral character or *virtue* is a language used to describe traits and dispositions or attitudes that are needed to be able to trust each other and to provide for human flourishing in times of stress, such as compassion, courage, honesty, faithfulness, respectfulness, humility, and other ways of being in the world that we want to be able to count on. These traits taken together and exercised regularly make up what we mean when we say a person is "of high moral character." These, too, are addressed more fully in later chapters of this book.

As a child, you acquired parts of your morality from parents, family, and friends; reading and television; your religious teaching; and experiences in school. Behavior was modified when knowingly or unknowingly you did something outside of what you had been taught is right and you were punished or shamed by others for what you did (or failed to do).

 Reflection

Consider some sources that have informed your own moral beliefs. Your answers can be personal reference points as you read on about morality.

1. Who or what have been five important influences on your understanding of right and wrong?

a. _____

b. _____

c. _____

d. _____

e. _____

2. Name three people who you admire for living exemplary moral lives. They may be people you know personally or only by reputation. What makes them admirable?

a. _____

b. _____

c. _____

Morality informs many decisions in your everyday experience, but you are so accustomed to moving through your life in accordance with your moral values and actions associated with moral duty that you have little conscious awareness of it. In short, it is safe to say that morality is habitual, shaping the character of individuals and communities, most of the time without them even realizing it.

As a student entering the health professions, you must reckon with at least three subgroups of morality: your personal morality, societal morality, and the morality of the health professions and its institutions. Fortunately, there are large areas of overlap. Whether as an individual among family members or friends, as a citizen, or as a professional, the sources of moral belief usually derive from similar understandings of value, of right and wrong, and of desirable character traits.

Personal Morality

Personal morality is a collage of values, duties, actions, and character traits each person adopts as relevant for his or her life. It is "who you are" as a unique moral being among others; you named some of the influences on you in the previous reflection. Everyone has a personal morality, and you must become intimately familiar with the particulars of your own. Doing so enhances the self-understanding that is essential to you as you begin to take on the responsibilities and tasks of your professional role. It is also a foundation stone from which you can step out to try to understand and respect the personal morality of patients, colleagues, and others with whom you come into professional contact. To illustrate, the health professionals treating Drew Harvey will not be successful if they are not aware of their own moral values and beliefs as they encounter the moral values and beliefs of the Harvey family. Without deep self-awareness, it is impossible to discern why you respond to another with the feelings, emotions, and judgments that arise in the course of your communications and decisions.

 Reflection

Identify five key components of your own personal morality (e.g., lying is wrong; I should be kind to myself and others; everyone deserves respect).

1. _____

2. _____

3. _____

4. _____

5. _____

Compare your list with a classmate's to discuss key differences and how you think they might affect your lives as future colleagues in the health professions. Also, identify areas of agreement.

Personal Morality and Integrity

One of the most essential resources in your professional life is your own integrity. Its components are embedded in the values that make up your personal morality; when you act in accordance with those values, you can be assured you have preserved your *integrity*. The term "integrity" comes from the Latin *integritas,* meaning unimpaired condition, sound, whole, undivided. It is easy to understand how living by the guidance of your personal morality helps you to maintain a clear sense of who you fundamentally are when challenges arise. The reward is that you can maintain a sense of unified purpose, direction, and action as different kinds of situations arise. Edmund Pellegrino summarizes it well:

> *"Classically, personal integrity has been understood as a person's commitment to live a moral life. The woman or man of integrity is honest, reliable, and without hypocrisy. He will admit mistakes, be remorseful, and accept the guilt that follows wrongdoing. The person of integrity fulfills the obligations of his private and his professional life, which are consistent with each other. He or she follows his conscience reliably and predictably. This pursuit is intrinsic to the person's identity. To violate it is to violate that person's humanity."*[2]

In short, *ethical* integrity is the awareness of doing the morally right thing. Often you are able to affirm your personal integrity by observing a breach of it in others. For instance, observing the effects of a friend who lies to cover a mistake helps you to understand why you do not want to take the same course. You will come back to the topic of integrity in Chapters 6 and 7, which deal with how to survive ethically during your student and professional years.

Societal Morality

Large components of personal morality are drawn from a morality that is shared with others in society. *Societal morality* contains values and ideas of duty that spring from deep religious, philosophic, and anthropologic beliefs about humans and their relationship with God (or the gods in some cultures), with each other, and with the natural world. Societal morality becomes codified in laws, customs, and policies. In the United States, the founding fathers and mothers who risked crossing oceans and leaving behind almost every security tried to capture the common denominator of their societal morality in a slogan that states that "all are created equal" and therefore everyone should have an equal chance at "life, liberty and the pursuit of happiness."

Almost always, some tensions exist between personal and societal morality. These tensions are played out in societal debates, with individuals and groups taking sides to try to influence laws and policies. Two current health care–related debates deal with the morality of abortion and assisted suicide. Appropriate limits of the use of the physical environment for human purposes; the moral rights of embryos, undocumented immigrants, prisoners, or others; and tax increases for the purpose of providing basic human services to poor people all are examples of other debates that present challenges at the level of social policy.

Group Morality: Health Professions, Codes, and Institutions

Every member of society, except perhaps the most isolated recluse, joins or is swept into one or more subgroups of society by virtue of being a member of a religious group, a workplace culture, a club, a service organization, an ethnic cluster, or other deep affiliation. The moral guidelines adopted by these groups constitute *group morality*. One such group you are in the process of joining is the health professions. Sociologists have written extensively on the moral and other assumptions governing *professional morality*.[3] Professional morality embraces moral duty, values, and character traits that do not apply equally or at all to others in society. For instance, citizens in general are not morally required to offer help to another in need of medical attention. You are. Citizens are not morally required to keep in confidence information they hear about another. You are. Citizens are not morally required to be nonjudgmental about another's character. You are, through your fiduciary duty discussed in other parts of this book, notably in Chapter 4.

 SUMMARY

> You are a member of a group in a special type of relationship with others in society because of your professional role; with this role comes special moral expectations that arise from that role.

One significant resource that describes the details of professional group morality as it applies specifically to your chosen field is the *code of ethics* of your profession.

Professional Codes of Ethics

Your professional code of ethics today has emerged from a historical understanding that professionals are in a position to have a powerful positive or harmful influence on others. The code highlights that you are in a special type of group that is given societal privileges, but with these privileges come the responsibility to conduct yourself in ways that are acceptable not only to members of your group but also to the larger society. The ancient oaths, such as the familiar *Hippocratic Oath* (Box 1-1), were statements swearing their group intent to practice in specific ways that reflected a commitment to human well-being. Although codes do not require the actual swearing in that characterized the ancient oaths, they serve the same general purpose and often are recited during ceremonies during a landmark in a student's progress towards becoming a professional.

Most codes are produced by your profession's organization and reflect the collective wisdom about how members should conduct themselves as professionals. This gives the items in the code an authoritative voice that represents the profession of which you will become a member.

BOX 1-1   HIPPOCRATIC OATH

I swear by Apollo the Physician, by Aesculapius, Hygeia, and Panacea, and all the gods and goddesses, making them my witnesses, that I will fulfill according to my ability and judgment this oath and this covenant:

To hold him who has taught me this art as equal to my parents and to live my life in partnership with him, and if he is in need of money to give him a share of mine, and to regard his offspring as equal to my brothers in male lineage and to teach them this art—if they desire to learn it—without fee and covenant; to give a share of precepts and oral instruction and all the other learning to my sons and to the sons of him who has instructed me and to pupils who have signed the covenant and have taken an oath according to the medical law, but to no one else.

I will apply dietetic measure for the benefit of the sick according to my ability and judgment; I will keep them from harm and injustice.

I will neither give a deadly drug to anybody if asked for it, nor will I make a suggestion to this effect. Similarly I will not give to a woman an abortive remedy. In purity and holiness I will guard my life and my art.

I will not use the knife, not even on sufferers from stone, but will withdraw in favor of such men as are engaged in this work.

Whatever houses I may visit, I will come for the benefit of the sick, remaining free of all intentional injustice, of all mischief and in particular of sexual relations with both female and male persons, be they free or slaves.

What I may see or hear in the course of the treatment or even outside of the treatment in regard to the life of men, which on no account one must spread abroad, I will keep to myself holding such things shameful to be spoken about.

If I fulfill this oath and do not violate it, may it be granted to me to enjoy life and art, being honored with fame among all men for all time to come; if I transgress it and swear falsely, may the opposite of all this be my lot.

From Edelstein, L. 1943. The Hippocratic Oath: text, translation and interpretation. Bulletin of the History of Medicine 2(Suppl), 3. © Johns Hopkins University Press, Baltimore. Reprinted with permission.

Why is it so important to know your code?

- Your code is your profession's most succinct statement of its professional (group) morality. It is literally a 'codified' shorthand of your larger moral role in society.
- It is a protector of your own best interests as a professional committed to a patient's well being. Patients or families, policy makers, or others may ask you to do things that you judge are not in accordance with your professional moral judgment. The code likely will provide support for your position if your deliberations fall within the common denominator of moral judgment in your profession.
- It also provides a measuring rod for you to engage in continual self-improvement in practice. In a given complex situation, you can refer to it to ask "How do I measure up against the moral standards and specific directives outlined in my code?" "How am I doing?"

 Reflection

Go to the code of ethics of your profession and be prepared to compare it with the Hippocratic Oath displayed in Box 1-1, an updated version of which still is taken by many medical students on graduation.

Note: You can usually find your code on the website of your professional association. For example, a nurse in the United States would go to the American Nurses Association website, a physical therapist to the American Physical Therapy Association website, etc.

What are the striking differences?

Where do you see areas of overlap between the ancient oath and your code regarding the core concepts presented as essential to the morality of the health professions?

Which items in your profession's code apply to the situation of the health professionals treating Drew Harvey? Would your code help them in the decision they have to make? If so, how could they use it?

_____

_____

_____

_____

Institutional Policies as a Resource

Today, in modern institutionalized society, the morality of the health professions should be embedded in the policies, customs, and practices of health care institutions. It would be a perfect world if members of the professions could rely completely on these policies. Fortunately, that does work for most of the decisions you will have to make. But understandably, the moralities may clash at times. For example, institutional policies regarding the performance of abortions are one issue that has caused deep consternation for some health professionals because of their personal morality. Many hospitals and clinics in the United States have adopted policies that commit the institution to enabling medically safe abortions to women under the conditions detailed in the U.S. Supreme Court decision for Roe v. Wade, and policies in other countries follow the same pattern. Realizing the moral sensitivity of this issue, society in the United States has developed mechanisms to protect personal moral convictions related to participation in abortion procedures (see the section "Moral repugnance"). However, protection from following policy is not always assured either. For example, health professionals who object to treating male homosexual patients with AIDS on the basis of a personal morality that rejects homosexuality are not exempted. Overriding an objection to treat is the professional duty to provide "due care" to everyone whose symptoms and other signs require intervention, and institutional policies almost always concur with this position.[4] The predicament that the health professionals found themselves in regarding Drew Harvey's care presents a traditional professional morality challenge because it is safe to assume that most of them would find it personally wrong to fudge details about his immediate rate of improved function. At the same time, their duty of due care for him means that some of them probably consider it because the institutional policies seem unfair.

These situations are by no means limited to the health professions. People through the ages have had to come to grips with institutional practices that grate against their personal or group moral values and duty.

 Reflection

The Christian Reformation in the 1500s took place when the personal morality of some religious leaders came into conflict with the customs and patterns of moral conduct in their religious institution. The famous statement, "Here I stand. I can do no other," exemplifies the moral breaking point persons sometimes reach. The phrase is attributed to reformist Martin Luther as he nailed 95 objections to the official church policy regarding a practice called "indulgences" to the door of All Saints Church in Wittenberg, Germany.

Name some other historical or contemporary examples of a moral breaking point between individual policies or practice.

_____

_____

_____

_____

The good news is that overall, the policies of health care and other institutions where you will find professional employment will likely help prevent you from having to participate in processes, procedures, or other activities that run counter to your personal and professional moral integrity. It is always a good idea before accepting a position to become well informed of job expectations outlined in policies.

 SUMMARY

> Moral values, duty, and expectations of character occur at the level of personal life, within one's society, and as members of various groups. For professionals, professional group morality is recorded in oaths, codes, and other practice guidelines. Institutional policies should be geared to fostering conduct consistent with high moral standards, although conflicts may arise in some instances.

From the Moral to the Ethical

You have learned that morality provides a basis for moving successfully through many daily actions: I will stop at this stop sign; I will not cheat on this exam. But occasionally, the naturalness comes to a gradual or screeching halt. Should I trust my feelings about what I am seeing in the treatment of this patient? How should I interpret my own thoughts on this? Does my experience count here? The authors have heard several metaphors that characterize this situation. "Suddenly the light went out and I couldn't tell where I was." "I was strolling along and turned my ankle. After that, I couldn't walk without thinking about it." "I thought I saw it clearly, but the edges went blurry and grey." "I was eating and bit my tongue. It took all the joy out of lunch." "I call it my 'oops!' moment!" "I felt like I was rowing without a paddle."

These "Stop—but don't stop, drop, and run!" reactions are a means of protecting ourselves against straying from the morality on which we have learned to rely. They signal that something in the way we have habitually structured our conduct and attitudes may not be fitting for this situation. Take them as healthy immune responses trying to reject something potentially harmful to your moral sensitivity and wisdom. Fortunately, these push-back reactions also can function in societies.

Reflection

In recent history, societal self-consciousness about the accepted
United States morality in regard to racial and other discrimination led
to the recognition that not all was well. The United States civil rights
movement, which required dramatic changes in personal, social, and
institutional behaviors, was one response to the dis-ease created by this
heightened awareness. Although by no means perfect, it has had its
positive effects. For example, in the middle of the 20th century, almost
no one in the United States would have anticipated a public law in
2000 that legislated against disability discrimination or that an African-
American president would be elected in 2008.

Can you name some other instances in which a reflection on current moral
    policies and practices opened up new ways of seeing and acting?

1. _____

2 _____

3. _____

4. _____

Ethics is the discipline that waits in the wings as a health-restoring
resource when moral guidelines fail to do the job alone.[5] Ethics provides
a language, some methods, and tools for evaluating the components of
personal, societal, and group morality to create a better path for yourself and
others. Some of its most important uses are to clarify, organize, and critique
morality to highlight what does and does not fit in a particular situation. It is
a process that holds up what "is" and asks, "OK! What really ought to be?"

Ethics: Studying and Reflecting on Morality

Ethics is a systematic study of and reflection on morality: "systematic study
of" because it is a discipline that uses special methods and approaches to
examine moral situations, and "reflection" because it consciously calls into
question assumptions about existing components of our moralities that fall
into the category of habits, customs, or traditions. Originally, the systems of
analysis were developed as areas of philosophy and theology. Today, the
social sciences and other disciplines have added to the number and types of
approaches that are useful for such a task. You will have an opportunity to
learn more about them in Chapter 4.

Ethics takes as its gold standard this question: What do human dignity
and respect demand? Some second level questions are:

• Do our present moral values, behaviors, and character traits pass the
  test of further examination when measured against this standard?

- In situations in which conflicts arise, which values, duties, and other moral guidelines are helpful and why?
- When new situations present uncertainty, what aspects of present moralities will most reliably guide individuals and societies on a sustainable path for survival and thriving?
- What new thinking is needed in such situations and why?

You were introduced to ethical codes earlier in this chapter. How they fit into the larger picture of ethics is important for you to recognize. Fundamentally, they are useful, essential starting points for ethical deliberation. As you will more fully see in Chapters 4 and 5, a description of moral duty and character traits along with statements about some situations you often will encounter (e.g., confidentiality, loyalty to the patient and society), your code is not in itself designed to do the full work of ethics for you. You must bring your own critical thinking and attention to morally complex problems with the help of ethical theory and methods.

The websites and professional literature of many health professions associations now offer case examples or opinion pieces that apply to your profession. Such adjuncts to ethical codes are superb learning opportunities for you.

Ethicists and Ethics Committees

Ethicists have as their primary career activity the work and teaching of ethics. At one level, they analyze issues. They help to clarify the moral values, duties, and other aspects of morality in specific situations. (Medical ethicists or health care ethicists specialize in areas of health care.) At another level, they work to help resolve issues if possible. They work as consultants in the design of ethical policies and practices. They often encourage individuals and institutions not to be driven solely by the pressures of efficiency so that more thoughtful conclusions can be reached in complex moral situations (Figure 1-1).

In many institutions today, *ethics committees* serve much the same purpose and usually include ethicists and thoughtful professionals and laypeople. But ethics is not the work of ethicists or ethics committees only. Ethics is the work of everybody.

---

⑤ SUMMARY

Ethics is the study of and reflection on everyday morality. It functions as a fundamental resource in every thoughtful person's life and takes specific forms when someone assumes a special role, such as health professional. Ethics codes are a starting point for insights, but you need to go beyond them too, to become a role ethicist capable of analyzing complex morality issues that face you as a health professional.

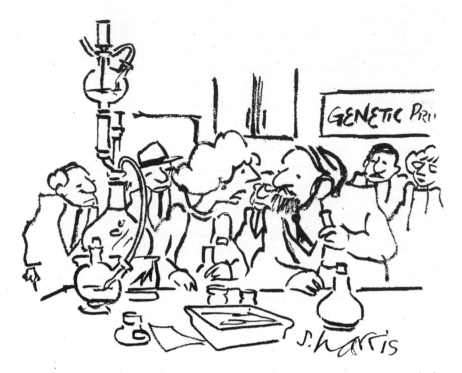

"I FIND IT HARDER AND HARDER TO GET ANY WORK DONE WITH ALL THE ETHICISTS HANGING AROUND."

Figure 1-1. (Courtesy Sidney Harris, with permission.)

The Moral and Ethical Thing to Do

You commonly hear someone say, "That's the moral and ethical thing to do." You hear the terms "moral" and "ethical" used interchangeably. We suggest you use them more purposefully, however, because after what you have just learned, that phrase should have more meaning for you. The "moral thing to do" means that the traditions, customs, laws, and other markers that an individual and society call on for habitual moral guidance allow you to proceed with confidence in your course of action. Conversely, the "ethical thing to do" means that the course of action that would be taken in the everyday moral walk of life has been reflected on and your moral judgment dictates that it still seems the right thing to do (or to refrain from doing in this particular situation). Fortunately, most situations allow you to act both morally and ethically!

Using Ethics in Practical Situations Involving Morality

The scholarly discipline of ethics has always been interesting from the point of view that its subject matter has immediate relevance for everyday life. Aristotle and others in the classical Greek era called ethics "practical philosophy." This interest has led to the development of ethicists and ethics committees discussed previously. But we now turn to your own formation as an ethicist. In this chapter, you read that ethics is about studying and reflecting on moral situations, such as the one the health professionals treating Drew Harvey face. In subsequent chapters, you will see how ethics tools help you analyze specific moral problems, work toward resolution of moral conflicts, and act in a manner consistent with high moral standards. *Analyze. Seek resolution. Act.*

Analysis

Analysis of morality allows you to stand back and identify ethical issues and challenges and to delineate aspects of morality that are involved in a situation. One type of analysis is the process you engage in when two parts of your own morality collide: "I shouldn't lie to my spouse, but the truth will be bitter and I shouldn't hurt her either." An analysis also requires you to pay attention to the human aspects of the situation.

 Reflection

The famous medieval physician Galen fled Rome during the plague. He analyzed his personal morality and decided he had to flee on behalf of his wife and children, whose lives he knew were threatened by the plague. We are told that for the rest of his life he had nightmares about his failure as a professional who had abandoned his patients. In other words, his beliefs regarding his personal and professional duty collided head on. Do you think his analysis served him well in resolving his dilemma? Did he do the right thing? Why or why not?

_____

_____

_____

_____

Answers to these questions require that your own analysis about his situation include reasoning about right and wrong, the psychological dynamics he had to navigate, and the practical consequences of his alternatives. Analysis uncovers relevant knowledge to help inform possible directions towards resolution and purposive action.

Seek Resolution

Ethical reflection geared to resolving complex situations that involve morality goes beyond analysis alone. The knowledge base derived from analysis is complemented by a process that works toward resolution. Obviously, this is what Drew Harvey's health care team will have to do. One approach to finding resolution is to try to build consensus among the various concerned parties (e.g., yourself, patients, families, the institution). Some ethics approaches focus on how to resolve issues when there is no consensus or when consensus does not seem to fully address the moral conflicts embedded in the situation.

Action

Purposive action stems from analysis and thoughtful work toward resolution of an ethical problem that you face. The health professionals involved with Drew Harvey's potential discharge from their care are looking for direction in order to act.

 SUMMARY

The recognition that ethics can be used for analysis, for moving towards resolution of complex situations, and ultimately as a guide for action has led to a resurgence of interest in ethics in practical contexts. Health care ethics is one such area of applied ethics.

Legal Protections for Your Ethical Decisions

Legal protections come in the form of case law *(Constitutional law)* as a result of court decisions from the lowest courts to the Supreme or High court of the land that set legal precedence for future similar situations; legislation *(statutory law* or *statutes)* passed through congress or parliament; and legally binding regulations *(administrative law)* promoted through a state's or national government's regulatory bodies, such as the United States Department of Health and Human Services.

How Does Law Factor into Professional Morality?

National and state or provincial laws are a big help for the most part. They embody and codify moral values and types of duty that should govern individual and institutional conduct related to the health professions and provide legal interpretations of key professional issues. Just a few examples: Laws outline the conditions under which health professionals have the "license" or "privilege" to practice in a state, province, or territory. Laws provide clarification about informed consent, confidentiality, and conditions related to a health professional's competence, among many other issues. Each of these is based on moral values relevant to the health professional and patient relationship, on an understanding of professional duty, and on societal expectations of the type of moral character professionals will cultivate and exhibit. Many health professions programs today wisely include a course on health care law governing their profession; if you do not have one in your program of study, web and other resources also are available for you to learn about the legal dimensions of your practice.

As a general rule, laws and moral standards of a society seem to support each other. But you should not expect the same guidance from laws or policies that you receive from ethical codes and vice versa. Each has its special function. For a succinct summary of major distinctions between law and ethics, you will find Jennifer Horner's chart helpful.

Morality*	
Law	*Ethics*
Defined by government	Defined by individual and community
Based on concepts of justice and equality	Based on how we define a "good," worthwhile, or meaningful life
Formal rules resolution of complex problems	Informal guidelines for resolution of complex problems
Uniform	Some uniformity; respectful of diversity
Minimum standard of behavior ("at least")	Ideal or aspirational ("better" or "best")
Coercive (penalties for misconduct)	Noncoercive ("dictates of conscience")
Rules of law enforced by regulatory authorities and courts	Standards and exhortations by custom, professionals standards, discussion, and persuasion
"Must"	"Should"

*Widely held societal values (universal, ultimate, impartial, other-regarding).
With permission from Horner, J. 2003. Morality, ethics and law: introductory concepts. *Seminars in Speech and Language* 24(4):269-273.

Protections

As you think about living within the dictates of your conscience and professional morality in seriously contended moral issues, keep in mind the following general resources available to professionals through laws and policies.

State Interests

Common law (i.e., law that comes into practice over time through the lived life of a community) dictates that there is a *state interest*, a responsibility to intervene on behalf of persons under four circumstances: (1) to save their life, (2) to prevent their suicide, (3) to protect them from harm as an innocent third party, or (4) to protect them as a bearer of the "integrity of the professions." This final cause for legal intervention obviously applies to professionals only. It has evolved because of circumstances in which health and other professionals have been faced with requests by patients or clients or have been dictated to by policies to act in ways that are believed by a court to be contrary to the true moral and legal social role of a professional. This protection must be appealed to on a case-by-case basis.

Licensing Laws

Professionals become certified, registered, or licensed to practice nationally and within a particular state or jurisdiction after the completion of all formal professional preparation requirements. Written into the *licensing laws* that govern professional practice are both responsibilities and protections or rights. Among the rights is your right to practice within the dictates of your practice guidelines and own convictions. This right is weighed against the reasonable expectations of patients or clients who come to you for professional help.

Moral Repugnance

As mentioned previously in this chapter, *moral repugnance* came into the health professions literature with the Supreme Court decision Roe v. Wade, which made abortion a legal right. It is written into a conscience clause that allows individuals who believe it is morally wrong to participate in abortion procedures to be exempt from having to do so. An important aspect of this provision is that the procedure itself is key to whether this exemption will be upheld. It is not a protection against, for example, your refusal to treat patients whose lifestyles are morally unacceptable to you. Therefore, it is a limited but important protection. Many have argued that a request to assist in the lethal procedures that cause death in capital punishment would fall under the protection of this notion. The same is true should medically administered euthanasia become legal in the United States as it is in the Netherlands. This conscience clause operates as a conscientious objection analogous to conscientious objection in situations of war.

Limits of Protection

In summary, society and, as we saw in a previous section of this chapter, many institutions that deliver high-quality health care are aware of the need for your personal protection in those hopefully rare circumstances in which you feel morally compromised. However, the final burden of proof regarding why you refuse to participate in an action or take a position contrary to the norm falls on you, but you may be able to find support in one of the previously mentioned legal mechanisms that have been developed. The best recourse is to know your own values and reasons for behavior and have good justifications to support them. Fortunately, most health professionals seldom experience the deep, troubling tension of being in a situation they believe will compromise their personal and professional moral convictions.

 SUMMARY

Protections that allow you to follow the dictates of your own conscience are provided through federal and state or other more local legal mechanisms, although in the end, the final burden of proof for your action falls on you.

Summary

This chapter is but one step into your lifelong journey in professional ethics. You have chosen a career path that requires complex moral judgments regarding patient care, health policy, and other aspects of professional life. This chapter has introduced you to some basic ways of thinking about the sources of morality on which you can draw, the general relevance of ethics to your everyday professional life, and some legal protections you can expect if you are faced with potential compromises of your convictions. You also have begun to make some basic distinctions about major approaches to ethics. As you study the subsequent chapters, you will be better able to appreciate the contribution of these considerations.

Questions for Thought and Discussion

1. Search your local or other national newspaper for an article about health care involving ethical issues.
   a. What is the basic point of the article? What is the reporter saying?
   b. What does the writer or reporter suggest are the main moral issues raised in this situation? Do you agree? Why or why not?
2. You learned in this chapter about personal, group, and societal moralities. Identify a value in your own personal morality and describe that value's relationship with the morality of a group or society you are currently living in. Use the following box to compare the moralities.

Personal Value	Group Value	Societal Value

Now compare your list with a classmate's.

REFERENCES

1. Beauchamp, T.L., Walters, L., Kahn, J.P., et al., 2007. *Contemporary issues in bioethics.* Wadsworth Publishing, Belmont, CA.
2. Pellegrino, E.D., 2009. Physician integrity: Why it is inviolable. In: Crowley, M. (Ed.), *Connecting American values with health reform: A publication of the Hastings Center.* The Hastings Center, Garrison, NY, pp. 18–20.
3. Friedson, E., 2001. *Professionalism, the third logic: On the practice of knowledge.* University of Chicago Press, Chicago.
4. Hughes, M.T., Marcozzi, D., 2004. Duty to treat versus personal safety. *Virtual Mentor* 6, 5.
5. Berlinger, N., 2009. Perspective: Helping people out. *Hastings Center Report* 39 (1), 53.

2

The Ethical Goal of Professional Practice: A Caring Response

Objectives

The reader should be able to:

- Identify how care is the goal of professional ethics activity.
- Describe the basic idea of "a caring response" and ways this response is expressed in a professional relationship.
- Describe what mastery entails within the health professional and patient relationship.
- List some types of claims encountered in a professional role and why the patient's interests must take priority when conflicting claims arise.
- Describe at least two important distinctions between the caring expressed in friendships or family life and the caring expressed in a health professional and patient relationship.
- Define patient-centered care.
- Discuss the relationship of compassion and technical expertise in achieving a caring response to a patient's needs.
- Identify the two components of professional responsibility and why both are essential for a caring response.
- Describe how the concept of rights enhances the understanding of what a caring response entails.
- Discuss some burdens and benefits of care giving as they arise in the health professional and patient relationship.

New terms and ideas you will encounter in this chapter

a caring response	technical	accountability
care	competence	ethical standard
mastery	compassion	responsiveness
claim	professional	right
patient-centered	responsibility	human rights
care	due care	

Topics in this chapter introduced in earlier chapter

Topic	Introduced in chapter
Code of ethics	1
Personal integrity	1

Introduction

The goal of professional ethics is to arrive at *a caring response* in situations you encounter in the course of carrying out your professional role and its functions. Obviously, a health professional must thoroughly grasp what a caring response looks like. Its shape is determined by the character of the health professional and patient relationship. Specific forms it takes depend on the activities in which you engage as you carry out the tasks of your chosen profession. Sometimes the *care* is offered on a one-to-one basis, but often it is offered as one member of the team providing diagnostic or treatment interventions. If you, the professional, pursue a lesser goal than a caring response, or a misguided one, the relationship becomes distorted and results in that patient being given short shrift. This is not surprising because all good relationships present certain "problems" or "challenges" that require caring attention. In this chapter, we present the idea of a caring response for close examination, but this is not the only opportunity you have to consider it. Looking ahead, in Chapter 3, you will be introduced to ethical challenges that present themselves in three major forms or prototypes: moral distress, ethical dilemmas, and locus of authority challenges. Each calls for you, the professional, to be guided by the goal of a caring response.

 SUMMARY

A caring response is the ethical goal of every health professional and patient relationship.

Caring is essential to the *mastery* of your professional identity. In general, when one speaks of mastery or expert practice, it refers to successfully having prepared to recognize, give considered attention to, and be able to fully address a challenge, with its resolution the ultimate ideal. In the health professions, your mastery is affirmed only when the patient experiences your response as a caring response insofar as it took the two of you as far as possible toward the ideal of resolving the problem that brought him or her into your life. This is not a new idea. In fact, a recent review article in a major medical journal traces a long history of care as the central feature that divides the mere science of medicine from its essential quality.[1] Moreover, the author shows that recent physiologic and neuro-imaging study results show positive findings in patients who experience personal engagement with a health professional as a result of the latter's attitudes and conduct characteristic of care. This author concludes that a caring response is fundamental to both the art and the science of effective health care interventions. In Chapter 4, you will learn some of the ethics approaches and theories that, over the ages, have been developed to help you gain mastery of the attitudes, skills, and knowledge that equip you to find a caring response that benefits the persons involved. After these introductory chapters, you will have many opportunities to consider different types of situations in which you are required to determine what a caring response involves in each instance. To get you started, consider the following story, which highlights some personal, professional, and societal moralities that you learned in Chapter 1, and the challenges that Pat Jackson, a physician assistant, is encountering as she goes about trying to live by her intention to promote a caring response.[2]

🐚 The Story of Pat Jackson and Mr. Sanchez

Pat Jackson was very excited about being invited into a rural group practice in her home state. During her hiring interview, she found the team of physicians, nurses, technologists, therapists, and others compatible with her own commitment to high quality health care. She told the team how she welcomed the opportunity to attend school in a large city but now was eager to return as a physician assistant to the type of setting she had so enjoyed as a child. The group was impressed with her enthusiasm and the several academic and humanitarian awards she had received during her training.

And so it was a terrible moment for her when with the honeymoon period barely over she misdiagnosed Mr. Sanchez's symptoms of asthma as a temporary allergic response attributable to the very high pollen count that month. He came into the clinic with the stuffy nose and watery eyes she had seen several times earlier in the week. That Friday evening, she was eager to get out of the clinic in time to serve at a community church supper down the road from where she lived; she was relieved that because he was another pollen sufferer she could quickly send him on his way with a prescription to relieve his respiratory stuffiness. When she asked him whether he had ever had such a reaction before, Mr. Sanchez said "no." She noted that he may or may not have completely understood her question, although his "no" seemed emphatic enough that she did not think it necessary to call in her colleague who could pose the question to him in his native Spanish.

She also knew that he, like many others who came to the area to work the fields during this time of the year, could be faced with allergies he had not encountered previously. But when he was brought in by his foreman 2 months later with obvious difficulty breathing, it dawned on her that maybe she should have probed deeper during his first visit. She was aware that the allergy medication she had prescribed probably would have done him no additional harm but also that untreated asthma can have dire, even fatal, results for a patient. She referred him to the attending physician who conducted tests that confirmed severe asthma. She found herself hesitating to tell Mr. Sanchez or his foreman that she had failed to make the correct judgment 2 months earlier, knowing from living in rural America that acceptance of new young professionals from "away" comes slowly and that word travels quickly. "Why am I hesitating?" she asked herself. "I am an honest person!" Pat knew that had his asthma been treated on the first visit, it would likely not have been so severe now. She concluded that part of her hesitance also stemmed from not wanting to disturb the trust she felt her clinic was building with Mr. Sanchez's ethnic community, many members of whom had been suspicious of the "white caregivers" and therefore failed to come for care or follow up on prescribed interventions. But even that explanation did not relieve her of a sinking feeling about how she had handled Mr. Sanchez's situation on that first visit.[2]

Many issues can be raised in this story, but your opportunity here is to focus on your opinion about how Pat's mandate to provide a caring response to Mr. Sanchez should have been achieved. Because you have not yet been introduced more formally to the idea of a caring response, we ask you to rely on your everyday understanding.

 Reflection
Do you believe that when Mr. Sanchez first came to the clinic Pat treated him with the full attention consistent with your idea of how a caring professional should respond?

Yes____ No ___

Most readers probably can see some aspects of Pat's situation that could lead to her devoting less than her full professional attention to Mr. Sanchez. If you do, what are they?

_____

_____

_____

_____

When Mr. Sanchez returned, Pat hesitated to share her misgivings with him or his foreman. In your opinion, do you think her sources of hesitance have sufficient weight to override her concern that she is being dishonest by withholding some information from him when in fact she is an honest person?

Yes____ **No** ___

Jot down some thoughts about your answer and how they help support your understanding of what a caring response would look like in this situation.

_____

_____

_____

_____

As in many ethical challenges, you may find yourself seeing two sides of the coin and realize that each has a pull on your moral sensibilities. We will discuss this at more length in Chapter 3.

The Patient as Focus of a Caring Response

A caring response does not always mean that you will be able to completely resolve the conflict of claims on you, but it does require you to put your priority to optimizing the positive results and minimizing damage to the patient. What do we mean by a "claim?" A _claim_ is a request made verbally or nonverbally by virtue of the expectations people have of your professional role. It says, "Give me your attention!" You know that your role will involve many types of relationships, with patients or clients and other times with families, professional team members, research subjects, policymakers, or the public. And the list is not complete if you fail to include your relationship with yourself and your own health! Each and every one of the parties you encounter will come with claims on your time, services, expertise, or other type of attention. From time to time, you will find yourself torn between more than one claim on your care, just as Pat did. She understood that her patient Mr. Sanchez had a strong claim on her to be treated with the best attention possible; but still, when she realized she may have been negligent in her treatment of him, some other claims on her also raised their head. For one thing, she knew the value of her clinic's services in this community and that her presence as an essential new addition on the health care team was a boost to the overall effectiveness of the clinic. She must not compromise that effectiveness. She cared about her colleagues and their heavy workloads, so she felt the need to reflect on the negative effect it might have if their load was increased because she was shunned by patients when the word got out that she was not competent. She was also sensitive to the bigger role of her clinic in providing quality care to a previously underserved Hispanic community in the area and wondered if her admission might undermine their trust in the clinic. Finally, she put into the mix the desire to be caring of herself by honoring her wish to participate in a social event on this Friday night in her newly adopted town. All of this was waging war with her personal value of honesty.

Reflection

Stop right here and think about your day so far. What conflicting claims on your attention have you already faced?

_____

_____

_____

_____

   Conflicting claims are part and parcel of everyday life. But Pat's professional role helps her to set priorities in relation to Mr. Sanchez. Her primary concern **must** be the well-being of the patient under consideration. At the same time, Pat's commitment to honesty, one part of her personal value system, tends to tip the scales in the direction of finding a way to share the information with Mr. Sanchez. This course of action not only keeps the patient in center focus but also allows her personal integrity to be honored.

How, when, and where it should be shared requires her to bring other character traits such as compassion and courage into play as she attempts to minimize possible deleterious effects this information may have on him, the clinic, or his ethnic community. She will be wise to engage the services of her colleague who can speak Spanish and comes from Mr. Sanchez's ethnic group himself.

Patient-Centered Care

Patient-centered care, or client-centered care, is a term adopted in the health professions' clinical and ethical literature to emphasize the imperative that professionals keep a focus on the well-being of the whole person. Nursing and medicine have led the way in developing the concept, but almost all health professions have adopted it in principle.[3] Entire models of the health professional and patient relationship have been built around this notion, and you likely will learn one or more of them in your professional preparation. The central concept that runs through these models is that patient's values, concerns, and preferences have moral weight in the everyday clinical decision-making process. Although the terms health care and managed care may have the term "care" embedded in them, they may simply mean dealing with patients in a technical or aggregate sense. For this reason, clinicians and ethicists add "patient-centered" as the orienting point on their moral compass that always brings the focus back to what matters to the patient and what the health professions have to offer.

You can easily see that patient-centered care is highly individualized, tailored to fit each patient. This focus of attention is frequently challenged in an era of clinical specialization and sophisticated medical technology. Clinical procedures often are so specialized that a particular disease, symptom, body part, or biologic system can become the focus of attention. The dehumanizing effect that a fragmented focus has on both the health professional and the patient is illustrated in Figure 2-1.

One important feature of patient-centered approaches is that they show how profoundly a lack of effective communication with the patient can throw the focus of care off center, away from the patient in his or her unique situation. For instance, Pat Jackson may or may not have communicated the basic information Mr. Sanchez needed, but a high probability exists that he would have felt more cared for as a person if she had engaged her colleague who knew Spanish, his primary language, and had asked more questions about his stuffy nose and watery eyes when he first came to the clinic. We devote an entire chapter to communication issues in Chapter 11.

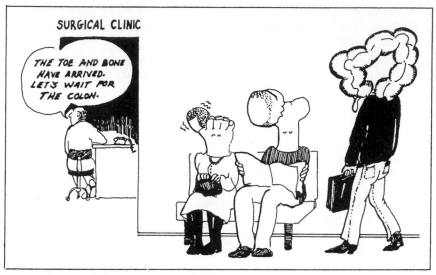

Figure 2-1. Professionals' view of patients. *(From Purtilo, R., 1978. Kapital II. Att upprätta en relation. In: Vård, vårdare, vårdad. [Translation: Care, care giver, receiver of care.] Stockholm: Esselte Studium, p. 139.)*

 SUMMARY

From time to time, you will be torn by conflicting claims on your attention. Your primary loyalty must be to the patient. "Patient-centered care" is a clinical phrase that is used to help remind you of this priority and that care must be tailored to each individual. Effective communication is not often thought of as an ethical activity, but it is essential for the goal of a caring response to be realized.

Three Characteristics of a Caring Response

The term "care" is used to convey many different things. Whole ethical theories are built on principles of care; you will become more acquainted with an ethics of care approach in Chapter 4. At present, we introduce you to the basic meaning and dynamics involved in professional caring, a concept that has several specific characteristics to be aware of in your professional role.

Navigation Between Friendly and Professional Conduct

A professional caring response includes aspects of conduct that are identical to the ones you show toward a friend or relative. So, let us begin with your own experience.

Reflection

If you have been to a physician, therapist, or other health professional for an ailment recently, what are some aspects of your exchange that were similar to those you might have with a friend or family member and that you would characterize as signs of their care for you?

_____

_____

_____

_____

If you listed some things you each did that were sensitive to making each other comfortable, or that showed mutual regard for the other, or that were light and in appropriate good humor, they are apt examples of everyday caring relationships. These are the human sensitivities, affection, and politeness that also bolster a patient's belief that you care about him or her.[4] This friendly caring can take the most mundane forms in your professional life, including taking time to attend to a patient's personal hygiene needs (e.g., putting a water glass and toothbrush of a bedridden patient with in reach), decreasing physical discomfort (e.g., offering a pillow or straight-back chair), or complimenting a patient. We have found that acknowledging a patient's birthday or anniversary can bring a smile. And the professional caring that is in common with other human relationships also goes deeper, of course, so that basic trust and appreciation develop between them. Given just the little we know about Pat Jackson and Mr. Sanchez think of some things you think she might have done to show basic human caring towards him.

At the same time, a health professional's relationships with patients are very different too, with moral and legal dimensions not fully applicable to other relationships. Therefore, a caring response must mean something more than common everyday expressions of affection, nurturance, or protectiveness associated with care.

 Reflection

Examine the picture of these friends in Figure 2-2. What do you see that may not seem appropriate for a health professional and patient relationship?

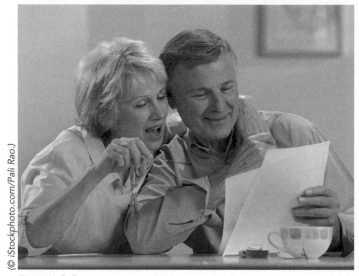

Figure 2-2.

_____

_____

_____

_____

Their physical proximity is one cautionary message. A governing characteristic of your professional caring response is that you must not cross psychological, physical, and sexual boundaries that would make the patient responsible or responsive to you in ways that go outside of (or create opposition to) the healing core of the relationship.[5] The form that your caring response must always take is to focus your interactions on the health-related matters that you are competent to address through extensive training in your field, distinguishing you from other caring people in the patient's life. One way to exercise this discipline is through the type of information you request from the patient. For instance, a helpful question to ask yourself is, "What do I need to know about the patient to provide the best care possible?" You will likely come to know other things too, but your intent should be guided by this need. In addition, if you pour your heart out to a patient like you would to a friend, it not only may take attention from his or her issues but also create a feeling that you are the one who came to be cared for instead of the patient.

Touching a patient also warrants your disciplined attention. As you learned in Chapter 1, you may have "license" to touch and, in some professional roles such as surgery or laboratory tests that require injecting a needle, to physically invade this stranger whom you know only because he or she is a patient. Such actions go well beyond what a nonprofessional can morally and legally do. Great respect for the privileges health professionals have earned through their professional preparation must be enveloped in an equally deep respect for the effect the physical contact may have on the patient. For instance, knowing that Mr. Sanchez is a farm laborer can provide Pat with clues about the environment in which he lives each day and may help to guide her in how to approach him. His age and ethnicity can provide more clues as to how he will feel about having a young woman palpate him on the face, neck, or trunk and ask questions he may feel are a private matter. More will be said throughout this textbook about the shape of the health professional and patient relationship. As various aspects are addressed, you will be able to further flesh out what it means to provide a friendly caring response tempered and shaped by professional role boundaries and how to exercise the discipline of staying focused on the patient.

Care Expressed Through Technical Competence

A caring response depends on competently and conscientiously carrying out your professional duties. It goes beyond a patient's hope that you will offer a kind or even generous response to the ailment, to counting on your technical skills to allow you to respond wholeheartedly to the diagnosis and symptoms. Without *technical competence,* the goal of a caring response cannot be achieved. One of the authors recalls a physician who year after year instructed the incoming class of medical students, "You will be driven to feel compassion, sympathy for the situation of many people who come to you. The first rule of compassion is [your technical] competence, competence, competence!"

Compassion often is seen as a human characteristic involved in **caring** for the patient, while applying one's technical expertise is the real stuff of **treatment.** We are among those who, like the experienced doctor mentioned previously, see this as an erroneous distinction. Compassion, which comes from the Latin meaning "to suffer with" the patient, is not only about feeling the patient's plight but also is a motivator to be able to relieve the suffering. Therefore, conscientious application of one's technical skills is in itself an essential component of a caring response.[6] Without integration, both become distorted in terms of what you are there to do for the patient. More specifically, your technical expertise places you in a unique position to aid that person in maintaining or regaining health (or relief of suffering or a peaceful death) in ways that he or she cannot achieve without you. At times, the most caring response also includes documenting shortcomings of practices that do not meet this goal and working with others to help change policies that fall short for a whole group of similarly situated persons. For example, Pat Jackson gradually became aware that Mr. Sanchez is a member of a minority group in which asthma is a serious health problem and that the reimbursement for asthma treatment and follow-up often falls short of assuring effective clinical management of the problem. Part of her reflection was based on whether she herself had done anything to undermine the clinic's attempt to provide the best care possible for this group and, if necessary, to document shortcomings in policies that are keeping the clinic from providing it. We can assume that their data could have an impact on policymakers once they saw the health compromises that such a shortcoming was engendering. In this regard, her anxiety was well founded because we have every indication that she was a well-intentioned and conscientious clinician committed to applying her expertise fully.

 SUMMARY

A caring response includes the exercise of compassion understood as the conscientious expression of a professional's technical competence.

Care as Professional Responsibility

The idea of a caring response is also partially captured in the common phrase *professional responsibility*. In legal language, professional responsibility can be summarized by the term *due care*. Due care specifies what is reasonably expected of you in your role as a provider of professional service to a particular purpose.[7] You can see how technical expertise applies to this idea. But you can probably also identify a justice component to this legal phrase, which suggests that it is your duty to give each and every patient what he or she rightly has coming. So, it goes beyond compassion and technical expertise to something more. Before going into more detail, take a minute to draw on your common sense idea of responsibility.

 Reflection

Pat was concerned by Mr. Sanchez's condition when he returned to the clinic partially because she was afraid she may have been negligent and had not in fact shown due care in her treatment of him. But her concern did not seem to end there. What else do you think was troubling her that might have been related to her feeling of what we are calling

professional responsibility? Jot down your ideas here to refer back to as
you continue through this section.

_____

_____

_____

_____

Accountability and Responsiveness

From an ethical point of view, the authors find that one of the most helpful
interpretations of professional responsibility is that described by theologian
Richard Niebuhr in his classic book *The Responsible Self*. [8]

> Professional Responsibility = Accountability + Responsiveness

Accountability. The most common understanding of professional re
sponsibility associated with the health professions grows out of the western
philosophical traditions that emphasize the individual's part in upholding
the moral life. Accountability, holding one to account for one's actions,
assumes that one is not only capable of acting in a certain way and has the
appropriate knowledge to do so but also is free to go ahead unimpeded. Once
those conditions are met, your decisions rest entirely with you.

Accountability also implies that there is an *ethical standard* or ideal
against which one's actions can be measured. If you go back to examine
your chosen profession's code of ethics through the lens of your being held
accountable, you will note that it is very duty oriented and describes the
basic ideals and standards expected of anyone in your profession. In that
regard, we could all benefit from having the sign that former US President
Harry Truman kept on his desk, "The Buck Stops Here," meaning "I am
finally the one who has to answer to what happens and if I am in touch with
the appropriate standards and ideals I deserve to be held to account."

Whether with a patient or sitting at the desk of a President, a caring
response requires being accountable. As you can quickly discern, accountability can also lead to abuse of the power invested in one by virtue of one's
societal role. Part of a caring response is not to take advantage of that
position. It is within this framework that Niebuhr proposes the necessary
complement of "responsiveness."

Responsiveness. An important contribution by Niebuhr often overlooked
in ethical discussions of responsibility is that it is relational. Responsiveness
requires willingness to engage with the other to gain a deep awareness and

understanding of the person or group to whom one is accountable and a willingness to adapt your conduct to honor it. More specifically, it turns the focus of attention to the other in the relationship. Accountability, taken alone, is unidirectional and does not allow for the enhanced understanding of what one is being accountable *to,* and *why*. The importance of adding responsiveness to the concept of responsibility is emphasized in this excerpt by ethicist Thomas Ogletree who also relates it to the idea of personal integrity as what is fitting introduced in Chapter 1.

> *"Responsive judgments are guided by the notion of what is fitting. The fitting action may be largely self-evident once we have grasped what is morally at stake in a situation. Yet it may emerge only gradually, through the thoughtful balancing of multiple variables in their negative and positive features. Moral imagination and discernment are as important to this balancing process as are conceptual precision and logical rigor. The reasoning involved, moreover, is often more akin to weaving a tapestry than to forging a chain."*[9]

 Reflection

Given these insights, jot down some aspects of Mr. Sanchez's situation to which Pat Jackson and her colleagues must be responsive to choose a course of action that is not only the most fitting for him but also allows them to be accountable in a manner that preserves their own integrity.

_____

_____

_____

_____

In Chapter 4, you will be introduced to some approaches to ethics that show how over time the field itself has seen the necessity of incorporating details of the patient's story into your deliberation about morally right conduct. The approaches include narrative ethics that is based on skillful interpretation of patients' narrative accounts of their condition, ethics of care that takes the ideas of care being discussed in this chapter and elsewhere as the central feature of professional responsibility, and still others that emphasize relationships and highlight the role of diversity in ethical decision making. Although "a caring response" is the goal of any bioethical theory regarding the health professional and patient relationship, you can begin to appreciate that caring is not a simple matter to be dismissed.

Rights and Professional Responsibility

As you know, the idea of rights plays prominently in ethical and legal deliberations regarding our responsibility toward each other, animals, and the environment. What is a "right?" Basically a *right* is a concept to identify stringent claims or demands of one person on another. If I present you with something that is my right, you must honor this quality or need in me. The weight of your demand creates a duty for me to respond to it. For instance, in the founding document of the United States, The Declaration of Independence, we find the phrase that Americans are "endowed" with the rights of life, liberty, and the pursuit of happiness. If I have a right to life, you have a duty to help protect it and you certainly must not rob me of it. Therefore, rights and duties are inextricably linked, although as you will learn in Chapter 4, not all duty-driven ethical theories or approaches rely (historically speaking) on the relatively recent concept of rights.

When rights are interpreted as applying to everyone alike, they are said to be *human rights*. The core idea of human rights is that it is one important means of expressing a common hope for humanity that flows beneath differences of culture, civilization, and ways of life, like the magma that flows beneath the earth's varied surface. We are born to nourish our life individually and as a society, and we have invented the idea of human rights to try to help us understand what we must do to make this nourishment available to everyone when we are different in so many external ways.

Some rights are associated with health care and the health professional and patient relationship in the United States and other countries. Health care itself is viewed as a right in many parts of the world.

 Reflection

If you think back to the relationship between Mr. Sanchez and Pat Jackson, what do you believe are some rights each of them has?

The patient Mr. Sanchez's rights:

_____

_____

_____

_____

The health professional Pat Jackson's rights:

_____

_____

_____

_____

Compare what you wrote with the following commonly cited rights of patients and health professionals.

The patient has a right to:
- respect from the health professionals and health care system,
- a clean and welcoming environment,
- high-quality care,
- confidentiality of sensitive information,
- shared decision making about course of treatment, and
- truthful information about one's condition to enhance self-determination about what to do in regards to treatment options.

Health professionals have a right to:
- respect from the patient,
- relevant information necessary for treatment to be effective,
- freedom to freely exercise clinical best judgment (i.e., professional autonomy), and
- fair payment for professional services.

Critics of rights approaches point out that an emphasis on rights in health care has the following shortcomings:
- Rights are highly individualistic, emphasizing the demands of one individual on another and thereby often obscuring their common interests or that others' interests also are relevant to the situation.
- When rights conflict, very little within rights approaches exists to help to resolve the problem.
- Rights often are too general for the responder to determine which duties would adequately meet the demand for a response. An example is the right to health care. My demand for health-related services based on my right to health care can be interpreted by you as anything from a right to a band aid to all the services and goods you can provide. Understandably, discussions of rights often entail a discussion of justice and how a particular good or service is distributed fairly.

We urge you to pay careful attention to rights language that you find in your ethics codes, policy statements, or institutional documents; in licensing laws; and in use by colleagues or patients. In each case, the language is designed to urgently summon a caring response to a request that is embedded in the demand. Your professional responsibility is to discern the shape of such a response. You will discover that no one formula for implementing human rights fits all patients, any more than it fits all nations, cultures, or civilizations, because each human experience and relationship brings its own history and values to the discovery of what to do to honor the rights claim.

 SUMMARY

Rights are stringent claims on someone else or society for a caring response to a person's or group's needs. Human rights usually are viewed as universally understood needs such as food, shelter, health care, and the protection of life itself. Rights claims may come from both health professionals and patients, helping to shape professional responsibility and summon a truly caring response.

Burdens and Benefits of a Caring Response

In the final section of this chapter, we ask you to join us in thinking about some aspects of professional care and care giving that all too often are not addressed in the health professions and bioethics literature A caring response is such a fundamental goal in the health professions that sometimes the real burden and benefits of engaging in the professional relationship are overlooked.

The Burden of Care

Although care giving is usually cast in a positive light for good reasons, it is easy to ignore the reality that searching for a caring response and acting according to what it requires of you is a burden at times.

 Reflection

Have you ever been in a personal relationship where your caring incurs a burden at times? These may be burdens that you willingly carry or that you find yourself wishing you could be free of. You may want to name the type of things that feel like burdens in that relationship for a reference point as you read on.

_____

_____

_____

_____

The burden of caring is not limited to personal relationships. In a graduate course of students in the professions, one author asked the students to be brutally honest with themselves about negative feelings they had at times about care giving. Some of their responses are:

REFLECTION ON PROFESSIONAL CARING RELATIONSHIPS

> Sometimes I find myself pretending to care, when in fact, internally, I don't care at all, and that makes me feel irritated with myself.
> Caring for others in their grief leaves me grieving as well, and I need to take time to absorb these losses.
> Sometimes I ask myself, "Do I care too much?"
> Without a doubt, my most difficult caring relationship is with myself.
> I wonder why at times when I don't care I am perceived as caring.
> How does care embody me and what do I do with that responsibility?
> I can't say I like having to be caring at times. Some patients are such babies.
> I am surprised and perplexed when I honestly feel, "I do not care."
> Some people know how to make you question, "Why do I show so much caring when they are so ungrateful?"
> Caring can be a drag if the patient is being difficult.

Are these health professionals expressing feelings that make them unfit for their professional role? Not necessarily. It goes beyond the purpose of this text to unpack all the underlying conditions that might lead a professional to make such statements regarding the feelings about caring that arise from time to time. The purpose of sharing their feelings here is to mark for you that professionals know they have to try to live up to their professional responsibility but there are personal costs associated with doing so at times. A caring response is not all sunshine and fresh air. In Chapter 7, where the focus is on caring for yourself, you will have an opportunity to explore how to overcome barriers to your own caring or live through them without letting them govern your responses to patients. For the time being, you have an opportunity to use this insight to prepare yourself for situations in which you do not automatically warm up to finding the caring response for a particular patient.

Benefits for the Caregiver

Fortunately, overall, the amount of negative burden the responsibility of a caring response incurs is small compared with the benefits. Developmental psychologists tell us that one of the most important ways adults gain a recognized place in society is through their contributions to that society's well-being. Professional care giving benefits you by putting you in a position to participate in activities that society respects. For most health professionals, care giving is also a basis for self-fulfillment and job satisfaction. Many can relate to the line in the prayer of Saint Francis of Assisi, "It is in giving that we receive." What do professionals receive? You often hear those who have been in the field for a long time recount how much their work has given them, including remarkable insights into their own humanness, in both its vulnerability and strengths; how they have been inspired by patients' "will to live" or gumption to continue on in spite of seemingly great challenges; and by patients' and families' kindness and gratitude that helps keep the professional going. What we hear, and as clinicians we have experienced, is that in the search for a caring response to a patient the health professional also stands to gain something wonderful.

How then does this understanding and awareness help to shape a truly caring response to a patient's situation? Your part in engendering mutual respect for what each offers the other as humans must burn at the core of the relationship. We can catch a glimpse of this when Pat Jackson began to take a second look at who Mr. Sanchez was when he came back a second time. One way to look at his return is that it became an occasion for her to learn something important about herself and the kind of professional she wanted to be. She had to move towards acknowledging that the only thing an individual professional or the professions as a whole really can offer is to somehow tap into a patient's or group's dream of healthfulness and try to support it. (We call it mutual goal setting.) When we fail in word or deed to get that part right, we lack essential evidence on which to build a caring response. Understanding that you and the patient are working together towards promoting a more healthful humanity can counteract mainstream society's error in believing that the technology and other tools of your profession govern the goodness that comes from your care giving alone.

 SUMMARY

The professionals' acknowledgement of caring that individual patients, their families, and the health professions environment often provide completes the web of care that surrounds the health professional and patient relationship.

Summary

This discussion on the ideals and functions of professional care, care giving, and the goal of a caring response has been added as a separate chapter for the first time in this edition of the book. The authors realized that the goal of a caring response is being explored by psychologists, sociologists, ethicists, the legal profession, and policymakers and therefore warrants special attention as health professionals continue to refine their unique and special contributions to individuals and societies. Fortunately, we have had to provide only the bare essentials for you because a copious amount of theoretical and practical material is already available in almost every health profession. You are now ready to take what you have learned about a caring response into the specifics of ethical reflection, analysis, and action.

Questions for Thought and Discussion

1. As a health professional, you will be expected to provide a caring response to all kinds of people. Who do you think will be the most difficult populations of patients to truly *care* for? Give some specific examples of behaviors or other characteristics that you think would make patients especially challenging.
2. Describe a medical or dental visit in which something happened to make you feel that the professional's attention was not patient-centered on you. What happened? What could the professionals and others in that environment have done to make you feel more like they were motivated by the goal of a caring response to you?
3. The emergency departments of major hospitals are a whirlwind of activity, with many life or death situations for patients who literally have just come through the door. A young nurse recently said to one of the authors, "There's no time for care here. We are too busy; it's life or death interventions 24-7."
   a. What are some examples of how emergency room professionals can demonstrate a caring response to patients?
   b. Now do the same exercise in an operating room setting.
   c. And finally, with a team working in a locked residence for patients with advanced Alzheimer's disease.

REFERENCES

1. Harris, J.C., 2009. Toward a restorative medicine: The science of care. *JAMA* 301 (16), 1710–1712.
2. Purtilo, R., 2009. *In: Handbook for rural health care ethics: A practical guide for professionals.* Nelson, W. (Ed.) Dartmouth College, Hanover, NH University Press of New England, Lebanon, NH. Available from: <http//dms.dartmouth.edu/cfm/resources/ethics>.
3. Lauver, D.R., Ward, S.E., Heidrich, S.M., et al., 2002. Patient-centered interventions. *Res Nurs Health* 25 (4), 246–255.
4. Kahn, M.W., 2008. Etiquette-based medicine. *N Engl J Med* 358, 19.
5. Purtilo, R., Haddad, A., 2007. Professional boundaries guided by respect. In: *Health professional and patient interaction,* 7th ed. WB Saunders, Philadelphia, PA, pp. 213–245.

6. Dougherty, C., Purtilo, R., 1995. The duty of compassion in an era of health care reform. *Cambridge Q* 4, 426–433.
7. Garner, B.A., 2009. *Black's law dictionary*, 9th ed. West Thomson Publishing, Eagan, MN.
8. Niebuhr, H.R., 1963. *The responsible self: An essay in Christian moral philosophy*. Harper and Row, New York.
9. Ogletree, T., 2004. Responsibility. In: Post, S.G. (Ed.), *Encyclopedia of bioethics*, 3rd ed. Macmillan Reference USA Thomson Gale, New York, pp. 2379–2384 [quote, p. 2383].

3

Prototypes of Ethical Problems

Objectives

The reader should be able to:
- Recognize an ethical question and distinguish it from a strictly clinical or legal one.
- Identify three component parts of any ethical problem.
- Describe what an "agent" is and, more importantly, what it is to be a "moral agent."
- Name three prototypical ethical problems.
- Distinguish between two varieties of moral distress.
- Compare the fundamental difference between moral distress and an ethical dilemma.
- Describe the role of emotions in moral distress and ethical dilemmas.
- Describe a type of ethical dilemma that challenges a professional's desire (and duty) to treat everyone fairly and equitably.
- Identify the fundamental difference between distress or dilemma problems and locus of authority ones.
- Identify four criteria to assist in deciding who should assume authority for a specific ethical decision to achieve a caring response.

New terms and ideas you will encounter in this chapter

clinical question	ethical question	moral residue
legal question	prototype	ethical dilemma
workman's compensation	agent	locus of authority
disability benefits	moral agent	
	moral distress	

Topics in this chapter introduced in earlier chapters

Topic	Introduced in chapter
Ethical problem	1
Integrity	1
Professional responsibility	2
A caring response	2

Introduction

You have come a long way already and are prepared to take a giant stride towards becoming skilled in the art of ethical decision making. The first part of this chapter guides you through an inquiry regarding how you know when you are faced with an ethical question instead of (or in addition to) a clinical or legal question. Then comes the further question: How do you know if the situation that raised the question is a problem that requires your involvement? This chapter helps you prepare to answer that question too. You will learn the basic features of any ethical problem and be introduced to three prototypes of ethical problems. To help you get started, we offer the story of Beulah Watson and Tiffany Bryant.

 The Story of Beulah Watson and Tiffany Bryant

Beulah Watson is a 46-year-old environmental services employee in a large hotel in town. She has been employed for 18 years in this position and by and large says she has enjoyed her work. In recent years, however, she has increasingly suffered from shoulder and neck pain that the physician employed by the hotel's health plan accredits to her many years of tugging and hauling heavy linens and cleaning equipment on the job.

Tiffany Bryant is the occupational therapist who has been treating Ms. Watson for the pain and stiffness in her upper body, which has caused her much discomfort and has increased her absenteeism. Beulah Watson originally was prompt in keeping her appointments, but recently she has missed almost all of her sessions. Tiffany is concerned about whether Beulah is taking the time off to do other things while telling her workplace that she has a therapy appointment. This idea starts to work on Tiffany, and she gets more and more annoyed with Beulah.

Finally, Tiffany calls the hotel looking for Beulah but instead she gets her supervisor, the environmental services manager. Tiffany tells her about Beulah's regularly missed appointments (five in the last 6 weeks). She also tells the manager that the hotel is being charged for the missed visits because Beulah has not called to cancel, which is the billing policy of the institution where Tiffany is employed.

The manager responds that Beulah does not qualify for release time from work for the visits, and because the clinic hours correspond with her work hours, she may not keep all her appointments for that reason. She adds that Beulah probably is worried about the salary loss, even though the treatments are paid for, because she is the sole breadwinner for herself, her disabled husband, and two small grandchildren. The manager says she will talk to Beulah about the unacceptability of her failing to let the occupational therapy department know when she decides not to keep her appointment. In fact, if Beulah keeps that up, the manager continues, she will find herself paying for the missed appointments because the hotel cannot be expected to pay for her lack of responsibility. Tiffany responds that maybe Beulah did not know about the policy. The manager replies, "It doesn't matter. She knows better than that. By the way, she has been here all the times you mentioned except one, when she did call in sick, so at least she wasn't off on shopping trips or anything like that."

A week goes by. At the scheduled time for Beulah's appointment, she again does not appear. Tiffany has been uneasy about the conversation with the manager, and when the time comes for her to fill out the billing slip for another missed appointment, she feels positively terrible.

 Reflection

Do you share Tiffany's feelings that something is not right? If yes, what do you think the problem is? You can jot down a few thoughts here and refer back to them as the chapter progresses.

_____

_____

_____

_____

Recognizing an Ethical Question

Health professionals face all types of questions in their clinical practice. Some are ethical questions, but others are not. Many times what might appear to be an ethical question is in fact something else, such as a miscommunication or a question about a strictly clinical fact or a legal issue. Often complex questions present with clinical, legal, and ethical problems.

The following exercise is designed to walk you through one example of an issue that includes clinical, legal, and ethical dimensions, with a description of why the last is an ethical question.

Is this an ethical question? Yes or no:

Can a person with early stage dementia drive?

If you answered "no," you are right. It is a *clinical question* because clinical tests and procedures can help answer it. Patients who pass various cognitive assessments and an on-road driving evaluation **have the clinical ability** to drive and those who fail do not. Refer back to the story at the beginning of this chapter. In the narrative about Beulah Watson, Tiffany Bryant, and the hotel manager, what additional clinical information would help you better evaluate the situation?

Now consider the following question. Is it a clinical, legal, or ethical question?

Must patients with early dementia comply with medical advice in this type of situation if they want to continue to drive?

If you said "a *legal question*," you are on the right track. A tip-off is the word 'must.' As you learned in Chapter 1, the laws of the state and other laws are designed to monitor public well-being and enforce practices that protect the public good. Almost all states include procedures to help assure road safety. Relevant information about people who are dangerous behind the wheel is found in part through clinical examinations. Clinical and legal systems are interdependent in that and other situations, so it is not always up to an individual patient to ignore clinical recommendations.

Now, go to the specific legal implications of Beulah Watson's situation. When the physician employed by the hotel referred Beulah for therapy, she had assessed that the patient's discomfort was from years of labor at the hotel. The time may come when Beulah wants to recover *workman's compensation* for her condition or apply for *disability benefits*. Workman's compensation and disability benefits are legally enforced national programs in the United States to help protect employees from financial duress when injured on the job. And so, a related legal question relevant to this situation is: Do patients have the right to benefits provided by the government if for any reason they miss prescribed treatment and the professional reports this?

Eligibility usually requires that a patient comply with treatments that are prescribed; the fact that Beulah missed so many treatments may compromise her case. The hotel management may choose to fight her claim for disability benefits now that Tiffany has contacted them with this information.

Finally, consider this question, which is an *ethical question*. As you read it, think about why it is.

Should people with dementia who refuse to take a recommended on-road driving assessment be allowed to continue driving? If so, under what circumstances?

The word "should" is the tip-off here. It points to something in society all have agreed to support and each individual has a responsibility to help do so. Tiffany's reflection on whether she should have talked with Beulah's supervisor and her ambivalence about having to charge for treatments that she did not administer are examples of ethical questions about the wrong-doing or rightness of her actions that she was pondering.

⊚ SUMMARY

Ethical questions can be distinguished from strictly clinical or legal questions, all of which often arise in health professional and patient situations. An ethical question places the focus on one's role as a moral agent and those aspects of the situation that involve moral values, duties, and quality-of-life concerns in an effort to arrive at a caring response.

To continue your learning, we invite you to familiarize yourself with prototypes of ethical problems into which many different everyday ethical questions can fit.

Prototypes of Ethical Problems: Common Features

What is a *prototype?* Prototypes are a society's attempt to name a basic category of something. Prototypes can be objects, concepts, ideas, and situations.[1] Prototypes of ethical problems are recognizable as a group by three features they have in common. Each of the prototypes you will learn about in this chapter appears different from the others, and in fact, each has a different role to play when ethical questions have arisen. That said, the first step into this venture is to become familiar with the same basic structural features you find in all the prototypes of ethical problems:

A: A moral agent (or agents)
C: A course of action
O: An outcome
Each feature will be discussed in turn.

The Moral Agent: A

Which of the following best describes your idea of a health professional as an agent?

 a. A person with more than one basic loyalty. A deeply divided loyalty (e.g., a double agent).
 b. A person who has the moral or legal capacity to make decisions and be held responsible for them (e.g., a signee on a contract).
 c. A person who plans schedules, events (e.g., a booking agent).

If you answered B, you are most clearly focused on the meaning of agency in the health professions roles you will assume. In ethics or law, an *agent* is anyone responsible for the course of action chosen and the outcome of her or his actions in a specific situation. Obviously, being an agent requires that a person be able to understand the situation and be free to act voluntarily. Acting as an agent also implies intention: the person wants something specific to happen as a result of that action. A *moral agent* is a person who "acts for him or herself, or in the place of another by the authority of that person, and does so by conforming to a standard of right behavior."[2]

 Reflection

> This book emphasizes your role as a moral agent in the health profession setting because as a professional you must answer for your own actions and attitudes. If you have observed a situation in which someone in your chosen field has had to act courageously, then you have observed a moral agent at work. Briefly describe what you observed and why you feel the responsibility fell to that person to be on the front line of the decision.

_____

_____

_____

_____

A moral agent intends the morally right course of action. You can probably see that the idea of responsibility that you learned about in Chapter 2 is in fact the description of what an agent does; with an ethical challenge in the health professions, the actor is assuming the role of a moral agent. Professional responsibility is exercised through moral agency. Tiffany, the physician employed by the hotel, and the hotel manager all are agents whose actions influence the outcome of Tiffany's efforts and affect Beulah's health. As a health professional, Tiffany is clearly in the role of being a moral agent.

Agents and Emotion

Both your reason and emotion operate as part of your internal website where you can go and search to find the appropriate tools to exercise your professional responsibility. Much will be said about ethical reasoning and problem solving in this book. Over the years, considerable debate about the significance of emotion in an agent's activity has taken place. Strict rationalists view emotion as too subjective and unpredictable to serve as a reliable guide. However, a burgeoning body of current professional and lay literature lends new knowledge about the role of emotion in decision making more generally to support the essential role of emotion in ethical decision making. Such well-regarded bodies as the Harvard Decision-making Science Laboratory conduct research on the mechanisms through which emotion and social factors influence judgment and decision making. From their work and the work of others, we find convincing arguments for assigning emotion at least two roles in ethics.

First, emotion is an "alert" system that warns that you may be veering off the road of a caring response. When you encounter a morally perplexing situation, you, who will be accountable, feel discomfort, anxiety, anger, or some other disturbing emotion. Nancy Sherman, a contemporary philosopher working on the place of emotion in morality, proposes that emotions are "modes of sensitivity that record what is morally salient and . . . communicate those concerns to self and others."[3] Sometimes, an emotional response to wrongdoing or tragedy or a heroic act stirs a person out of lethargy and into moral action on someone else's behalf.[4] In other words, your emotions help grab your attention and motivate you to "do something."

Second, according to current research, emotion kicks in again at the point of decision making to complete the human picture of what is happening.[5] Even if you have been logical in your assessment of the ethical problem, emotion puts the last strokes on the canvas, bringing this decision into focus as one example of how humans actually conduct their lives all around. In the end, each of us can be ethical only about what we see, feel, loathe, or love. In short, ethical responsibility devoid of life infused into it by emotional responsiveness in specific situations is vacuous and can deter you from your best intent to be an effective moral agent.

 SUMMARY

An agent has responsibility for an action. A moral agent has responsibility to act in a way that protects moral values and other aspects of morality. An ethical problem requires attention to both reasoning and emotion in the process of decision making. Emotion alerts, focuses attention, motivates, and increases one's knowledge about complex situations.

The Course of Action: C

The course of action includes the agent's analysis, the judgment process of discerning the best likely resolution to the problem, and the decision to act in accordance with that judgment. The next two chapters spell out how this process works within the context of ethical problem solving using ethical theories and approaches, so we need not go into more detail about that now. Tiffany Bryant used the information she had to analyze the situation. One attempt at resolution was to call the hotel looking for Beulah. Her emotional response afterwards reflected a concern for this patient's well-being even though she was irritated when she made the call because her discomfort suggests she was not sure she had exercised the correct moral judgment in saying what she did to the supervisor. As we know, Tiffany also felt a sense of responsibility to continue to bill the hotel for treatments Beulah did not receive although she did not like this policy in her workplace. This back and forth reflection about what she was feeling and doing kept the course of action alive to the possibilities of what should happen.

The Outcome: O

The outcome is the result of having taken a particular course of action. Of course, the goal is that a caring response is achieved in what actually happens as a result of the whole process. We would need to have more information about what actually happened as a result of Tiffany's conversation and what she thought about it to know whether she would consider it a good outcome for her patient Beulah Watkins.

Some ethical approaches you will learn to use in the next chapter place much more weight on the outcome; others place moral priority on the course of action. In everyday descriptions of ethics, this is sometimes referred to as the tension between the "means" one employs and the "ends" achieved. The important point here is that applying yourself to real-life professional situations requires your full participation in all three features of an ethical problem. Deciding which of the features takes precedence in a particular ethical problem depends in part on the approach or theory you adopt.

 SUMMARY

The three prototypes of ethical problems share three features in common: a moral agent (or agents), a course of action, and an outcome.

Three Prototypes of Ethical Problems

Having acquainted yourself with the common features of all prototypes, you are ready to learn more about the prototypes themselves: moral distress, ethical dilemmas, and locus of authority problems.

Moral Distress: Confronting Barriers to Moral Agency

Moral distress focuses on the agent (A) herself or himself when a situation blocks her or him from doing what is right. Moral distress is a term that came into the ethics literature primarily through nursing ethics and has become more generalized because of its usefulness in understanding ethical problems that all health professionals experience. Moral distress reflects that you, the moral agent, experience appropriate emotional or cognitive discomfort, or both, because of a barrier from being the kind of professional you know you should be or from doing what you conclude is right. Your emotional response and feelings play a major role in helping you recognize that you have moved from striding confidently along in your moral life to experiencing that something is going wrong. You can see that your response to the situation is coming from an awareness that your integrity is threatened because a threat to integrity arises when you cannot be the person you know you should be in your professional role or cannot do what you know for certain is right. Health professionals find that these emotional signals give rise to physical expressions that warn something is wrong: a knot in the pit of their stomach, a catch in the easy stride, or being awakened in the early hours of the morning with the haunting feeling that something is awry. Again, we are reminded that emotions and feelings are critical data of the moral life, trying to say, "Stop! Wait! Don't! Think twice!"

Moral agents in the health professions encounter two types of barriers that create moral distress: type A and type B.

Type A: You Cannot Do What You Know Is Right (Figure 3-1)

A common problem today is barriers to adequate care of individual patients created by the mechanisms for the delivery and financing of health care, although there are also other sources. A recent survey of occupational

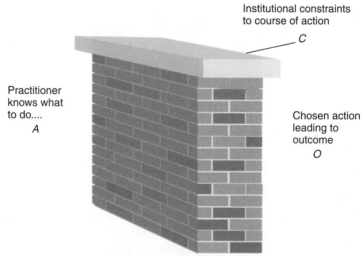

Figure 3-1. Moral distress: type A.

therapists found that the highest percentages of moral distress in descending order of occurrence were reimbursement constraints, conflict with organizational policies, excessive pressure to meet productivity standards, lack of administrative support, questionable or unrealistic clinical decisions by others, patients who decline treatment, decision making regarding patient discharge, excessive pressure to increase billable hours, and compromised care as a result of pressure to decrease costs.[6] For example, a hospital policy may be to refuse admission of patients who do not have insurance to fully cover the cost of their treatment or to discharge patients that physicians, nurses, therapists, or others judge to be unsuited for the rigors of transition to the home environment. Here the morally right course of action (C) leading to the desired outcome (O) is blocked by policies and practices. The moral distress comes precisely because of the repercussions the professionals believe they may have to endure. Institutional and traditional role barriers keep them from exercising their moral agency for the good of patients.

This does not mean that you will never take into account the larger social context in which you are practicing. For instance, health professionals must always attend to the larger public health considerations in the case of a patient with a serious highly infectious disease. The patient may experience forced quarantine or be placed in isolation. The health professional's emotional discomfort in such a situation that requires acting for the good of many other individuals is not an example of moral distress. The patient himself or herself still can be the recipient of the best care possible. Only when you are quite sure you cannot be faithful to the basic well-being of the patient is there legitimate reason for moral distress.

Another powerful barrier to doing what is right is suggested in the previous paragraph but all too often fails to be included in discussions of moral distress. Moral distress often occurs because of internal barriers such as the fear of repercussion of one kind or another—real or imagined—that looms in the professional's awareness, blocking action. Wanting to do the right thing and not having the inner strength to do it while under the weight of anxieties and fears often results in heightened moral distress rather than leading to freedom through action (Figure 3-2). This process, faced time after time, can result in *moral residue*, an accumulation of compromises that takes a heavy toll on one's integrity.[7]

To face those uncomfortable feelings and emotions and remain motivated to do the right thing requires that each and every one of us receive support from others to step up, speak out, or stand firm as the occasion calls for it. In some other parts of this book, you will be introduced to team and institutional supports that can help you navigate out from under the burden of these internal barriers.

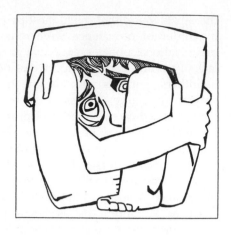

Figure 3-2. Internal barriers.
(From Purtilo, R., Haddad, A,. 2002.
Respect: the difference it makes.
In: Health professional and patient
interaction, *7th ed. WB Saunders,*
Philadelphia, p. 12.)

Type B: You Know Something Is Wrong But Are Not Sure What (Figure 3-3)

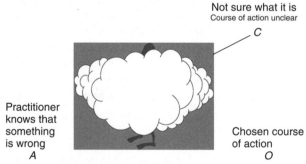

Figure 3-3. Moral distress: type B.

The barrier may not be policies practices or internal anxieties and fear but instead may be that the situation is new or extremely complex. Your only certainty is an acknowledgment that something is wrong; the rest is a big question mark. You may question how to arrive at the morally correct course of action (C) or how to work toward a specific outcome (O) that is consistent with your professional goal of achieving a caring response in this The ethical challenge is to remove the barrier of doubt or uncertainty as much as possible, sometimes achieved through probing deeper into the facts of the situation. When there is high uncertainty, doubt requires that the moral agent must seek advice and critically problem solve through the situation to better understand how to address its complexity. As you can readily see, emotions often play a major role in this type of situation too.

Reflection

Think about Tiffany Bryant's moral distress. We asked you to think about why you might feel uneasy too if you were in her situation. What subtype of moral distress is she facing? Explain your answer in a few words here.

_____

_____

_____

_____

We assume that Tiffany's discomfort partially stems from wanting to do what is best for Beulah Watson but not being sure what because it's likely she has not been faced with this set of issues before. She wants to show a caring response that befits a health professional, but she is not sure how to do that under the circumstances. Understandably, she also wants to honor the rules and policies of her workplace but is distressed about charging for Beulah's missed treatments. Her moral distress is more of type B, as we read her situation.

---

⑥ SUMMARY

Moral distress occurs when the moral agent knows what the morally appropriate course of action is but meets up against external barriers, internal resistance, or a high level of uncertainty.

As she analyzes the situation, Tiffany thinks about whether her distress also is related to the fact that she is facing an ethical dilemma. So, join her now in that reflection, as we turn to the second type of prototypical ethical problem: the *ethical dilemma.*

Ethical Dilemma: Two Courses Diverging

Many people call all ethical problems ethical dilemmas. More correctly, an ethical dilemma is a common type of situation that involves two (or more) morally correct courses of action that cannot both be followed; that is, to take course C_1 precludes you from taking course C_2. As a result, you (the agent, the responsible one) necessarily are doing something right and also wrong (by not doing the other thing that is also right). You are between a rock and a hard place, between the devil and the deep blue sea (Figure 3-4).[8]

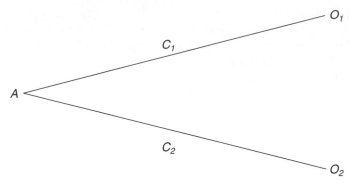

Figure 3-4. Ethical dilemma.

Ethical dilemmas involve both ethical conflict and conduct. Suppose that Tiffany Bryant has just read the previous paragraph and realizes that she had an ethical dilemma but did not recognize it at the time. She was aware of her moral distress and that further analysis was needed. Here is why she now knows she had a dilemma.

On the one hand, Tiffany is an agent (A) who has a professional duty to look after her patient, Beulah Watson, and to take the course of action (C_1) that will demonstrate her attempt to give Beulah the best treatment possible. The desired outcome (O_1) is the relief of the patient's pain and stiffness. On the other hand, Tiffany is an agent (A) who has a duty to abide by the policies of her place of employment. The course of action (C_2) that will express that duty is to charge for all treatments that are given or are not officially canceled. The desired outcome (O_2) is the financial solvency of the occupational therapy clinic. Both outcomes are ethically appropriate, taken alone. However, Tiffany Bryant probably caused some negative repercussions for Beulah in her course of action that included sharing potentially damaging information to Beulah's supervisor. The supervisor did not sound pleased, either by Beulah's absenteeism from scheduled treatments or that the hotel was being charged for the missed treatments. In charging for the treatments, Tiffany maintained fidelity to her workplace at the price of protecting Beulah Watson from exposure that may cause her additional problems.

Of course, Tiffany might have thought that charging for missed appointments is wrong under any circumstance, a position being examined in the health profession literature because this practice is increasing in health care institutions.[9]

In subsequent chapters, you will have ample opportunity to work with several types of dilemmas because they are the most commonly confronted type of ethical problem.

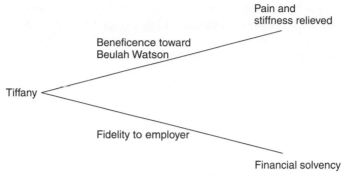

Ethical dilemma in story of Tiffany and Beulah.

Justice Seeking as an Ethical Dilemma

A special ethical dilemma arises in regards to searching for ways to allocate societal benefits and burdens fairly and equitably. As in all ethical problems, the agent (A) makes a judgment to take a course of action (C) that results in an outcome (O). The situation is this: competition exists for a cherished but scarce resource such as a medication, health professionals' time, money to pay for health care, or an organ or other types of lifesaving or quality of life–enhancing procedures. The agent's (A) morally right course of action (C) is to give everyone a full measure of the resource to the extent their needs warrant it. In so doing, the outcome (O) is that the patient's legitimate claims are honored. The scarce supply, however, requires that the agent take difficult, even tragic, courses of action, the outcome being that some claimants get the cherished good and others do not.[10] In short, it is morally right to give your own patient everything he or she needs to benefit from your interventions. It is also morally right to spread resources around to the benefit of others. The question of how to treat each person fairly, and to treat groups equitably, becomes a challenge that involves a dilemma of justice, a problem that physical therapists in an important study of the meaning of caring in their professional practice found increasingly difficult in a health care system that values cost control and a high margin of profit.[11] This dilemma is by no means limited to one profession; in fact, it is a common theme in health professions literature today. You will study this more extensively in later chapters of this book and how you can optimize your efforts in the face of contemporary justice dilemmas.

 Reflection

Describe an example in your chosen field of how you might become involved in a dilemma that requires you to make tough decisions because of scarce resources. One way to approach this is to think of the setting in which you are likely to work and the special, sometimes expensive, procedures that may be available to a range of patients. Another is to imagine conditions under which your worksite is short staffed and you must make difficult choices about where to cut corners.

_____

_____

_____

_____

---

⑤ SUMMARY

An ethical dilemma occurs when a moral agent is faced with two or more conflicting courses of action but only one can be chosen as the agent attempts to bring about an outcome consistent with the professional goal of a caring response. A special case of a dilemma involves justice issues when there is not enough supply of a needed resource or service.

Locus of Authority Problem

A *locus of authority* ethical problem arises from an ethical question of who should have the authority to make an important ethical decision. In other words, **who** is the rightful moral agent (A) to carry out the course of action (C) and be held responsible for the outcome (O)? Locus of authority problems most often arise when ambiguities exist about who is in charge (Figure 3-5). Schematically, the situation looks like this:

$$A_1 \text{————————} O_1 \quad \text{vs.} \quad A_2 \text{————————} O_2$$
$$\quad\quad C_1 \quad\quad\quad\quad\quad\quad\quad\quad\quad\quad C_2$$

Figure 3-5. Locus of authority problem.

Note that two people assume themselves to be appropriate moral agents (A_1 and A_2) and proceed along parallel (or even conflicting) courses of action (C_1 and C_2). As each analyzes the situation, they may come to different conclusions about how to achieve the best outcome (O_1 versus O_2) for a patient.

This kind of ethical problem highlights that it does matter who has decision making authority and say-so.

Reflection

In the story of Tiffany Bryant and Beulah Watson, who do you think should make the decisions about whether to charge for missed treatments?
The health professional providing the service?
The supervisor of the unit?
The institutional administrator?
The government or some other, larger societal regulating body?
The patient?
    Give a brief explanation for your thinking that supports your position.

_____

_____

_____

_____

Sometimes no ambiguity exists, but reflection on the issue reveals that the wrong person has the authority. In that case, the situation creates moral distress. The challenge of determining the appropriate locus of authority is the topic of thoughtful reflection by ethicists and other individuals. In the context of the health professions, there are at least four ways of thinking about authority in health care decisions.

1. Professional expertise: You are in a professional role along with other people in different professional roles. This is the essence of teamwork that characterizes so much of health care today. The role differences mean that you bring different spheres of expertise to the situation. In some areas of the patient's care, each professional is an authority on some part of the whole picture. That alone should be a vote for the person who has the most relevant knowledge about the patient's condition and other relevant facts.

2. Traditional arrangements: Traditionally in the health care system, the physician has been the authoritative voice in health care decisions. The physician is considered to be *in* authority because of his or her office or position rather than (or in addition to) being *an* authority because of special expertise. From this perspective, the medical director of the unit would unquestionably be the one to make a decision about what to do, although he or she may choose to invite advice and counsel from other individuals.

3. Institutional arrangements and mechanisms: Sometimes the decision about the authoritative voice comes from special institutional arrangements. For example, some tasks may be delegated to committees. In these instances, the committees or designated individuals assume specific

task-related roles. This is really a variation of the first two roles, the designated individuals being in authority both because of their expertise and the positions they hold. For example, it is possible that the authority for making a decision regarding billing for missed treatments may be referred to a committee designed to deal with humane treatment of patients in unusual situations rather than treating billing solely as a financial issue.

4. The authority of experience: A voice of authority may emerge because of the insight that comes from experience. There are always those situations in which we seek the advice of people who have been in similarly perplexing situations and defer to their judgment. Tiffany Bryant may wish to seek advice for the next step from a supervisor, senior member of the professional staff, or other person judged to have the benefit of experience. This is seldom institutionalized as a formal mechanism for dealing with locus of authority challenges and is a variation of the professional expertise approach, which assumes that expertise often is refined with experience in a wide range of situations.

None of these sources should be taken for granted as the appropriate authority for all situations. The ethical gold standard remains what will result in a caring response for the patient.

 SUMMARY

Locus of authority situations focus on problems determining the appropriate moral agent in a situation. Conflicts often can be resolved with an analysis of who has the most expertise, the traditional practices regarding who makes what decisions, an appeal to policies, and respect for experience. The goal is to achieve an outcome consistent with a caring response.

Summary

This completes your introduction to three prototypes of ethical problems that will help you be ready to act as you face complex situations in your roles as clinician, administrator, researcher, teacher, or team member. The prototypes of moral distress, ethical dilemmas, and locus of authority situations will guide you as you analyze and decide which course of action is the most likely to achieve an intended outcome consistent with honoring your professional responsibility as a moral agent.

Questions for Thought and Discussion

1. Jane is a pregnant health professions student who does not want to treat a patient with AIDS in the intensive care unit. Thinking it is because of her pregnant condition, her clinical supervisor assures her

that she is safe as long as she uses the universal precautions designed to make the treatment of patients with infectious diseases safe for everyone. Jane still hesitates, saying, "I know it's irrational, but I'm afraid I will not be effective because I'm so afraid of hurting my baby." She pauses and then adds, "To be honest, I also feel it is God's will if some people get AIDS."

Are either or both of Jane's reasons sufficiently compelling to warrant her being excused from assignment to this patient? Why or why not? What type of ethical problem faces her clinical supervisor? Describe how you have arrived at this conclusion using the three features of any ethical problem.

2. Loretta is a physical therapist specializing in diabetic foot care. She sees Louise monthly. Louise is quite down when she hobbles into the clinic today, her ankles bandaged, with blood oozing through the gauze. She tells Loretta, "I'm sure my feet are much worse this month. I haven't been so good about my sugar, and it didn't help that my husband hit my ankles with his cane twice last week. I think he is upset about my taxi fare to get here. I think I'll stop coming." She begins to cry.

   What are the clinical, legal, and ethical questions that face Loretta in this case? What should she do?

3. Describe an ethical dilemma that you or someone you know has faced. This does not have to be a problem that arose within the health care context. What did you have to take into consideration as you moved toward a decision about which of the two or more courses of action available to you should be taken? Did it result in a good outcome?

References

1. Lakoff, G., 1987. *Women, fire and dangerous things: What categories reveal about the mind*. University of Chicago Press, Chicago, p. 12.
2. Taylor, C.R., 2008. Right relationships: Foundation for health care ethics. In: Pinch, W.J.E., Haddad, A.M. (Eds.), *Nursing and health care ethics: A legacy and a vision*. American Nurses Association, Silver Spring, MD, pp. 163–164.
3. Sherman, N., 2004. Emotions. In: Post, S. (Ed.), *Encyclopedia of bioethics*, 3rd ed. vol. 2. Thomson Gale, New York, pp. 740–748.
4. Purtilo, R., 2000. Moral courage: Unsung resource for health professional as friend and healer. In: Thomasma, D., Kissell, J. (Eds.), *The health professional as friend and healer*. Georgetown University Press, Washington, DC, pp. 106–112.
5. Bechara, A., 2004. The role of emotion in decision-making: Evidence from neurological patients with orbitofrontal damage. *Brain Cognition* 55, 30–40.

6. Slater, D., Brandt, L., 2009. Combating moral distress. *OT Practice* 2, 13–18. Available from: <www.AOTA.org>.
7. Hardingham, L.B., 2004. Integrity and moral residue: Nurses as participants in a moral community. *Nurs Philos* 5 (2), 127–134.
8. Beauchamp, T.L., Childress, J.F., 2009. Professional-patient relationships. In: *Principles of biomedical ethics*, 6th ed. Oxford University Press, New York, pp. 288–331.
9. Fay, A., 1995. Ethical implications of charging for missed sessions. *Psychol Rep* 77, 1251–1259.
10. Freeman, J.M., McDonnell, K., 2001. Making moral decisions: A process approach. In: *Tough decisions: Cases in medical ethics*, 2nd ed. Oxford University Press, New York, pp. 241–246.
11. Greenfield, B.H., 2006. The meaning of caring in five experienced physical therapists. *Physiother Theory Pract* 22 (4), 175–187.

4

Ethics Theories and Approaches: Conceptual Tools for Ethical Decision Making

Objectives

The reader should be able to:
- Distinguish between an ethical theory and ethical approach.
- Understand the process of clinical reasoning in the health professional.
- List the different modes of clinical reasoning.
- Describe ethical reasoning as a distinct mode of clinical reasoning.
- Describe the usefulness of the basic ethics theories and approaches as tools in analyzing ethical problems and attempting to resolve problems by arriving at the most caring response.
- Name five types of ethical theories and approaches that help illuminate what a "caring response" entails.
- Describe a narrative and what it means to take a narrative approach to an ethical issue or problem.
- Assess the contribution of psychologist Carol Gilligan and others who stress relationships.
- Relate the basic features of an "ethic of care" to "a caring response," introduced in Chapter 2.
- Describe the role of moral character or virtue in the realization of a good life and its significance for health professionals faced with the goal of arriving at a caring response.
- Describe ways the various story or case approaches help one understand what a caring response involves.
- Describe the function of a principle (norm, element) in ethical analysis and conduct.
- Identify six principles often encountered in professional ethics that can help guide one in trying to arrive at a caring response to a professional situation.
- Discuss the meaning of autonomy in Kant's and Mill's theories and the relevance of each to ethical conduct.

- List five reasonable expectations a patient or client has because of the health professional's responsibility to act with fidelity.
- Describe the principle of veracity as it applies in the professional context.
- Describe the basic difference between deontologic and utilitarian ethical theories of conduct and the role of each in the health professional's goal of acting in accordance with what a caring response requires.

New terms and ideas you will encounter in this chapter

clinical reasoning	character trait	justice
ethical reasoning	moral character	deontology
theories and approaches	principles	deontologic theories
normative ethics	principle-based	teleology
metaethics	approach	absolute duties
story or case	nonmaleficence	prima facie duties
approaches	beneficence	conditional duties
foundationalist based	autonomy and self-	teleologic theories
narrative approaches	determination	utilitarianism
postmodernists	fidelity	rule utilitarian
ethics of care approach	veracity	
virtue theory	paternalism	

Topics in this chapter introduced in earlier chapters

Topic	Introduced in chapter
Three uses of ethics in everyday life	1
Moral duty and character	1
Codes of ethics	1
A caring response	2
Patient-centered care	2
Professional responsibility	2
Right(s)	2
Prototypes of ethical problems	3
Moral agent	3
Moral distress	3
Ethical dilemma	3

Introduction

In this chapter, you will be introduced to a whole "toolbox" of conceptual tools you can use to accomplish your professional goal of arriving at a caring response in the wide variety of challenges you may encounter. These tools are presented in the form of ethical theories and ethical approaches. An ethical theory is researched and well developed and provides us with an assumption about the very nature of doing right and wrong. Most are historically based and have evolved for current usage according to a society's or group's development and need for interpreting or addressing current moral challenges. In contrast, an approach does not propose to be a complete system or model but an aid to existing theories. For instance, the principle-based approach to which you will be introduced in this chapter is quite recent and has roots in ancient Western ethical theories. Both ethical theories and approaches provide you with a framework for diagnosing, communicating, and problem solving ethical questions you encounter in your clinical practice.[1]

If you are like us, you probably take a look at how many pages you have ahead of you for your assignment and you quickly conclude that this is a very long siege of reading! The idea behind this chapter is to provide you with a "mini book" of ethical theory. Depending on your course of study, your professor may add to these pages with another more theoretic text or may split the chapter into smaller parts. We encourage you to work your way through the chapter carefully so that the rest of your study of this book is easier and your preparation in ethics more complete.

In Chapter 1, we suggested three general ways that ethical tools have usefulness in your everyday life: (1) to analyze moral issues, (2) to help resolve moral conflicts, and (3) to move toward action when faced with a problem. In Chapter 2, you learned about the caring response as the goal of professional ethical practice. In Chapter 3, you had an opportunity to learn the basic varieties (i.e., prototypes) of ethical problems you will encounter in your professional career. In this chapter, you will gain more knowledge and tools that enable you to move skillfully from the identification of a problem, through its analysis, and, hopefully, to its resolution through action that achieves your goal of a caring response. Chapter 5 provides a simple six-step process you can follow as you apply everything discussed in this and the previous chapters. To help set the stage for your thinking, consider the story of Elizabeth Kim, Max Diaz, Melinda Diaz, and Michael Leary.

🐿 The Story of Elizabeth Kim, Max Diaz, Melinda Diaz, and Michael Leary

A speech and language pathologist, Elizabeth Kim, works in a large urban school system. She is responsible for performing many student evaluations and interventions each day and takes her job seriously. Elizabeth services the Richards Elementary School and two other schools in the Lakeview district. Students and parents who meet Elizabeth quickly learn that she is a bright spot in the otherwise anxiety-producing ordeal of navigating services for children with learning disabilities. Elizabeth prides herself on being thorough and always explains everything to both the students and parents in language they can understand.

Two weeks ago, Elizabeth had an experience that upset her, and she is not sure what to do about it. A young student, Max Diaz, had met Elizabeth for his speech and language pathology evaluation at Richards Elementary School. Max has an expressive language disorder, and Elizabeth felt strongly that he would benefit from an augmentative communication device. She has used these devices in the past and has seen great success with them. Elizabeth has her quarterly supervision meeting with Michael Leary, the school principal, that afternoon. She talks about Max in the meeting because she is intrigued by his case. She tells Principal Leary her evaluation results and that she will be recommending the augmentative device. Principal Leary tells Elizabeth "Please do not put that recommendation in your written report. Max's mother has not been overly involved in advocating for his needs. If we can hold off on meeting with her for Max's education plan until the end of the school year, I won't have to buy the device until the next academic year. Those devices are really expensive, and I don't know if we have the money right now. Besides, who knows if it will really even work for him, given English is his second language." Elizabeth leaves the meeting feeling uncomfortable.

The speech and language pathology evaluation report was completed and submitted to the administration. Elizabeth did include the recommendation for the augmentative device in the report because she knew that it was in Max's best interest. She was eager to train Max in how to use this type of device. All that was needed now was administrative and parental approval. As soon as the individualized education plan (IEP) could be scheduled, they could move forward. A copy was sent to Principal Leary, Max's homeroom teacher, and his mom, and one was placed in his academic record in the administrative office.

Several weeks later, Elizabeth asks Principal Leary when Max's IEP is going to take place. She wants to get his mother's and the team's approval to move forward with various interventions, including the augmentative device. He tells her that Melinda, Max's mom, has been slow to respond to the school's request for a meeting, saying "We offered her a date, but she could not make it. Since then we have not been able to coordinate with a

Spanish interpreter. I may just try to schedule her without one. Actually, the longer it is put off, the better, as we won't have to bear the cost of the device you recommended on this year's school budget."

Knowing that the longer the meeting took to arrange, the longer Max would go without service, she wanted to say, "Aren't you going to follow up and encourage her to get in soon?" but she didn't. She knew Principal Leary would have to schedule the meeting and was also was afraid he may have been insulted by such a question.

Today, 3 months after the evaluation was completed, Elizabeth is walking another student to the after school program when she sees Max with his mom, Melinda Diaz, in the corridor. Melinda says, "Oh you must be the speech therapist. Thanks for the papers you sent to me about Max. It's too bad that you and the teacher couldn't meet a couple months ago. I was looking forward to talking with you all. I can't read English that well so I had a hard time understanding the papers."

"Oh. Did Principal Leary talk with you about setting another meeting time sooner rather than later?" Elizabeth asks, feeling tense.

"No, he didn't. He just keeps saying, 'Don't worry.'"

"Well," Elizabeth says, "You have the right to set another meeting time sooner rather than later and to have an interpreter there if you want to."

Melinda immediately looks concerned. Elizabeth wants to say something to reassure her, but the words fail her. The school bell rings, and Elizabeth says a hurried goodbye. She feels a gnawing in the pit of her stomach, but she cannot immediately figure out what, if anything, she should do next.

That Elizabeth Kim is distressed is not surprising because something definitely is wrong. In fact, we might wonder about a health professional who felt no emotion at all about this situation: a young child with a learning disorder who is not performing to his potential and communication between his mother and the school staff appears to have broken down. Maybe Elizabeth has said too much—or too little—to help this family and school, both of whom have had some difficult discussions to confront. She is not sure how far she should go in advocating for her client and taking on the system.

Reflection

What is the caring, morally responsible action in this type of situation?

_____

_____

_____

_____

We return to this story throughout the chapter, so keep your response in mind.

Ethical Reasoning: A Guide for Ethical Reflection

Clinical Reasoning

As a health professional, you must learn to blend your knowledge, skills, and attitudes in response to varying clinical situations that require your professional judgment.[2] As you have read in the previous chapters, being a health professional means you must learn to be responsible for your actions on others, both clients and the public. So, before we highlight theoretical parts of ethical study that take you deeper into addressing situations, we must discuss clinical reasoning. You may be familiar with the terms critical thinking or practical reasoning. These terms are similar to clinical reasoning.

Clinical reasoning is the complex thought process that health professionals use during therapeutic interactions. Schell defines this process well by stating that clinical reasoning is used by practitioners to "plan, direct, perform and reflect on [client] care."[3] Most significantly, clinical reasoning is used to guide action. Health professionals use clinical reasoning to analyze and synthesize information that they have gathered in the care of a patient.

You have likely already been trained to develop your clinical reasoning. Throughout your educational process, has a professor, clinical instructor, or supervisor ever asked you "why" when you gave an answer to a clinical question? If so, they are trying to understand your reasoning. They want to ensure that you not only know the answer to the question but that you have thought about and analyzed the situation from a broad perspective. The process of clinical reasoning is important because it guides your decision making in the care of the patient. The more complex the clinical case, the more demands placed on your reasoning.

Modes of Reasoning

Health professionals use different modes of reasoning in response to particular features of a clinical case (Table 4-1). Many modes of clinical reasoning are used simultaneously to solve a clinical problem. For a caring response to be actualized, health professionals must use clinical reasoning to ensure that their decisions have meaning for the client. At various points in your clinical practice, you should stop and ask yourself, "Why am I doing what I am doing?" This helps you reflect on your clinical reasoning. Your reasoning is one of the strongest foundations you can have as a professional. It must continue to grow throughout your career to meet the demands and challenges of our ever-changing patient population and service delivery environment.

Table 4-1   Forms of Clinical Reasoning

Forms of Clinical Reasoning	Description
Scientific Reasoning	A framework for understanding the condition of the patient. Involves the use of scientific methods such as hypothesis testing, cue and pattern identification, and evidence as related to a diagnosis. Scientific reasoning includes both diagnostic and procedural reasoning. The focus is generally on the diagnosis, procedures, and interventions for a specific condition. Data are systematically gathered, and knowledge is compared.
Narrative Reasoning	A framework for understanding the patient's "life story" or illness experience. This type of reasoning helps clinicians make sense of the patient's past, present, and future. Includes an appreciation of how his or her life story is influenced by culture, condition, and experiences.
Pragmatic Reasoning	A framework for consideration of the practical issues that impact care. Such issues include treatment environments, equipment, availability of resources (including training of individual providers), and other realities associated with service delivery.
Interactive Reasoning	A mode of reasoning that is used to help clinicians better interact with and understand their patient as a person. Highlights the interpersonal nature of the therapeutic relationship (e.g., the use of empathy, nonverbal communication, therapeutic use of self).
Conditional Reasoning	A blending of reasoning that involves the moment-to-moment treatment revision based on the patient's current and future context. Used to anticipate outcomes over short or long periods of time.
Ethical Reasoning	A mode of reasoning used to recognize, analyze, and clarify ethical problems that arise. Helps clinicians make decisions regarding the right thing to do in a particular case. The moral basis for professional behaviors and actions. The focus is not on what *could* be done for the patient, rather on what *should* be done.

Adapted from Schell and Schell (2008), Mattingly and Fleming (1994), and Leicht and Dickerson (2001).[4-6]

Ethical Reasoning

Ethical reasoning is a key component of clinical reasoning. It is about norms and values and ideas of right and wrong. You use ethical reasoning when you ask yourself, "What is the morally correct action to take for this client?" Ethical reasoning helps guide the provision of professional care with an emphasis primarily on conduct. When you recognize the morally significant features of a clinical scenario, you are using your ethical reasoning. Ethical reasoning requires that you be able to gather relevant information and correctly apply your ethical knowledge and skills in the process of ethical reflection. This requires great attention to the details of each case.[7] Ethical reasoning is not only concerned with recognizing, gathering, and applying ethical knowledge but also emphasizes the process one goes through when reasoning about the situation. We successfully engage ethical reasoning when we not only recognize that x is good and y is bad but when we articulate reasons for *why* x is good and y is bad.[8] Some *theories and approaches* to ethics today use modes of reasoning outlined in Table 4-1 (e.g., narrative or interactive reasoning) that complement strictly ethical reasoning. Even the theories that focus mostly on character traits, narratives, or relationships must be reflected on. More will be said about this as the chapter unfolds.

 SUMMARY

Clinical reasoning requires that you be able to gather relevant information and correctly apply your knowledge and skills in a way that meets your desired goal of a caring response.

Metaethics and Normative Ethics

The ethical theories and approaches you will use for situations like that with Elizabeth Kim and Max Diaz fall within the dimension of ethics called *normative ethics*. Almost all the ethical reflection you do relevant to everyday life problems is in the area of normative ethics, so several approaches and theories are described in detail in this chapter. However, each theory also is part of a larger approach called metaethics. *Metaethics* tries to discover the nature and meaning of ethical reasons we propose as valid for making judgments about morality. How do we know whether there are ultimate truths about morality? Does the certainty about what Elizabeth Kim should do come from lived experience? From revelation or Scripture? From reasoning? Is there a "natural law" from which humans can discern truths about right or wrong? These are just some questions with which metaethics deals. An understanding of metaethics requires that you become more aware of your beliefs—religious, philosophic, what you have been taught or told—to recognize that they influence you regarding what is right or wrong, virtuous or blameworthy, whenever you face a situation with troubling ethical issues.

Normative ethics asks more concrete questions related to morality. When you assessed the situation described earlier in this chapter, you were using the concepts of normative ethics if you wondered, what would be an appropriate expression of care toward Max and Melinda Diaz? What types of acts are morally right or wrong and therefore should be considered in this case? What are the morally praiseworthy or blameworthy character traits (virtues) needed for the individuals or institutions involved in this story to arrive at a caring response? What values are morally good or bad for the harmonious functioning of this group of individuals? Your encounters with real situations involving patients, colleagues, other people, rules, policies, or practices are what will motivate you to engage in normative ethical reflection and ethical problem solving.

 SUMMARY

Normative theories and approaches deal with methods for ascertaining right and wrong actions and morally praiseworthy or blameworthy attitudes and behavior. Metaethics deals with the *source* of the reasons we give for our positions. Acquaintance with metaethics helps you gain insight into your own and others' basis for moral judgments.

The Caring Response: Using Theories and Approaches to Guide You

You have already learned that the goal of your ethical deliberation is to answer the question: "What does it mean to provide a caring response in this situation?" You have also learned that although you will be faced with legitimate competing loyalties as a health professional, your primary loyalty must always be patient centered. But all these insights beg for further description about how to actually arrive at the ethically appropriate caring response in a particular situation.

Several ethics theories and approaches are relevant to your work of putting together this caring response. Your ethics work differs from an academic philosopher's because you must not only apply clear thinking to ethical problems, which a philosopher must do as you learned in Chapter 3, but also decide on purposive action. You will not use all the theories or approaches covered in this chapter for any one situation. Just as you need to select the correct tool for building anything, the same is true for the tools we are describing.

The first two types, story or case-driven approaches and virtue theories, emphasize the importance of the kind of person you should strive to be (i.e., your attitudes and dispositions), so that you are well positioned to enact a caring response. Taken together, the several varieties share the common themes of paying attention to the details of stories for their moral content, becoming aware of one's emotions in relation to what is happening in the story, and development of character traits that allow one to be prepared to act in a caring manner. Collectively, they also stress the moral relevance of relationships, both between individuals and with the institutional structures of society.

The last three approaches and theories, principle-based approaches, deontologic theories, and teleologic theories, are geared to forms of ethical conduct itself. Principle-based approaches have been developed to help people understand general action guides for ethical behavior, some of which are related to duties or rights, others related to consequences. Regarding deontologic and teleologic theories, these mouthfuls can be broken down into more digestible pieces by looking at their roots: the root word "deonto" means duty; the root word "telos" means end. Already you can see a distinction developing. Deontologic theories delineate duties (actually duties, rights, or other forms of action), whereas teleologic ones rely on an assessment of the ends or consequences to determine right or wrong. You have heard the expression, "Do the ends justify the means?" Deontologists would say "no"; teleologists would say "yes." As noted previously, some principles guide you toward duty, others toward the "telos" or consequences. Are you ready to delve into these five theories or approaches in more detail?

Story or Case Approaches

In professional ethics, the story is the inevitable beginning point of ethical reflection because you encounter ethical problems in everyday life with everyday patients (or others). In *story or case approaches,* the assumption is that morally relevant information is embedded in the story.

In professional ethics, you also are equipped with foundation stones of ethical codes, a tradition, and societal expectations of how you will respond to legitimate requests for your professional services. Therefore, although the appropriate starting place for ethical analysis is the story, there are standards, principles, and other moral guides against which your opinion must be tested when you are deciding on a caring response. It is not simply, "You hold your view and I hold mine and they are on equal footing, morally speaking." Therefore, professional ethics also is *foundationalist based* by nature.

Narrative Approaches

Narrative is the technical term applied to the story's characters, events, and ordering of events (e.g., the plot), although in health care ethics and legal circles you will more often see the term "case." *Narrative approaches* are based on the observation that humans pass on information, impute and explore meaning in theirs and others' lives, commemorate and celebrate, denounce, clarify, get affirmation, and, overall, become a part of a community through the hearing and telling of stories. Stories help us make sense of experiences. They are passed down from generation to generation among families or whole communities.[9] Sometimes, the stories have been fictionalized in novels, poems, plays, songs, or other literary forms. Narrative ethicists conclude that good moral judgment must rely on the analysis and understanding of narratives. Kathyrn Hunter, a contemporary leader in narrative approaches to ethics within health care, reiterates this point, noting that through narratives:

> *"[W]e spin and untangle explanatory accounts of the way the world works and how we and our fellow human beings act in every conceivable circumstance. Memories of the past and ideas of the future are expressed in narrative accounts of how the world was and how it will, or should, become."* [9]

Her emphasis on "should" underscores the narrative ethicists' position that future moral choices of individuals and communities are shaped through understanding and taking seriously the information and lessons embedded in stories.

Elizabeth Kim's situation is revealed to you as a narrative. One thing probably disturbing to her is the fragmented narrative she herself has received. She lacks certain information about the student's mother, the principal, and their exchanges that she would need to be confident of the moral challenges in the situation. This means that she is not only without all the facts and details but may feel she lacks pertinent information to make a valid ethical judgment about the real significance and meaning of the events unfolding before her. From the standpoint of ethical problems, Elizabeth is in a situation of moral distress.

Narrative approaches also highlight that in complex situations, there is not just one but several accounts. Suppose this story simply was titled "The Story of Principal Leary." What different concerns might Principal Leary express regarding his role, his relationships with the student Max, Max's mother (and all students and parents), and Elizabeth, or anything else? It may be a different story than the one told by Elizabeth. Or suppose this story was titled "The Story of Melinda Diaz." Surely this mom's account would include details about her personal life and experiences, her response to her son's learning disability, and her hopes, dreams, and fears. These details would alter inexorably what Elizabeth's story taken alone conveys. Narrative ethics approaches require your diligent effort to consider as many "voices" as possible before interpreting the situation for its moral significance.

 SUMMARY

Narrative ethics requires attention to the details of the story and that all voices be considered before the situation is assessed for its moral significance.

Approaches Emphasizing Relationships

Some ethical approaches that rely on narrative search for the central moral themes of human relationships revealed in the story. You can immediately see the importance of this insight for health professionals because almost all your work involves relationships. In this approach, ethical issues or problems are embedded in the relationships, not just the individual's situation. Patient-centered understanding of clinical situations is an example of such a relationship. Being patient-centered in your professional orientation means that you always take the patient (and his or her network of support) deeply into account regarding your ethical decisions. Not surprisingly, this approach has been promoted and refined by psychologists, particularly those working in the area of moral development.

Carol Gilligan became an important leader in this area in the 1980s, her work having been drawn from a widely accepted model of children's moral development advanced by Harvard psychologist Lawrence Kohlberg. He hypothesized that children go through stages of moral development similar to cognitive development and that children become more independent and autonomous as they mature as moral beings. His work became a, if not the, dominant moral development theory in the early 1980s.[10] At that time, Gilligan, working as Kohlberg's graduate student, noted that his work depended on studies of boys and young men. She repeated some of the work with girls and young women, only to discover that her subjects conceptualized ethical issues and problems differently than their male counterparts. Girls had a high sensitivity to how various actions would affect their important relationships (i.e., with parents, friends, teachers, or other authority figures) and concluded that girls' "awareness of the connection between people gives rise to a recognition of responsibility for another."[11] Moral maturity was not characterized by an increasing independence from everyone else but rather by decisions that would result in deeper and more effective connections and relationships to significant others and the larger community.[11]

Gilligan's work has become one vital basis for ethicists to emphasize how relationships figure into morality. Many have worked to refine their understanding of the ways relationships are central within various social settings, including professional relationships. Moreover, further examination has shown that although girls and women may be socialized to think in terms of sustaining relationships, the significance of Gilligan's findings are by no means gender specific.

Postmodernists assert that because there are radical differences among people and cultures, according to gender, age, ethnicity, or other differences, no one set of moral rules or values is a valid guide "across the board" or even "across a relationship."[12] They highlight that mainstream society fails to respect how deep the diversity of human morality goes, so it simply imposes its own morality to its own advantage, distorting relationships.

Institutional and other social arrangements of a society influence individual action and relationships too. Ethical reflection requires recognition of the powerful influence of each player's and some groups' socially assigned "place" in society and how relationships are affected by the assumptions regarding social status.

If you noted the difference in power between Elizabeth Kim and Melinda Diaz or between Elizabeth Kim and Principal Leary because of their relative power and status within the delivery of care, you were correctly paying attention to social or institutional influences on relationships as relevant considerations in ethical analysis.

In summary, in story-driven approaches, the first major task is to be attentive to the details of the situation. How is this accomplished? You must not only be humble in the face of rich diversity but also respectful of deep differences and, to the extent possible, show respect for those differences in your relationships with others. You also must take seriously the larger social and institutional forces that influence relationships, a topic covered in more detail in Chapter 8.

Ethics of Care Approach

So far you have been introduced to ethical approaches you can use to:
- Discover the areas of moral relevance by paying attention to the details of a narrative;
- Highlight the moral significance of relationships in the situation;
- Remember to be attentive to deep differences among persons or groups; and
- Appreciate the power of institutional and other social arrangements to influence a situation.

In this subsection, you will have an opportunity to examine some ethical approaches that take the idea of care itself as their central feature. There are many varieties of a "care ethic" at this time, but generally speaking, in an *ethics of care approach*, the major question is "What is required of a health professional to be best able to express, 'I care'?" As you noted in Chapter 2, taken in its richness, care is the language adopted in the health professions, ethical literature to emphasize the imperative that professionals must keep a focus on the well-being of the whole person. It is within this context that we have emphasized the goal of professional ethics as being a caring response. Bishop and Scudder describe the core of an ethic of care as residing in the health professional's "caring presence" as follows:

"Caring presence does not mean an emotive, sentimental, or maudlin expression of feeling toward patients. It is a personal presence that assures others of another's concern for their well-being. This way-of-being fosters trust, mutual concern, and positive attitudes that promote good health. When caring presence pervades a health care setting, the whole atmosphere of that setting is transformed so that not only is sound therapy fostered, but patients appreciate, take pride in, and feel part of the health care endeavor."[13]

At least two aspects of a care ethic approach are implied. First, it is dependent on making real contact with the patient as a person; that is, it is deeply relational. Second, it fosters trust. Baier[14] places trust as one of the central notions for an ethics approach that derives from a perspective of care. That, in turn, suggests that you as the health professional must bring trustworthiness to the relationship, a notion that is discussed in greater detail later in this chapter.

As nursing ethics became more sophisticated, the idea of care emerged as a central theme in studies designed to characterize the profession's identity.[15] In an ethics of care approach, the caring relationship serves as a frame to evaluate ethical issues.

Some ethicists worry that an accent on the silver thread of care may deflect attention from injustices woven into the basic warp and woof of the health system, placing all the responsibility to care on individual professionals in the face of policies, practices, and institutions that are unjust. At the same time, Andolsen[16] holds that there is much more overlap in the two themes than many theorists admit.

Story and Ethics of Care Approaches and a Caring Response

Story or case approaches combine to illuminate several facets of the overall picture of care. For instance, the vigilance directed to the details of the story and its narrator(s), the emphasis on relationships that shape the story, and a deep respect for the differences that exist among peoples and cultures all are important tools in understanding what it means "to care." Continue to watch for articles and other opportunities to refine your own interpretation of what a full theory of an ethics of care would involve in your relationships with patients. It will be extremely important for you in your quest for a caring response to a wide variety of professional challenges.

We turn now to *virtue theory*. The appropriateness of giving your attention to this theory is expressed by a health professional who in thinking about her profession said, "caring behavior involves the integration of virtue and expert activity of . . . [professional] practice."[17] In other words, "being" and "doing" are both involved and deeply related. An understanding of virtue theory provides an important link between the motivation to find a caring response and the ethical acts or behaviors that follow from the character traits we cultivate.

Virtue Theory

Many varieties of virtue theory have been developed over the ages. We want to provide you with some basic threads that have created the general tapestry of varieties called virtue ethics. Looking back on the early Western development of those theories, Aristotle can be credited with providing us with a basic framework for this thinking.[18] Within the Judeo-Christian theologic tradition that has deeply influenced Western ethics, the virtue dimensions of Thomas Aquinas's theories have had a profound impact on the shaping of virtue theory.[19] Within the health professions and early medical ethics writings, the idea of virtue also was dominant. For example, authors of the Hippocratic School wrote approximately 70 essays on health care in addition to the Oath, several of which discussed character traits. For example, The Decorum enjoins that a physician "should be modest, sober, patient, prompt, and conduct himself [sic] with propriety in professional and personal life."[20] In short, the professional caregiver will have the moral fiber necessary to carry out the various duties outlined in the Oath.

Maimonides was a highly respected and renowned Jewish philosopher of the 13th century who wrote extensively about the relationship of medical issues to Jewish law. The prayer of Maimonides is based directly on the belief that the development of certain character traits enables the caregiver to exhibit appropriate moral behavior. In making this promise, the physician calls on God for help to have the right motives worthy of this high calling:

> *"May neither avarice nor miserliness nor thirst for glory nor for great reputation engage my mind, or the enemies of truth and philanthropy could easily deceive me and make me forgetful of my lofty aim of doing good to my patients. May I never see in a patient anything but a fellow creature of pain."*[21]

Maimonides believed that important character traits of the health professional are sympathy for the patient's plight, humility, and a devoted commitment to helping others.

From those early influences, many normative versions of virtue theory have evolved so that the tapestry of thought today is splendid indeed. The easiest way into the understanding of virtue theory is through the basic idea of character traits and moral character.

Character Traits and Moral Character

A *character trait* is a disposition or a readiness to act in certain ways. Some character traits are supportive of high ethical standards. Some people exhibit character traits that lead an observer to judge that they are of a high *moral character*. In other words, they are a type of person who habitually acts in a manner that will be praised by others because it upholds high standards. To some extent, our society is measured by the type of people in it, and professionals are judged on this basis more than on any other criterion. Your oaths, codes, and standards of practice declare it. Your state licensing laws require it of you.

Certain character traits enable you to be the kind of person you want to be as a caregiver.[22] For example, honesty will manifest itself in your trying to refrain from deceiving others for your own comfort or protection. Courage may be needed to speak out against injustice or other wrongdoing. Courage combined with honesty will be needed for a therapist to admit that she or he mistakenly took the wrong treatment approach to a patient. Compassion can help motivate you to refrain from thoughtlessly harming vulnerable people.

Recall the health professionals involved in Max Diaz's case. Honesty taken alone would dispose you to encourage Elizabeth Kim to tell the mom about the intentional delay in her son's IEP. Honesty and courage taken together would dispose you to telling her but also to take every step to ensure that she actually receives the correct information. This may involve some risk-taking conduct if Elizabeth believes a cover-up is going on. In other words, the two virtues together will drive her to take measures that ensure Principal Leary is held accountable. These two character traits combined with compassion would motivate her to make sure the information is transmitted in a way that shows respect for everyone involved. Taken together, the habitual practice of exercising these traits would create a high moral character that prompts her to do everything possible to diminish harm and foster a morally healthy work environment.

 Reflection

Patients are very different in their responses to personality types of health professionals. But more fundamentally, they almost all have strong feelings about the kind of person you as a health professional are. Character traits of respect, compassion, and honesty are high on the list of character traits that most patients want to be able to count on. What other character traits do you feel are necessary for health professionals?

_____

_____

_____

_____

Probably the most widely esteemed traits are those that convey an attitude of respect for individuals who come to you as patients. The underlying ideal is that individuals should be treated as ends, not as means to some other end.

Both individual and institutional virtues are important within the health professions. In this respect, one can speak of the moral character of an individual health professional and the moral character of health care institutions. In addition to the elaboration of specific virtues that should be cultivated, you will need to know several other points about the cultivation of virtue.

First, experience is extremely important. Only through experience can we ultimately learn exactly what contributes to a morally good life (the goal of exercising virtue in the first place).

Second, because the cultivation of virtue depends on experience, we cannot simply think ourselves into being virtuous or knowing what virtue consists of. We must add feelings. Emotions must be attended to; as you learned in Chapter 3, they are the motivators toward certain kinds of actions and not others.

Third, in the process of experiencing and feeling what is happening in the situation, we ourselves become transformed. When we follow the inclination of virtue, we are working at becoming more virtuous. We grow into virtue by acting in accordance with what virtue counsels us to do.

Fourth, a community of persons is vital for discerning virtue in a situation. In this regard, the health professions are one community where such discernment takes place.[23]

Character Traits and a Caring Response

Several positive character traits may be called into play at one time or another to prepare you attitudinally for the action you will have to take to achieve a caring response. Understandably, the development of habits that allow you to move easily into a caring response will serve you well. Being able to live a life of moral excellence requires exercise, but we believe Aristotle was correct in saying that high moral character is the key component to a good life overall. Morality is about the pursuit of good; along the way, we all struggle with the balance. We must understand the duties that we uphold as agents and uphold these duties for the right reasons. But good character traits help us build good moral character for the tasks we face.

 SUMMARY

The early crafters of the idea that professionals must exert high moral character through the cultivation of virtues make good common sense when viewed through the lens of the professional's moral task of achieving an outcome consistent with a caring response.

We have come a considerable distance already in this chapter. Although the professional ethic takes the story and your attitudes to what you learn from it as the fundamental starting point, the ethical challenge does not end there. You must now link virtue with action. The caring response requires that you become a certain type of person (i.e., of high moral character) to do what is right. Therefore, because professional ethics requires action, and dispositions and character traits, we turn now to ethical theories and approaches collectively termed action theories. They include principle-based approaches, deontology, and teleology.

Principle-Based Approach

When you move to purposive action, it is helpful to be able to say, "Toward what end?" Moral agent Elizabeth Kim will ask, "What guidelines can I use to help know if my course of action is in the (morally) right direction to achieve the right outcome?" This concern, and the recognition that guidelines are needed, led to the development of methods that emphasize ethical *principles* and therefore are termed a *principle-based approach*. In most professional ethics literature (and modern social ethics writings), these methods are called principles, but we also think of them as elements because they do for ethical theory what the basic chemical elements do for chemistry theory: they provide a way to see something concretely that is quite abstract. As you know, a chemical element can be combined with other elements. Sometimes, they combine to form a new compound that looks and acts differently than each of the units taken individually. Sometimes, they clash. Often, two or more elements have different relative weights so that one is heavier than the other(s). Key principles are shown in Table 4-2 for your future reference.

There is more to the story than Table 4-2 indicates because "I" may be a person, a group, or even an institution. Principles can help you know how an individual, group, or institution stands in relationship to other people, morally speaking. The British philosopher David Hume[24] justified this position in his belief that we incur obligations to act in certain ways because we

Table 4-2 Ethical Principles

Principle	When Applicable
Nonmaleficence (refraining from potentially harming myself or another)	I am in a position to harm someone else.
Beneficence (bringing about good)	I am in a position to benefit someone else.
Fidelity	I have made a promise, explicit or implicit, to someone else.
Autonomy	I have an opportunity to exercise my freedom in a situation.
Veracity	I am in a position to tell the truth or deceive someone.
Justice	I am in a position to distribute benefits and burdens among individuals or groups in society who have legitimate claims on the benefits.
Paternalism	I am in a position to decide for someone else.

have received positive responses to our own needs to be treated humanely: "I have benefitted from society, and therefore ought to promote its interests." Some philosophers argue that principles help to identify what we should do in special relationships regardless of whether we have received benefits from the other person (or from society). Some such relationships, Hume says, are between parent and child, spouses, faculty and student, or citizen and society. The health professions are another source of special relationship, with patients.

Several principles are extremely important in the health care context. For example, the principle of nonmaleficence, or "do no harm," was an explicit theme in the ancient Hippocratic Oath and ever since has been viewed as an overriding moral principle guiding health professionals' conduct toward patients. Because of the importance of these principles, you have this opportunity to examine several in more detail.

Nonmaleficence and Beneficence

Primum non nocere ("First, do no harm") is thought to be at the nexus of traditional health care ethics and often is attributed to the authors of the Hippocratic Oath. It is at the very heart of what is meant by a caring response! The principle of *nonmaleficence* is the noun used today to talk about this type of action. You can figure out the general meaning of the term by breaking it into its prefix, non, and the root, maleficence ("mal, bad, or evil"). The difference in power between professional and patient alone helps to support the instinctive wisdom of this strong call to refrain from abuse. Furthermore, Western societies in general usually attribute greater significance to a harmful act done out of deliberate intent than out of neglect or ignorance. It is difficult to believe that a society could survive if people went around trying to harm each other, and the laws of our land take seriously the necessity of stemming the potential for harm to go unchecked. The early purveyors of professional ethics left nothing to chance, warning health professionals that there is no room whatsoever for acting in ways designed to bring about harm.

In professional ethics, not harming and acting to benefit another *(beneficence)* are treated as separate duties. Sometimes, philosophers treat them as different levels of the same principle or element. When duties are thought of in this latter fashion, at least four types fall along the continuum of the same principle:

Do no harm.

Prevent harm.

Remove harm when it is being inflicted.

Bring about positive good.

Professional ethics limits beneficence to the last three on the list.

Reflection

Consider the principles of nonmaleficence and beneficence in relation to the story in this chapter. Elizabeth is worried about the direction of Max Diaz's care. She believes his learning and academic progress is being delayed, causing harm to his overall success at school. Is Elizabeth following the principle of nonmaleficence by her actions so far? The principle of beneficence?

_____

_____

_____

_____

What evidence do you have that she is or is not?

_____

_____

_____

_____

In your opinion, what would she have to do to be beneficent in this case, given the level of her authority and her knowledge, skills, and compassion?

_____

_____

_____

_____

Because these two principles are so pervasive in the everyday decision making by a professional, you are well advised to think about their relevance in every new situation you encounter.

Autonomy

The principle of *autonomy* is the capacity to have the say-so about your own well-being, "the capacity to act on your decisions freely and independently."[25] Some call this the principle of *self-determination*. Obviously, the principle applies to you whether you are acting in your professional role (professional autonomy) or as a citizen (social autonomy) or have become a patient (patient autonomy). Professional autonomy points out that a health professional must be free of encumberments to act in his or her best judgment on behalf of patients. Much of the discussion that follows focuses on the important arena of patient autonomy.

We know that patients' basic health care needs have not changed significantly over the decades, but the idea of what fully constitutes a caring response has changed. Today, so many clinical interventions are possible that the type and number of interventions alone may lead to suffering. A few years ago, the health professional who did everything clinically possible for a patient was seen as beneficent. Today, that same professional could find that the process leads to moral regret; the patient or patient's family may charge that harm has resulted because the interventions have gone beyond what the patient wanted or could tolerate.

In light of this situation, the last several decades have seen the emergence of the patient as a more active negotiator regarding health care decisions. The patient's autonomy, say-so or self governance, has come to be accepted as a legitimate moral claim to be placed in the balance with the health professional's independent judgment about what is beneficent. Again, we are reminded that the emphasis today on "patient-centered" care is dependent on shared decision making in the relationship. Some suggest that autonomy has too much emphasis, creating a monopoly on our moral attention.

The principle of autonomy (or self-determination) and its role in morality have been developed from the views of diverse and colorful figures in philosophy. Two who have been especially influential are the deontologist, Immanuel Kant, and one of the crafters of a consequence-oriented theory, John Stuart Mill (both of whom are discussed further later in this chapter). Both of their interpretations of the principle of autonomy have been adopted in health professions usage. Kant[26] emphasized the role of being in control of making one's own choices in accord with a moral standard that could be willed valid for everyone. Therefore, his main contribution was his discussion of self-legislation: the reasons for actions. Conversely, Mill[27] focused his thought more on the context of the freedom of action, arguing that an individual's actions legitimately can be restricted only when they promise to harm someone else. Up to that point, he contends, each person should be permitted to act according to his or her own convictions. Therefore, his main contribution was to highlight the social and political context in which the exercise of autonomy can thrive.[27] The two interpretations together point to our assumption today that a patient's input can be rational and that the context of decision making must be conducive to the patient's exercise of his or her real and informed wishes. Anything less fails to meet the criterion of a caring response (Figure 4-1).

Figure 4-1. This statement was written on a pad of paper by a 27-year-old hospitalized woman with ovarian-breast cancer syndrome. She could not communicate verbally because she had a tracheostomy and therefore could not speak. The physician had explained that he wanted to reimplement chemotherapy for a tumor that had appeared in her remaining ovary. She had already undergone an oophorectomy and hysterectomy and had received radiotherapy and chemotherapy for the previous tumors before their removal.

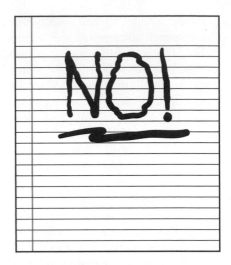

Gilligan, whose studies were introduced earlier in this chapter, is among those who criticize a focus on autonomy because it requires that a person be treated as an isolated unit standing alone, over and against all other people, whereas, as you recall, she emphasizes the importance of relationships for the moral life.[28] This is a serious criticism. She is correct in her observation that we understand ourselves as moral beings largely within the context of our relationships. Be that as it may, we also live in a society that is highly individualistic in its behavior and laws. The principle of autonomy provides direction in those situations in which an individual is in a position to make a claim on others to respect his or her selfhood. In fact, sometimes the claim for autonomy is given the power of a right.

Currently, there is much discussion about autonomy in regard to decisions about the timing and type of death one will have, a topic you will encounter again in Chapter 14. Underlying the idea of a right to die is the more fundamental belief in the right to autonomy or self-determination. But the principle of autonomy has much broader applications than end-of-life situations.

 Reflection

The principle of autonomy (or self-determination) is a helpful principle, but, like all of the principles, it is not absolute in the delicate complexity of real life situations. Liberty and agency are both essential to autonomy. Many patients experience restrictions to these conditions when their health and functioning is compromised. An elder with advanced Alzheimer's disease who lacks decision making capacity is one such example. Can you think of others?

You will revisit the principle of autonomy several times later in this book. Watch for it.

Fidelity

The principle of *fidelity* comes from the Latin root *fides*, which means faithfulness. It is about being faithful to one's commitments. Being faithful to the patient entails meeting the patient's reasonable expectations. Patients come with all kinds of expectations. What can be counted as a reasonable expectation?

First, there is a reasonable expectation that basic respect will be shown to anyone, anywhere. Sometimes, health professionals have been criticized for failing to show basic respect, such as respecting the modesty of a patient.

Second, the patient has reason to expect that you will be competent in what you do.

Third, the patient has a reasonable expectation that you will adhere to statements you have subscribed to as a member of a profession. The most public of these statements is your code of ethics.

Fourth, the patient has a good basis for believing you will follow the policies and statements adopted by your place of employment, and laws that are designed to protect patient well-being.

Finally, the patient has good reason to expect that you will honor what the two of you have agreed to, such as the promises involved in any informed consent form the patient has signed, verbal agreements, or serious conversations.

Can you think of others? A caring response cannot be affected if you fail to meet the reasonable expectations of your patients and others.

Veracity

The ethical principle of *veracity* binds you to honesty. Veracity means that you will tell the truth. This principle is more specific than, say, beneficence or fidelity. For this reason, some call it a second-level principle that directs you to engage in a specific type of behavior, which in turn can support your intent to be beneficent or to maintain your fidelity in relationships with patients and others. Kant gave veracity a central role, taking the position that veracity is an absolute to which no exception can be made. The lie, he argues in one place, always is wrong because the practice of lying is something that weakens the entire human fabric.[26] Most others weigh veracity heavily regarding its potential for benefiting others but do not make it the absolute or governing duty above all others.

In our story, Elizabeth Kim understandably seemed disappointed about the possibility that Melinda, Max's mom, was not being told the truth about Max's status and the IEP process. The situation was made more complex by the different professional roles of the principal and the speech and language pathologist.

Paternalism

Sometimes an ethical issue presents itself in this manner: The patient's deep preferences conflict with the health professional's judgment of what is best for the patient on the basis of the professional's values, which are not necessarily those of the patient. In other words, the conflict is between the patient's choice and the professional's judgment of what is best for the patient. In this situation, the principle of *paternalism* or *parentalism* may come into play. Paternalistic or parentalistic decisions are those in which a health professional acts as a parent with all of its negative and positive connotations. Paternalism limits patient autonomy; when evoked, the health professional makes a decision *for* the client instead of *with* the client.

Justice

Patients do not always get all the treatment and attention they deserve or need because of a lack of resources, and anyone who worries about that is worrying about the principle of justice in the situation. Discrimination against some individuals or groups may appear to be shortchanging them, and anyone who worries about that is worrying about the justice of the situation. A lack of due process regarding who receives priority in situations of conflict may cause concern, and anyone who worries about that also is worrying about the justice of the situation. In general, their concern is that all similarly situated individuals receive their fair share of benefits and assume their fair share of burdens. The caring response is achieved when individuals or groups are treated fairly and equitably.

Justice can be thought of as an arbiter. It serves to ensure a proper distribution of burdens and benefits when there are competing claims, not all of which always can be met fully. As you recall, a dilemma of justice is one variety of an ethical dilemma problem. The principle is called on when there are problems regarding what is rightfully due a person, institution, or society. Three types of justice have particular importance in professional ethics situations: distributive, compensatory, and procedural. We take up the complex issues of justice more fully in Chapters 15 and 16.

Principles and a Caring Response

This concludes our list of the ethical principles you will most often encounter in your professional roles. As you can see, they still are very general but they do move you in the direction of action according to some guidelines. In their particularity, they are instrumental in helping you further delineate the conditions that must be met if you are to show a caring response toward the patient. For instance, you know that you must honor the patient's reasonable expectations, you must do it truthfully, and so on. In short, the principles themselves force you to consider who the patient is as an individual different from all others.

 SUMMARY

Principles provide general moral guidelines in the search for a course of action that will result in an outcome consistent with a caring response.

You may have noticed that some principles are more oriented toward a duty-driven ethic. They include fidelity, autonomy, truthfulness (veracity), and justice. Others, namely beneficence and nonmaleficence, require you to weigh the most favorable (or least damaging) consequences in a situation. Does this sound vaguely familiar? It should. The "duty" theory of *deontology* naturally appeals to principles that help delineate what a particular duty (e.g., veracity) entails. The consequence-oriented theory of *teleology* uses the principle of beneficence or nonmaleficence as a guideline.

Both deontologists and teleologists express the need for individual or group actions to be guided according to principles. However, you have not yet had the opportunity to look more closely at these two major theories that have been highly influential in traditional professional ethics approaches. We turn to them now.

Deontologic and Teleologic Theories

Taking Duties Seriously: Deontology

Elizabeth Kim faces a perplexing situation regarding balancing loyalty and honesty. One approach would be to identify whether she has a duty that can help her decide what to do. In her search for a duty (or duties), she is appealing to *deontologic theories.*

One place where duties are codified is in codes of professional ethics. For example, currently you will find statements such as "respect a patient's dignity" or "honor the patient's [or client's] right to consent to a potential treatment." When you look more closely, the statements imply fundamental ideas about humans—namely, that we stand in relation to each other in a number of morally significant ways. In this regard, deontologists agree with Gilligan and others discussed in this chapter who emphasize the centrality of relationship and the importance of paying attention to the details of a patient's (or another's) story. Deontologists hold that there are basic concepts that individuals and societies recognize and agree on that give rise to a shared sense of duty or right. These could be arrived at through reasoning about such things or, others might argue, we intuit them. Although a narrative approach correctly helps to focus attention on particular details of a story, the deontologist goes further to say there is a concept of duty informing (or at least available to) all individuals.

Deontologic theories hold that you are acting rightly when you act according to duties and rights. In other words, duties and rights are the correct measuring rods for evaluating a course of action and its outcome. There are many versions of deontology. The person most often identified with deontologic approaches is Immanuel Kant, whose philosophies were introduced in the discussion of the principle of autonomy. His basic premises still figure strongly in arguments within health care ethics today. He held that every person has an inherent dignity and on that basis alone is entitled to respect. Respect is shown by never using people to achieve other goals or consequences that do not benefit them. He thought that duties help to determine how respect toward others can be expressed. It follows that the morally correct thing is always to be guided by moral duties. He concluded that some actions are intrinsically immoral, no matter how positive and beneficial one might judge the consequences to be, and that other actions are intrinsically moral, no matter how negative the consequences might be. In short, he said that one cannot judge the moral rightness or wrongness of an act on the basis of its consequences alone.[29] Whatever Elizabeth's conclusion about what Melinda Diaz or Principal Leary should do, Kant would arrive at his decision by a process of determining what their duty should be, not simply whether there would be a better consequence overall achieved by one type of act or another. Their professional responsibility would be guided by accountability more than responsiveness in the range of consequences.

 Reflection
Do you think that this appeal to duties is the correct moral tool to use in the situation Elizabeth Kim and Principal Leary find themselves? Yes or no?

Yes____   No____

What important moral considerations are taken into account in this approach?

_____

_____

_____

_____

What could be overlooked if they appealed to their sense of duty alone?

_____

_____

_____

_____

As you can begin to see, there are some challenges to applying this approach in its "pure" form. For instance, the idea that we ought to do the right thing, informed by duty, is general. How to show respect for individuals still needs further interpretation in any situation. What do we do when duties or rights themselves come into conflict? Deontologic theories require that a method of weighing be available to determine what to do when conflicts arise, and critics charge that there is no obvious way to weigh them (Figure 4-2). Such a process is not self evident. Thus, the appeal to principles discussed in the previous section is one attempt to provide further detail and interpretation to the general idea of duty and to order, or give varying weight to conflicting duties and rights.

Absolute, Prima Facie, and Conditional Duties

We have seen that from a deontologic viewpoint, principles can assist in interpreting one's duty. Principles that carry the weight of duties may be absolute, prima facie, or conditional. _Absolute duties_ are binding under all circumstances. They can never give way to another compelling duty or right. _Prima facie duties_ or rights allow you to make choices among conflicting principles. For instance, the prima facie duty of veracity is actually binding if it conflicts with no other duties, or rights, that are weightier in a given situation. But it is not an element that is absolute either because other elements may be more compelling. In the discussion of the primacy of "do no harm" over "beneficence" in the clinical ethics context, it was suggested that each is being treated as a prima facie principle, and the mandate not to

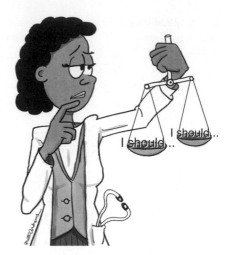

Figure 4-2. Weighing duties.

harm is more compelling than the mandate to bring about some positive good. A *conditional duty* is a commitment that comes into being only after certain conditions are met. For example, the Americans with Disabilities Act outlines certain duties and rights that apply solely to individuals who have disabilities.[30]

However binding a principle or element is deemed to be, it has the role of providing a marker to guide the conduct of individuals and groups wanting to live a good moral life.

Paying Attention to Outcomes: Teleology

Partially because of some of the criticisms of deontology, *teleologic theories* emerged, placing the focus on the ends brought about and the consequences of actions. The most important teleologic theory for our consideration of health care ethics is *utilitarianism*. This word takes its root from the idea of utility or usefulness.

Utilitarianism

In utilitarianism, an act is right if it helps to bring about the best balance of benefits over burdens, in other words, the best "utility" or consequences overall. The original approach was developed first by two English philosophers, Jeremy Bentham (1748-1832)[31] and John Stuart Mill (1806-1873).[32] Note that they are roughly contemporaries of Kant. In fact, they were vigorous opponents of Kant's position.

From a utilitarian point of view, as a moral agent, you must consider what several different courses of action could accomplish, the goal being to fit the action to the outcome that brings about the most good or least harm overall,

all things considered. In the case of Elizabeth Kim, you might say, "The goal is to treat Max Diaz in such a way that everyone else will be able to have the same type of care he gets" or "The goal is to be able to live with my own conscience." If both of these goals can be attained by taking one single course of action, it should be taken. If this is not possible, the course of action you believe will bring about the best consequences or "outcomes" overall should take priority.

One important task of this approach is to distinguish alternate paths of action and then predict as accurately as possible the consequences of each path. *Rule utilitarians* are sometimes thought of as a hybrid of deontologic and utilitarian approaches. Pure utilitarians weigh the consequences solely in the specific details of each situation. A rule utilitarian holds that you will always bring about more good consequences by following certain "rules" or duties. What the rules should be then becomes the task for these theorists.

Duties, Consequences, and a Caring Response

The deontologic and teleologic normative theories have been helpful tools for health professionals because they set a general framework for thinking about specific moral issues and problems in health care settings with a focus on the action that needs to take place. Probably as you were reading you were thinking, "Well, both the idea of courses of action consistent with duties and rights and the idea of consequences or outcomes are important in my attempt to arrive at a caring response." In fact, most of us do draw on both to make practical everyday moral decisions. Only occasionally does it make a big difference in what you judge to be right if you follow solely a deontologic line of reasoning or appeal to consequences only. Fortunately, most of the time, you can take action that is in line with your sense of duty, honor others' rights, and consider the outcomes you are bringing about without any conflict among the three. But it is in the occasional moment during which the means and the ends seem to be competing that it may become necessary to plant your feet firmly in one theory or the other and be able to justify why. See Table 4-3 for a brief summary of deontology and teleology.

Table 4-3   Theories of Deontology versus Teleology

Deontology	*Teleology*
Duty driven	Goal driven
Means count	Ends count
Kant	Bentham, Mill (utilitarians)

Summary

This chapter introduces you to ethical theories and approaches, the conceptual tools that will help you the most when faced with ethical problems in your role as a health professional. The ability to absorb a narrative for its moral content and the development of moral character will help you to be ready for the hard times when no answers seem to be forthcoming or when you are confronted with something that is not easy to face. You also have learned the most important principles, or norms of ethics, that you need to understand the ethical aspects of your life as a professional. Duties and rights are tools for recognizing and working to resolve problems that arise in your everyday practice. They must be balanced with values so that a caring response can be achieved. Although traditionally much of the language of health care ethics has been that of what is owed the patient (i.e., the language of duties), the importance of character traits and attitudes and, more recently, the ideas of patients' (and professionals' and society's) rights have enriched the understanding of professional ethics with its goal of ascertaining a caring response. With these basic frameworks at your disposal, you are well positioned to engage in the six-step process of ethical analysis and decision making introduced in the next chapter.

Questions for Thought and Discussion

1. This is an opportunity for the class to create a narrative of a patient, Esther Korn. It is a group exercise about a health care situation that came to the attention of the hospital ethics committee. The whole class can participate in the discussion as members of the ethics committee, and five people will assume various important roles.

   The ethics committee has been asked to give advice on whether Esther Korn should be sent back home or to a nursing home.

   Esther Korn, a 72-year-old woman, has been admitted to the hospital with a diagnosis of dehydration and serious bruises from a fall sustained in her home. She was found by a neighbor, Anna Knight, who says she stops by Esther's home daily because Ms. Korn has lived alone with her eight cats since being discharged from a state hospital with a diagnosis of paranoid schizophrenia, which is believed to be under control with medications. From the degree of dehydration, the health professionals believe that Ms. Korn was very dehydrated before she fell and that she had been lying on the floor for at least a day. The emergency medical technicians who brought her to the hospital described her home as "filthy, full of dirty dishes and clothes strung all over, with cat droppings everywhere."

Now, 5 days later, Ms. Korn seems confused about where she is, but she does know her own name. She says over and over, "Let me out of here! I want to go home!" Her sister, whom she has not seen "for several years" (according to Anna Knight), does not return the nurses' calls or voice messages. The nurses are not in complete agreement, but most of the staff believe that Esther would be better off placed in a supervised setting for her own safety. Anna Knight and the local priest, who visits her regularly, also have strong opinions about where Esther should live.

Five people will be "storytellers" to provide some missing parts to her story: one will be Esther, the other four will be significant others in her life. Together the class can create a fictional story that fills in information about who she is and what may, in fact, be in her best interest in this difficult question facing the ethics committee.

Person A: Write a few paragraphs about Esther from her neighbor Anna's perspective and what Anna thinks should be done.

Person B: Write about her from the Episcopal priest's perspective and what she would recommend.

Person C: Write about her from the perspective of her long-lost sister and what she would recommend.

Person D: Write a report from the point of view of the primary nurse and what he thinks.

Person E: Speaking as Esther, give some background as to what kind of person she believes herself to be, what is important to her, and so on.

When each of the five storytellers has completed this part of the exercise, read the notes aloud to the ethics committee (i.e., rest of the group). After everyone has heard the "bigger picture," answer the following questions:

- What should be done?
- What ethical approaches or theories influence your thinking the most?
- Which values do you think are the most prominent in this discussion?
- Did anything that was said in these stories change your mind about your initial thoughts regarding what should be done? If so, explain.
- Discuss what the health professionals must do to show caring in their relationship with Esther Korn.

2. Cite an example from health care in which a conflict could arise between your sense of duty to the patient and the negative consequences your act might have on someone else.

3. Elva, a 370-lb, 62-year-old woman, is in a nursing home after complications of diabetes and several small strokes. Although she has been overweight all her life, she now is at a weight where it is impossible to move her without a bariatric lift. Elva, however, refuses to be moved by it, claiming, "I'm not a piece of meat."

It is possible to transfer her to a chair using four or five of the staff. The administration, however, is worried that the staff could be injured while moving her physically. Her daughter insists that it is a violation of Elva's dignity and an unnecessary compromise of her autonomy to submit her to "the indignity of the mechanical lift."

You are the supervisor of the unit. What ethical principles presented in this chapter can help you to assess what to do in this situation? What should you do?

4. Walter is a resident in the same nursing home with Elva. He is a 78-year-old widower who has been on antidepressants since the sudden death of his wife 5 years ago. He, too, is visited often by his daughter. The staff of the nursing home inadvertently threw out his dentures with the sheets while making his bed. He had a habit of leaving them on the bed, and although the staff usually noticed them, a new employee failed to do so.

   Since then, Walter has adamantly refused to have his teeth replaced. The nursing home administration is more than willing to fit him with a new set of dentures and to pay all costs. His daughter is very much in agreement with the administration that he should have his teeth replaced. They are all aware that his nutrition is suffering, as is his ability to be understood when he tries to talk.

   Should Walter be allowed to continue without his dentures? What principles and other considerations of ethics should you, as a nursing home administrator, bring to bear on your decision on how to proceed in this situation? What should you do?

References

1. Doherty, R.F., 2008. Ethical decision making in occupational therapy practice. In: Crepeau, E.B., Cohn, E.S., Schell, B.A. (Eds.), *Willard and Spackman's occupational therapy*, 11th ed. Lippincott, Williams and Wilkins, New York.

2. Sullivan, W.M., Rosin, M.S., Shulman, L.S., 2009. *A new agenda for higher education: Shaping the life of the mind for practice*. Wiley, New York.

3. Schell, B., 2003. Clinical reasoning: The basis for practice. In: Crepeau, B., Cohn, E., Schell, B.A.B. (Eds.), *Willard and Spackman's occupational therapy*, 10th ed. Lippincott, Williams and Wilkins, Philadelphia, PA, p. 131.

4. Schell, B.A.B., Schell, J.W., 2008. *Clinical and professional reasoning in occupational therapy*. Wolters Kluwer/Lippincott Williams and Wilkins, Philadelphia, PA.

5. Mattingly, C., Fleming, M., 1994. *Clinical reasoning: Forms of inquiry in therapeutic practice*. F.A. Davis, Philadelphia, PA.

6. Leicht, S.B., Dickerson, A., 2001. Clinical reasoning, looking back. *Occupational Ther Healthcare* 14 (3/4), 105–130.

7. Hunter, K., 2004. Narrative. In: Post, S.G. (Ed.), *Encyclopedia of bioethics*, 3rd ed. vol. 4. Macmillan, New York, p. 1875.

8. Devettere, R.J., 2000. *Practical decision making in health care ethics*, 2nd ed. Georgetown University Press, Washington, DC.

9. Hunter, K., 2004. Narrative. In: Post, S.G. (Ed.), *Encyclopedia of bioethics*, 3rd ed. Vol. 4. Macmillan, New York, pp. 1875–1876.

10. Kohlberg, L., 1981. *The philosophy of moral development: Moral stages and the idea of justice.* Harper and Row, San Francisco, CA.

11. Gilligan, C., 1982. *In a different voice—Psychological theory and women's development.* Harvard University Press, Cambridge, MA.

12. Aylesworth, G., 2008. Postmodernism. In: Zalta, E.N. (Ed.), *The Stanford encyclopedia of philosophy.* Available from: < http://plato.stanford.edu/archives/win2008/entries/postmodernism/>.

13. Bishop, A., Scudder, J., 2001. Caring presence. In: *Nursing ethics: Holistic caring practice*, 2nd ed. Jones and Bartlett Publishers, Sudbury, MA, pp. 41–65.

14. Baier, A., 1995. The need for more than justice. In: Held, V. (Ed.), *Justice and care.* Westview Press, Boulder, CO, pp. 47–58.

15. Fry, S., Killen, A.R., Robinson, E.M., 1996. Care-based reasoning, caring and the ethic of care: A need for clarity. *J Clin Ethics* 7 (1), 41–47.

16. Andolsen, B.H., 2001. Care and justice as moral values for nurses in an era of managed care. In: Cates, D.F., Lauritzen, P. (Ed.), *Medicine and the ethics of life.* Georgetown University Press, Washington, DC, p. 41–56.

17. Bradshaw, A., 1999. The virtue of nursing: The covenant of care. *J Med Ethics* 25, 477–481.

18. Aristotle, 1984. Nichomachean ethics. In: Barnes, J. (Ed.), *The complete works of Aristotle*, vol. 2. Princeton University Press, Princeton, NJ, p. 1729.

19. Aquinas. 1945. Summa theologica. In: Pegis, A.G. (Ed.), *Basic writings of St. Thomas Aquinas.* Random House, New York.

20. Hippocrates, 1923. Decorum. In: Jones, W.H.S. (Trans.), *Hippocrates II.* Harvard University Press, Cambridge, MA, Loeb Classical Library, pp. 267–302.

21. Maimonides, 1927. Prayers of Moses Maimonides (H. Friedenwald, Trans.). *Bull Johns Hopkins Hosp* 28, 260–261.

22. Loewy, E.H., 1997. Developing habits and knowing what habits to develop: A look at the role of virtue in ethics. *Cambridge Q Healthcare Ethics* 6 (3), 347–355.

23. Marton, M., 2002. Personal communication. *National Endowment for the Humanities Seminar on "Justice, equality and the challenge of disability."* 24 June 2002, Bronxville, NY.

24. Hume, D., 1976. On suicide. In: Gorowitz, S., Macklin, R., Jameton, A. (Eds.), *Moral problems in medicine.* Prentice Hall, Englewood Cliffs, NJ, p. 356.

25. Beauchamp, T., Childress, J.F., 2008. *Principles of biomedical ethics*, 6th ed. Oxford University Press, New York.

26. Kant, I., 1963. *Lectures on ethics* (L. Infield, translator). Harper and Row, New York, pp. 147–154.

27. Mill, J.S., 1939. On liberty. In: Burtt, E.A. (Ed.), *The English philosophers from Bacon to Mill.* Random House, New York, pp. 1042–1060.

28. Gilligan, C., 1982. *Psychological theory and women's development*. Harvard University Press, Cambridge, MA.

29. Kant, I., 1949. In: Beck, L.W. (Ed.), *Critique of practical reason and other writings in moral philosophy*. University of Chicago Press, Chicago, IL, pp. 346–350.

30. Americans with Disabilities Act, 1990. H.R. Rep. No. 485 (II), 101st Congress, 2nd Sess. at 22 12.

31. Bentham, J., 1939. An enquiry concerning human understanding. In: Burtt, E.A. (Ed.), *The English philosophers from Bacon to Mill*. Random House, New York, pp. 792–856.

32. Mill, J.S., 1939. Utilitarianism. In: Burtt, E.A. (Ed.), *The English philosophers from Bacon to Mill*. Random House, New York, pp. 895–1041.

5

A Six-Step Process of Ethical Decision Making in Arriving at a Caring Response

Objectives

The reader should be able to:

- Identify six steps in the analysis of ethical problems encountered in everyday professional life and how each plays a part in arriving at a caring response.
- Describe the central role of narrative and virtue theories in gathering relevant information for a caring response.
- List four areas of inquiry that will be useful when gathering relevant information to make sure you have the story straight.
- Describe the role of conduct-related ethical theories and approaches in arriving at a caring response.
- Describe why imagination is an essential aspect of seeking out the practical alternatives in an ethically challenging situation.
- Discuss how courage assists you in a caring response.
- Identify two benefits of taking time to reflect on and evaluate the action afterward.

New terms and ideas you will encounter in this chapter

six-step process of ethical decision making	chemical restraints rounds

Topics in this chapter introduced in earlier chapters

Topic	Introduced in chapter
Ethics	1
A caring response	2, 3, 4
Moral distress	3
Ethical dilemma	3
Locus of authority problem	3
The importance of story or narrative	4
Paternalism	4
Deontology	4
Teleology	4
Utilitarianism	4
Character traits	4

Introduction

You have come a long way in laying the foundation for identifying proto-types of ethical problems and in identifying the ethical tools available to you for analysis in your search for resolution of conflicts consistent with a caring response. In this chapter, you will have an opportunity to apply what you have learned using a problem-solving method to analyze and move toward resolution of such problems. The story of Anthony Carnavello and Alexia Eliopoulos is a good starting point for this discussion.

⚕ The Story of Anthony Carnavello and Alexia Eliopoulos

Alexia Eliopoulos, a physical therapist, has just begun working in a munici-pal nursing home. The facility has a reputation for maintaining high standards of care. When Alexia interviewed for the position, she made a thorough tour of the home and talked with several employees and residents. Everything seemed "in order," and she took the job.

It is now near the end of her second week of work. Alexia goes to the nursing home office to read the personal record of a resident who may be transferred to another facility because of his apparently worsening mental status. She learns that Mr. Anthony Carnavello is 76 years old and has diabe-tes. Recently, his left leg was amputated because of complications from a fracture of his left femur sustained in an accident. According to the record, he fell in the corridor of the nursing home after tripping over a chair. Report-edly he is "confused" most of the time and is kept quite heavily sedated "to keep him from becoming violent." He is almost blind as a result of diabetic retinopathy. No neurologist's report is found in the record.

Alexia decides to introduce herself to Mr. Carnavello before she goes to lunch. When she finds Mr. Carnavello's room, she is surprised to see a shriveled-up, frail little old man lying in bed staring at the ceiling. Alexia introduces herself and tells Mr. Carnavello that she will be coming back to treat him in the afternoon.

Mr. Carnavello squints in an effort to see Alexia. Abruptly he raises up on one elbow and says, "I'm so scared! They keep giving me shots and pills that make me crazy! Can you get them to stop?"

Just at that moment, a nurse comes into the room with a syringe on a tray. "Anthony!" she says in a firm, loud voice. "Turn over on your side, please. It's time for your shot!"

Mr. Carnavello protests that the pills and shots are making him "crazy as a hoot owl." But the nurse has exposed one loose-skinned buttock and is deftly injecting the solution before Mr. Carnavello succeeds in resisting. He tries to take a swipe at her, but she backs off quickly. She pats his bony hip, saying, "There now, you're okay, Tony," and leaves immediately. Mr. Carnavello lies back on the pillow and sighs. He grabs the rail, pulls himself up toward Alexia, and says, "See what I mean!" Alexia thinks that Mr. Carnavello seems to be in genuine anguish. She reaches out to pat his hand, but he pulls it away and falls back against the sheet.

Alexia is angry and confused. There is a gnawing feeling in her stomach that something is wrong in the way Mr. Carnavello is being treated. At lunch, she shares her concern with Annette Carroll, the nursing supervisor for the entire home. Annette is highly respected by residents and staff alike. Alexia tells Annette it seems that Mr. Carnavello is not being treated with the dignity that the residents deserve. She doubts that Mr. Carnavello is "violent" but cannot put her finger on why she felt so much anger at the nurse who efficiently and without undue harshness gave him the injection. Maybe it is because she believes the medication is being used to "dope" Mr. Carnavello unnecessarily. As she recounts what happened, she can feel a seething rage rising up in her. She decides, on the spot, that she will talk to the nursing home administrator and announces that intention to Annette.

Annette listens attentively. When Alexia pauses for a few disinterested bites of her sandwich, she says, "Alexia, you have been here only 2 weeks. I can understand your uneasiness at what you thought you saw happening. And maybe you are right—maybe Mr. Carnavello is not being treated with the respect he deserves. But remember, being new here, there is much that you don't know. We are doing for him what we think is best, as well as trying to protect our staff from his dangerously aggressive behavior. He was worse before we started him on Haldol."

Alexia does not feel any better after lunch. She would like to talk to someone and decides to call a social worker who works in another nursing home.

As in most actual situations, Alexia's first encounter with what appears to be an ethical problem has left many questions unanswered. The path from Alexia's first perception to possible action consistent with a caring response traverses a *six-step process of ethical decision making*.

The Six-Step Process

Ethical decision making requires your thoughtful reflection and logical judgment (i.e., "ethical reasoning" discussed in Chapter 4) even though the situation usually presents itself in a mumbo jumbo of partial facts and strong reactions. The following steps allow you to take the situation apart and look at it in a more organized, coolheaded way while still acknowledging the intense emotions everyone may be experiencing about the situation and how these feelings factor into addressing the problem.

In Chapter 1, you learned that ethics is reflection on and analysis of morality. This step-by-step process is, overall, a formalized approach to both. In the context of health care, your professional ethics dictates that your reflection is directed toward arriving at a caring response in a particular situation. As a moral agent, your reflection and ensuing judgment are geared toward action.

Step 1: Get the Story Straight—Gather Relevant Information

The first step in informed decision making is to gather as much information as possible. Anyone viewing this situation might ask the following types of questions:

- Does Mr. Carnavello have organic brain disease or other central nervous system dysfunction that might explain his behavior?
- What tests have been conducted to confirm the type and degree of neurologic involvement?
- What does his "violent" behavior consist of?
- Is he at risk of injuring himself or others?
- What might have happened in Mr. Carnavello's history to make him afraid of the nursing staff or the whole setting and, therefore, to react in a hostile manner?
- Has the medical director been made aware of Mr. Carnavello's complaints about the effects of the medication?
- What is the recent history of the exchanges between Mr. Carnavello and the staff?
- What other approaches (besides medication) to Mr. Carnavello's ostensibly violent behavior have been—or could be—attempted?
- What evidence is there that approaching the nursing home administration will create problems for Alexia, Ms. Carroll, or others?

What other information about physical and *chemical restraints* (i.e., medicines that sedate the patient) in nursing homes should Alexia seek out?

1 *Reflection*

Are there other questions you thought of as you read the story?

_____

_____

_____

_____

The necessity for close attention to details takes you back to Chapter 4, which introduced you to the importance of the story or narrative. Without knowing as much as possible about the story line, it is impossible to ascertain the attitudes, values, and duties embedded in it. As you probably recall, the theories and approaches to ethics have important clues about how each of these is an important consideration if you are going to be able to arrive at a caring response. The fact-finding mission is absolutely essential as a safeguard against setting off on a false course from the beginning.

Some of the benefits of seeking out the facts in the situation described earlier are that you may be able to determine whether Alexia's perception of Mr. Carnavello's treatment is accurate and to understand why the various players in this drama are acting as they are. Although Annette Carroll's comments are difficult to interpret, she may be implying that Alexia's response would be tempered by more knowledge of the situation. Often, what initially appears to be a "wrong" act is, after all, a right or acceptable one once more of the story is known.

Fact finding also could help Alexia identify the focus of her anger more specifically. What triggered the response? Was it Mr. Carnavello's apparent helplessness in the situation? The nurse's actions? What Alexia has read about misuse of chemical restraints?[1-3] Why has Mr. Carnavello been labeled as "confused" and "violent" when Alexia believes he showed no signs of being either? Fact finding is an essential step in Alexia's ethical reasoning process. She must clarify the known facts of the case versus the beliefs. All of the facts are needed to make a judicious and well-reasoned decision.

The following general checklist for data gathering and adding specific questions will help you organize your thoughts around your specific situation. They are adapted from a handbook designed for clinicians.[4]

1. Clinical Indications
   a. What is the diagnosis or prognosis?
   b. Is the illness or condition reversible?
   c. Is life-saving treatment medically futile?
   d. What is the present treatment regimen?

  e. What is the usual and customary treatment for this type of condition?
  f. What is needed to relieve suffering or to provide comfort?
  g. Who are the primary caregivers?
  h. What can you learn about this patient's medical and social history?
2. Preference of the Patient
  a. What does he or she want in this situation?
  b. Who has communicated the realistic options to the patient?
  c. What was the patient actually told?
  d. What evidence do you have that what the patient said has been heard by key decision makers?
  e. Is he or she competent to make decisions about this situation?
  f. If not competent, does the patient have a living will, advance directive, or other document indicating his or her considered preferences?
  g. If not competent, is another person speaking as a legitimate legal substitute for this patient?
3. Quality of Life
  a. What are the patient's beliefs and values that make up his or her personal value system?
  b. What quality-of-life considerations are the decision makers bringing to this situation, and how are their biases influencing the decision processes?
  c. Is there any hope for improvement in the patient's quality of life?
  d. Are there any biases that might prejudice the clinician's evaluation of the patient's quality of life?
4. Contextual Factors
  a. What institutional policies may influence what can be done?
  b. What are the legal implications (court cases, statutes, and so on) regarding this issue?
  c. Are scarce resources an issue?
  d. How will these services be paid for?
  e. Are there family issues that may influence the plan of care?

Reflection

This general checklist is extensive but not exhaustive. Jot down some other types of information you think will help Alexia to accurately analyze this situation.

_____

_____

_____

_____

SUMMARY

Gathering as much relevant information as possible sets the essential groundwork for analysis and action consistent with arriving at a caring response.

When you have searched out the information you and others deem relevant or are convinced no additional helpful information will be forthcoming, you are ready to proceed to the next step.

Step 2: Identify the Type of Ethical Problem

Even while the initial fact finding is taking place, Alexia can begin to determine the type of ethical problem (or problems) she is facing and in that regard make significant progress toward arriving at a caring response. You know that in the beginning her worry was something like this:

Mr. Carnavello is a human, and humans always should be treated with dignity. Part of being treated with dignity includes allowing a person to take part in his or her own treatment decisions whenever possible and, in Mr. Carnavello's case, includes at the very least being treated with sensitivity to the anguish that he appears to be experiencing. To ignore his distress shows a lack of compassion, if not outright cruelty, and reduces him to the status of an object. Mr. Carnavello is not being treated as a person ought to be treated.

This is where the prototypes of ethical problems you encountered in Chapter 3 begin to work for you.

Moral Distress

You know that Alexia is experiencing emotional distress. She has witnessed a scene that baffled her, and she finds herself unable to forget about it. Our guess about the fundamental basis of Alexia's distress is her perception that Mr. Carnavello is not being treated with the dignity he deserves as a human. The distress, then, is consistent with Alexia's role as a professional with a moral responsibility to help uphold human dignity. In other words, she is a moral agent in a situation that she surmises involves morality and that, because it is worrying her, merits further attention. If she tries—but fails—to put more information in place, she may confirm that her distress is, in fact, moral distress type B. You also can presume that she has the virtues of a compassionate person. Otherwise she would not be worried about what she witnessed.

Ethical Dilemma

Goaded by her emotional responses, character traits, and the awareness that she is experiencing moral distress, Alexia is well positioned to assess whether she also has an ethical dilemma (or dilemmas). Do you think there is an ethical dilemma here?

Alexia learns that quite a few of the staff (but not all) believe the medications are being used disproportionately to the amount of "violence" Mr. Carnavello has been demonstrating. In fact, some of the staff confide that they believe he is being sedated not to benefit him but to keep him more in line with the conduct of the other more docile and cooperative residents. Mr. Carnavello has seemed very agitated and suspicious at times, and the medication has helped to improve his feeling of security, so that raises the possibility that it *is* benefiting him in that way. Of course, the nursing home is shorthanded, and the administrator points this out when Alexia finally goes to talk with her. Her argument is that if everyone took as much time and extra attention as Mr. Carnavello does (when without medication), no one would receive a fair amount of treatment. The principle of justice is an issue.

Finally, the administrator mentions that some of the staff are afraid of Mr. Carnavello, and she has a responsibility for their safety, too. There are several issues here that Alexia, as an employee and team member, may be implicated in as partial agent. Foremost of these is whether the employees, as a team, are acting ethically in the use of restraints under any circumstances. The one ethical dilemma that falls squarely on Alexia's shoulders at the moment, however, is this:

Alexia's dilemma arises from the fact that she has become more persuaded that she was right about what she saw happening to Mr. Carnavello. She believes the principle of beneficence to him is being compromised. But also she can agree with the points made by the administration and some of the staff regarding fairness to other residents. She is experiencing difficulty in deciding what to do that will honor the several principles guiding professional action in this situation. In summary, she has an ethical dilemma.

Locus of Authority Problem

If Alexia decides someone other than herself, the administration, or the team should be making decisions regarding any aspects of Mr. Carnavello's treatment (or the nursing home policies regarding treatment), she also faces a locus of authority ethical problem. For instance, although the story does not give you the benefit of knowing whether Mr. Carnavello's input is being included in the decision, Alexia could decide that the authority for this decision should rest with Mr. Carnavello. From what we have been told, we can assume that the staff and medical director have determined that the patient is not competent to make such a decision and therefore they are acting paternalistically.

 SUMMARY

An essential step in analysis is to identify the type or types of ethical problems that you face.

Step 3: Use Ethics Theories or Approaches to Analyze the Problem(s)

In Chapter 4, you were introduced to normative ethical theory and approaches. You have seen in the preceding pages that the narrative approach, which keeps relevant details of the story at the center of Alexia's deliberation, is the most crucial for her eventual decision to be consistent with professional ethics. She also needs certain basic attitudes to help guide her on the path of a caring response as she deals with her own anger about what she observes. Therefore, virtues such as compassion are among her most fundamental resources. You learned that situations requiring the health professional to be an agent (i.e., take action for which she or he is morally accountable) draw on ethical theories that focus on principles, duties and rights, or consequences. In other words, they are the tools for action.

To jog your memory, take a minute to review these action theories:
1. Utilitarianism
   Focuses on the overall consequences
   Is a particular type of teleology
2. Deontology
   Focuses on duty
   Alexia's story may make it easier to compare the two theories than when they were presented in Chapter 4.

It agent (A), Alexia, is like most health professionals guided by the principles of duty and rights in her professional role, she probably will decide that her weightier (i.e., more compelling) responsibility is to Mr. Carnavello.

If agent (A), Alexia, approaches it from a utilitarian standpoint, she will spend less time thinking about duties and will be guided by the desire to bring about the overall best consequences in this situation. The overall best consequences may be to "leave well enough alone" and not to make waves with the nursing home administrator or others.

1 *Reflection*
Which approach do you find yourself leaning toward in Alexia's and Anthony Carnavello's situation? Why?

_____

_____

_____

_____

 SUMMARY

In Step 3, the tools of ethical analysis further help move you toward resolution and action that are consistent with a caring response.

Step 4: Explore the Practical Alternatives

Alexia has decided what she should do. The next step is to determine what she can do in this situation. She must exercise her imagination and confer with her colleagues regarding the actual strategies and options available to her. Suppose she decides that her initial perceptions were correct and that she must act on behalf of Mr. Carnavello, even though the staff sees no problem?

At this juncture, many people oversimplify the range of options available to them. They tend to fall back on old alternatives when under stress, a behavioral pattern you can probably recognize from your own stressful situations. Therefore, imaginative pursuit of options is a big challenge—but an invaluable resource—in resolving ethical problems. In recounting Alexia's story, we learned that she believed her range of options was to confront the nursing home administrator or do nothing. A diligent search for other options can now make the difference between her doing the right thing and allowing a moral wrong to go unchecked.

 Reflection

Applying your own imagination to her situation, list all the alternatives you believe Alexia has. Try to identify at least four.

1. _____

2. _____

3. _____

4. _____

Having listed them, which one do you think is the best? Why?

Often, it is a good idea to try out some of the more far-fetched alternatives with a colleague whom you trust and with whom you can share the situation without breaching the patient's confidentiality. Alexia did this with the nursing supervisor. We do not know how the supervisor's counsel helped in the end, but we are sure that her words led Alexia to further examination of what her next step should be.

SUMMARY

Imagination enhances ethical decision making by allowing you to think more creatively and expansively about the alternatives.

Step 5: Complete the Action

Think of all the work Alexia has already done. She responded to her initial feeling that something was wrong, followed her compassionate disposition that motivated her not to let the matter go unnoticed, reasoned about and decided on the type of ethical problem(s) she was encountering, carried out an analysis using one or more of the ethical theories and approaches, and exercised her imagination to identify practical options needed to effect a caring response. She also shared her worry with at least one other person she knew commands her respect and that of others. Now she has one more task, but it is the crucial one, and that is to act.

If Alexia fails to go ahead and act, the entire process so far will be reduced to the level of an interesting but inconsequential philosophic exercise or, worse, may result in harm to Mr. Carnavello. Of course, Alexia may consciously decide not to pursue the situation any further, but insofar as it involved her deliberate intent, it is different than simply failing to follow what seems a correct course of action. If harm comes to Mr. Carnavello or others because of Alexia's inaction or unnecessarily narrow focus, she will be an agent of harm by her own omission or neglect. The solid ethical foundation she laid in Steps 1 to 4 will have been of no use.

Why would anyone fail to act in this type of circumstance? Mainly because it is sobering to be an agent in such important matters of meaning and value in others' lives.

 SUMMARY

The goal of your analysis is finally to act!

Some decisions are literally life and death decisions; all are of deep significance to the people facing the particular situation. Although the previous step required imagination, this final step requires courage and the strength of will to go ahead, with the knowledge that there may be risks or backlashes. As Alexia becomes more experienced, she will be increasingly aware that her integrity of purpose must be supported by her compassion and courage.

Step 6: Evaluate the Process and Outcome

Once she has acted, it behooves Alexia to pause and engage in a reflective examination of the situation. The practical goal of ethics is to resolve ethical problems, thereby upholding important moral values and duties. The extent to which Alexia's decision led to action that upheld morality, however, is knowable only by reexamining what happened in the actual situation. This evaluation is germane to her growth and development as an ethical professional and is essential if the outcome she hoped for was not realized.

In the medical model, a widespread mechanism for addressing interventions that go awry in the clinical setting is morbidity and mortality ("m and m") rounds. If you have not yet been in the clinical setting, the term "rounds" may be new to you. *Rounds* is the general term used for meetings of clinicians. Some are held sitting in a room (sit-down rounds), and others are held walking from patient to patient (walking rounds). Morbidity and mortality rounds allow health professionals whose interventions did not yield the hoped-for results to present the case to their peers for further evaluation. Sometimes ethical committees or your own unit staff meetings conduct ethics morbidity and mortality rounds to have a group review of a particularly difficult situation that seemed not to meet the ethical goal of a caring response. Rounds are a means for reflective discernment. They are an explicit way for the health professional to reflect on practice. This type of activity promotes ethical reasoning and helps ensure that care is individualized, just, and benevolent.[5]

Alexia's case is not unique. Studies have shown that the topics of conflict around goal setting and dual obligations are amongst the most frequently cited ethical issues encountered by rehabilitation practitioners.[6,7] Given this, suppose you, like Alexia, have just been through the process of arriving at a difficult ethical decision and have acted on it. Some questions you might ask yourself are the following:

- What did you do well?
- Why do you think so?
- What were the most challenging aspects of this situation?
- How did this situation compare with others you have encountered or read about?
- To what other kinds of situations will your experience with this one apply?
- Who was the most help?
- What do the patient, family, or others have to say about your course of action?
- Overall, what did you learn?
- What would you do differently if you were faced with the same situation again?

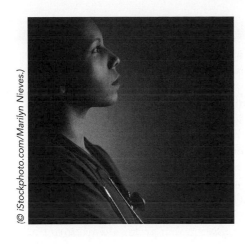

(© iStockphoto.com/Marilyn Nieves.)

Figure 5-1. Critical reflection = clinical growth.

All of these will serve you well in your preparation for the next opportunity to decide what a caring response entails in that new situation. When you reflect, you advance your ethical reasoning and are better prepared for the next time you are faced with a challenging situation (Figure 5-1).

SUMMARY

Reflection on your action prepares you for how you can continue to learn from your experience.

Summary

If you studied this chapter carefully, you will have identified the six-step process that anyone faced with an ethical question can apply in searching for a caring response.
1. Gather as much relevant information as possible to get the facts straight.
2. Determine the precise nature of the ethical problem (if Step 1 confirms that there is one).
3. Decide on the ethics approach that will best get at the heart of the problem.
4. Decide what should be done and how it best can be done (explore the widest range of options possible).
5. Act.
6. Reflect on and evaluate the action.

Questions for Thought and Discussion

1. The first step in ethical decision making is to gather as much relevant information as possible. The information-gathering process, however, can become so extensive that it becomes an end in itself and could actually deter one from proceeding to action at all. What types of guidelines would you use to decide that you have as much information as you need or can obtain?
2. A necessary step in ethical decision making is to act on one's own conclusions about what ought to be done. Under what conditions, if any, would you decide not to act according to your own best moral insights and judgment? That is, what, if any, are the limits to your willingness to act ethically?
3. In your professional practice, you would much prefer always to act ethically. What type of supports or assurances within your work setting would enable you to so act?

REFERENCES

1. Fletcher, K., 1996. Use of restraints in the elderly. *AACN Clin Issues* 7 (4), 611–635.
2. Farrell-Miller, M., 1997. Physically aggressive resident behavior during hygienic care. *J Gerontol Nurs* 23 (5), 24–35.
3. Omnibus Budget Reconciliation Act PL100-203. 1987. *Subtitle C. Nursing home reform*. United States Government Printing Office, Washington, DC.
4. Jonsen, A., Siegler, M., Winslade, W., 2002. *Clinical ethics: A practical approach to ethical decisions in clinical medicine*, 5th ed. McGraw Hill, New York, pp. 1–12.
5. Rashotte, J., Carnevale, F.A., 2004. Medical and nursing clinical decision-making: A comparative epistemological analysis. *Nurs Philosophy* 5, 160–174.
6. Foye, S.J., Kirschner, K.L., Brady Wagner, L.C., et al., 2002. Ethical issues in rehabilitation: A qualitative analysis of dilemmas identified by occupational therapists. *Top Stroke Rehabil* 9 (3), 89–101.
7. Triezenberg, H.L., 2005. Examining the moral role of physical therapists. In: Purtilo, R.B., Jenson, G.M., Royeen, C.B. (Eds.), *Educating for moral action: A sourcebook in health and rehabilitation ethics*. F.A. Davis, Philadelphia, PA, pp. 85–98.

Ethical Dimensions
of Professional Roles

6

Surviving Student Life Ethically

Objectives

The reader should be able to:
- Describe some opportunities for and barriers to achieving a caring response through ethical decision making peculiar to the student role.
- Describe academic integrity and its relationship to professional integrity.
- Identify two criteria of academic misconduct and cite some examples.
- Identify six areas where students have moral agency in the professional practice setting.
- Discuss two types of wrongdoing students may encounter and what should be done in each case.
- Assess the availability and usefulness of policies, procedures, and practices designed to enhance students' ethical development and decision making.

New terms and ideas you will encounter in this chapter

academic integrity	conduct	plagiarism
academic misconduct	cheating	legal fraud
intent		

Topics in this chapter introduced in earlier chapters

Topic	Introduced in chapter
Integrity	1
Caring response	2
Moral distress (types A and B)	3
Role of emotion	3
Ethical dilemma	3
Moral agent	3
Utilitarianism	4, 5
Ethical elements, principles	4
Veracity (truth telling)	4
Beneficence	4
Nonmaleficence	4
Six-step process of ethical decision making	5

Introduction

The ethics foundation presented in Section I of this book will serve you well during your student days and throughout your life. This chapter and Chapter 7 focus on your personal moral development and your opportunity to exercise appropriate ethical decision making throughout your career, beginning with the time you are a student. It is especially important to include your role as student and some of the particular opportunities and stresses of this period because no matter your age, the student years are the time your approach to ethical decision making in your professional role takes shape.

Special Challenges of Student Life

As a student, you have the advantage of coming into a situation with a fresh perspective and can raise issues that more seasoned professionals could miss or might gloss over. At the same time, a situation sometimes is misjudged solely because some students do not have the advantage of having served in a professional role or in a particular setting for a long time.[1] Your professional judgment is developing in your student experiences.

The story in this chapter highlights some ethical problems inherent in your role as a student.

The Story of Matt Weddle, Madeline Notch, the Bedacheks, and the Botched Home Visit

Matt Weddle is a nursing student in his next to last year of professional education. He has enjoyed his professional training, especially being in the actual patient care environment. Today, however, he went to bed discouraged and wondering if he has made the correct career choice.

Matt is on a home health care rotation. He has an excellent supervisor, Madeline Notch, who has tried to provide him with a wide range of learning experiences and proper supervision during his time with her. This has not been an easy task; the census for the home care association is high, and with major cutbacks in professional staff, she has been busier than usual. He is sorry to learn that she is going on vacation tomorrow and that his supervision will be turned over to another nurse, Eugenia Cripke.

Today Ms. Notch asks Matt if he would stop by Mrs. Bedachek's apartment to check on her son Tom and be sure his wound is healing well. "The wound may need debridement and a bandage change. You can make the judgment about whether to change the bandage, since I changed it myself yesterday on my way home from work." He is somewhat uncomfortable about going alone to see a patient he has not seen before. He also remembers being told by his academic clinical coordinator at school that under no circumstances should he go into a patient's home unsupervised. But he agrees to do so, not feeling free to question Ms. Notch about whether this is correct procedure. Instead, he assures her that he has done this procedure enough times under her supervision that he feels he should be able to do it. She agrees.

When he knocks at the Bedacheks' door, a large woman in a filthy house dress peers through a crack in the door. At first, she does not want to let him in, but when he shows her his name tag as identification that he is "the nurse," she admits him. He introduces himself with his name and says he is a student nurse. Mrs. Bedachek is already walking laboriously across the room toward the other occupant, an equally large man who appears unable to comprehend what is going on. The man strains to peer at Matt from a large armchair set up in the midst of the clutter in the small living room. Matt knows the man's name is Tom, but he is unprepared for the greasy-skinned person drooling onto the front of a mucus-stained shirt.

When Matt tells the patient what he has come to do, the man grunts. The woman says, "I don't want you to touch that bandage. It's fine." She draws up the man's shirt for Matt to see. Matt is surprised at the size of it and concerned about the dark seepage around the bottom edge. Mrs. Bedachek says, suspiciously, "Who are you again?" Matt repeats his name. "At least you're not a student," she says. "They're the worst." Matt says nothing. He feels uncomfortable about this whole situation.

He reaches toward the bandage to touch it, and she suddenly pulls the shirt back down over her son's trunk. The stench is making Matt feel woozy.

"I *said* it's fine," she says firmly.

Matt replies, "Okay," and leaves.

When he gets back to the office, Madeline Notch is there, clearing off her desk. "How did it go?" she asks. "Fine," he says. "Oh good," she replies. "I didn't want to tell you, but most people can't get through the front door. I went myself yesterday. I thought the wound looked really good except for that distal edge."

Matt had meant to tell her immediately about the whole scene, but for some reason, her comments unnerve him and he feels like a failure. He says, "Yeah, I agree."

She comes over to him. "Thanks so much for getting me through that squeeze. I knew you could handle that bandage change, and I was worried about letting it go." She continues, "Sometimes I think it's not worth trying to go on vacation!" She pauses and extends her hand, saying, "I have enjoyed working with you as a student. You will make a fine nurse. And you will enjoy working with Eugenia Cripke."

She leaves hurriedly, saying she has to pick up her son at daycare and get packed. Matt takes Tom Bedachek's record from the drawer and writes, "Wound debridement, bandage change. Purulent exudate around the distal rim of wound."

Almost everyone would agree that both Ms. Notch and Matt Weddle exercised poor ethical judgment.

Reflection

As you look at the story through Matt's eyes, what do you think are the reasons he is feeling discomfort after the day's events? Jot them down here.

_____

_____

_____

_____

During Matt's clinical education experience, he is facing an ethical problem, and clinical and legal ones, that have features very similar to those he will encounter in his eventual professional practice. Many times we are faced with unexpected situations that are unsettling for one reason or another. However, the opportunities to use his ethics knowledge and skills have presented themselves from the time he set foot in his educational program. We will briefly introduce you to some ways to survive student life ethically in the classroom and then compare them with resources for your experiences as a student in the clinic setting. In the latter, we will return to the story and you will have an opportunity to walk in Matt's shoes to explore the ethical implications of his situation.

The Goal: A Caring Response

You have already learned in Chapter 3 that for a person to be held responsible for her or his actions the person must be the moral agent in the situation. The health professional's agency revolves around being able and willing to provide a caring response in a variety of health-related situations. The conduct and attitudes for realizing this goal are embedded in your classroom experience. When you entered your program, you may have had to sign a student honor code or statement of *academic integrity*. Many universities have such codes and other ethical guidelines that detail the range and scope of your moral agency and responsibility and the responsibilities of the faculty toward you. If you study it carefully, you will see that the items taken together are designed for the positive outcome of your being able to maintain your integrity and the integrity of your profession. When integrity is being honored in the classroom setting, it is said that the student has exercised academic integrity. Breaches of this integrity constitute serious examples of *academic misconduct* that carry practical, including sometimes legal, sanctions against the student.

Recognizing Academic Misconduct

Undoubtedly professional educational programs are among the most rigorous and demanding of any type of education. Although the vast majority of students abide by the high ethical standards of honesty, respectfulness, and other conduct consistent with maintaining their own integrity and that of their chosen profession, a few find it too tempting to refrain from taking advantage of others' work to lessen their own burden. Their conduct conveys dishonesty, cheating, and other deceit and lack of respect for or fairness to others. In these cases, the reasonable expectations of the latter are not honored. It is correct to say that the person taking advantage of the situation has lost sight of his search for a caring response in regards to peers. Programs of professional preparation make the assumption that students who engage in unethical conduct in the classroom have a much higher likelihood of continuing this behavior in their professional career because the pressures on them will be even greater in their role over many years. They will have ignored the opportunities in their educational years to appreciate the power they have for doing harm to patients and others, and the opportunities for them to ethically flourish in their role. Breaches of academic integrity can begin with plans for how to cheat to improve one's grade, cut corners by using someone else's material, or lift someone's information without giving it the appropriate credit (i.e., plagiarism), to name some. *Intent* is a part of misconduct because it means that a person has set his or her sites on wrongdoing, but for an act to be judged as outright academic misconduct requires *conduct* that follows through on the intent.

Academic Misconduct = Intent To Engage In Wrongdoing + Action

The following straightforward exercise, based on the activities of five health professions students in the classroom who are faced with a midterm examination, helps to highlight some ways that academic integrity can be honored or compromised.[2]

 Reflection

Guido, Shivani, Karl, Aliana, and Jasmine are friends who always study together. On Thursday, they have an important midterm examination that includes about 10 pages of written material analyzing several clinical cases. They are very nervous about this examination because it brings together a large amount of material and they have been feeling overloaded with all of their coursework.

Which of the following constitutes academic misconduct?

1. The five of them study together and all agree to use the same sources and approach the problems in the same way. Yes____ No____
2. The five of them agree to text message each other during the examination if one signals to another that help is needed and the faculty member happens to leave the room. A set of codes will help them know which question the friend needs help with. Yes____ No____
3. They plan to sit in the examination room in such a way that they can see each other's answers if necessary. Yes____ No____
4. Aliana gives the secret signal that she needs help with examination question 4b. Guido uses text messaging to alert Aliana of her problem when the faculty member leaves the room. Yes____ No____
5. Karl goes to a website on his handheld device and copies a description from a similar on a case analysis but does not attribute this source. Yes____ No____
6. Jasmine is glad for plan # 3 because she is stuck on one of the questions and is able to get back on track by something she sees on Guido's paper. Yes____ No____

7. Karl has made some notes on the back of the label of his water bottle and uses it to help make sure he is covering the key points. Yes____ No____

We will walk through these responses with you. Plan #1 is not a breach of academic integrity, although it has the potential to rob each student of the opportunity to fully take advantage of preparation for the clinical issues they will face. Plans #2 and 3 are borderline activities, although neither constitutes misconduct solely on the basis of the students' intent to position themselves so that they can engage in *cheating* of various types. They would constitute a breach if the students actually take action on this intent. Plans #4 to 7 include both criteria of academic misconduct, intent and conduct. Plan #5 is a blatant act of *plagiarism*. As moral agents, the students have sacrificed their academic integrity for other ends.

There is a related issue that is extremely important for you to know. In plan #4, Guido chooses to assist Aliana according to the plan set out in plan #2. Just as the law has the idea of "accomplice," academic misconduct criteria require that you not only refrain from wrongdoing yourself but also report clear instances of wrongdoing by others. This idea carries through into your professional role. If you know that a classmate or professional colleague is engaged in wrongdoing, you are ethically and legally responsible for reporting it.

Fortunately, your professional education program with its honor codes, modeling by professionals, and other guidelines that are being offered to you allow you to fully appreciate the opportunities for refining the character traits and ethical conduct consistent with a caring response that you brought with you from your everyday life. The stakes grow higher when students enter the environment of their future professional activities. That is where Matt Weddle's ethical challenge takes place, in this instance, in a home care visit as a student. Some factors in his degree of moral agency are the nature of his role as a student, the character of the student-professor relationship, and his inexperience regarding some types of life situations more generally.[3]

 Reflection

Consider Matt Weddle's experience and write down some areas where he has moral agency as a student.

What is he ethically responsible for?

What is the minimum he would have had to do to constitute a caring response? This will give you a good basis for comparing your judgments about a student's moral agency with the suggestions in the paragraphs that follow.

_____

_____

_____

_____

Overall, you have an ethical responsibility to take full advantage of your student role to refine your ethical decision making under supervision. Most of Matt's experience was characterized by this type of situation. Until their last day together, Madeline Notch gave him ample opportunity to practice his skills under her supervision in a variety of settings. He had the benefit of continual discourse and feedback from her. By actually taking the opportunities seriously, he was acting responsibly by learning as much as he possibly could before having to make such decisions on his own. Once you graduate, you will no longer have the formal clinical, ethical, and legal supervision that you have as a student to help protect you from making poor judgments.

The Six-Step Process as a Student

As Matt's experience also illustrates, things do not always go smoothly. In the next few paragraphs, we will walk through the six steps of ethical decision making so that you can see an example of how each step is involved in highlighting where moral agency resides in your role as a student. Taken together, these examples can be summarized as follows. You have a moral responsibility to:

1. Gather relevant information from the patient or family, the patient's clinical record, and your supervisor, expressing serious doubts about your qualifications to your supervisor if you have been given the authority by that person to act independently and you feel ill equipped to do so.
2. Openly share what you know about the patient and other aspects of the situation with the health care team in an attempt to identify clinical symptoms and ethical problems.
3. Use the knowledge and skills you do have, including ethical theory and approaches, to participate in arriving at a caring response. Refrain from acts that would be wrong for anyone to commit.
4. Be ready to help identify the best alternatives possible for patients and others who are faced with ethical problems.
5. Remain faithful to your own convictions and exercise the will and courage to act on them.
6. Give yourself the opportunity to reflect on your action with your supervisor and others.

Having listed these six guidelines, let's go back to the story to give you an opportunity to move step by step through Matt's situation.

Step 1: Gather Relevant Information

As you recall, the first step in ethical decision making is to gather all of the relevant facts. As a student, you are practicing under supervision because it is assumed that you will have little knowledge gained from experience and likely also have partial classroom knowledge and skills. You probably have had some training in what to look for and how to interview and also have had an opportunity to observe others' conduct. But if you have doubts about either your knowledge or skills, it is your responsibility to express it at the outset.

In retrospect, you can see that Ms. Notch used poor judgment in sending Matt Weddle to the Bedachek's home alone. Although she thought he was capable of completing the technical procedures competently and independently, she had not thought through all the ramifications of the situation he might encounter. For instance, she was not being responsive to the literature that warns how differently patients might react to an unexpected visitor in the home care treatment environment, the environment in which most patients' autonomy is at its greatest.[4] It was her responsibility to do so, especially in her role as supervisor, and in that respect, she failed to exercise it well. In fact, if Matt's actions (or in this case, failure to act) led to litigation against the caregivers, she would be held legally responsible for what "her" student did or did not do.

Nonetheless, that does not leave Matt Weddle in a position of having no ethical responsibility. Students' moral agency extends to the point of telling a supervisor if he or she feels a serious lack of knowledge or capabilities. Likely this awareness is also one of the reasons Matt feels so disquieted at the end of the day. Moreover, by the time he has completed his first visit, Matt Weddle knows how Mrs. Bedachek feels about students. He knows how hard it will be for other students to go into the Bedachek home and be able to do what they are supposed to do for Tom. He also knows that he deceived the Bedacheks by not clarifying that he was a student when Mrs. Bedacheck made it known that she was confused on this point. This may seem like a minor detail to Matt, but it has the potential to erode all trust between the home care agency and this family. That fact alone could be critical information for the home health care team as they plan their schedules. During this one visit, what other information did Matt gain that you consider relevant to good patient care for the patient? For other patients?

Step 2: Identify the Type of Ethical Problem

A second step in ethical decision making is to be on alert for ethical problems in the situation. You have a responsibility to share what you do know with others who are accountable for and must be responsive to the patient's well-being. Sometimes students are great reservoirs of information. Although some patients may be hesitant to let students treat them, the converse often is true as well. And some patients feel safer telling a student what they do not want to say to a professional. In such moments, you are a key member of the team in regard to planning optimal treatment approaches, including providing insight into ethical issues.

This is your opportunity to identify some ways Matt's situation fits the prototypical ethical problem of moral distress.

One structural barrier to Matt's doing the right thing is that apparently he does not feel at liberty to question his supervisor's request to go to the Bedachek's home alone. This external situation is accompanied by the interior barrier of anxiety. But why? Ms. Notch has not presented the situation in such a way that he has reason to fear her disfavor; she does not appear to be motivated to wield her power unfairly or to be punitive. His anxiety and subsequent behavior may be at least partially explained by the nature of the student-teacher relationship in which the imbalance of power between the two is built into the structure. Matt's situation is an example of why some of the approaches you encountered in Chapter 4 place so much stress on imbalances of power within institutional structures themselves. This explanation fits the prototype of moral distress type A, in which there is a "structural" barrier to Matt's doing what his better moral judgment dictates.

He also may be experiencing moral distress type B. He knows a lot but is still in training. Understandably, there are unknowns related to the limited professional experience Matt brings to the setting. He knows how to change a bandage and to débride a wound. But the larger narrative of the story leaves many gaps for him to fill in as he goes along. For instance, perhaps he has had limited experience talking with people like the Bedacheks. He may never have seen a person with the degree of cognitive impairment Tom Bedachek manifests and may not know what type of impairment it is. He is not sure how to instill enough confidence in either of them to get on with the wound debridement. He also is being forced to reckon with his new realization that in home care a professional is going into the private "sanctuary" of a person's home and that adaptation to their home environment is essential if a caring response is going to be possible.[5] In Chapter 3, you studied about the role of emotion in ethical decision making and how emotion can be both helpful and a barrier to moving ahead. Matt is frustrated, afraid, and angry, but those responses do not indicate that he is uncaring. His being overwhelmed by the enormity of the unknown and being insecure in his judgment about what to do are not unusual student responses. As a student yourself you may recognize a tendency to discredit your own feelings, intuitions, and judgments. Students often are reticent to show their clinical supervisor their emotions for fear that they will be judged as weak. The worst outcome of this student-related stress is that you may assume you are completely unable to evaluate a situation correctly or even to get enough information to make a sound ethical assessment of it.

In contrast, the best outcome is to use emotion as an opportunity for support and discussion. The student years are the time to become as well prepared as possible.

 SUMMARY

As a student, you may be faced with moral distress and not effect an adequate caring response because of structural and knowledge barriers to your acting on what is right, compounded by anxiety and other emotions.

Let us continue to analyze Matt's problem, considering whether he also has an ethical dilemma.

Reflection

Does Matt have an ethical dilemma? If so, describe it briefly here.

_____

_____

_____

_____

We believe a dilemma that seems directly related to his student nurse status arises around Mrs. Bedachek's comment about how students are "the worst." When Matt first introduced himself, he identified himself as a student nurse. We do not know his motivation for remaining silent when she later made the derogatory comment about students. He had an opportunity then to reaffirm his student status, which clearly would have been the right thing to do. Let us give him the benefit of the doubt, however, and assume that his reason for remaining silent was that he truly believed this was the only way he could hold on to the little bit of confidence Mrs. Bedachek had in him and that allowing this deceit would benefit Tom Bedachek.

Sometimes patients are less comfortable with students than with others; therefore, Matt's judgment to remain silent as a way to allow the patient the benefit of feeling comfortable is consistent with his duty of beneficence.

Of course, the motivation might also be to bolster his own confidence, which is not in itself a bad thing. However, it does not place the needs of the patient first.

Step 3: Use Ethics Theories or Approaches to Analyze the Problem

A third step in ethical decision making is to apply the principles and other ethical guidelines available to you in your role. Again, as a student, your first response might be that you are not sure how to apply them in your new role. At the same time, if you look closely at Matt's situation, you can conclude that his actions include morally wrong or illegal acts. As a student in the clinical setting, he has not refrained from the exercise of hurtful character traits such as dishonesty and cheating the patient, which are harmful in any relationship. A bottom line regarding your moral agency as a student is that you have a responsibility to refrain from acts that are wrong for anyone to commit.

 Reflection

What are examples of Matt's failure to exercise his moral agency and take responsibility for his actions that are similar to any relationship where one person has an ethical responsibility not to harm the other? Jot your examples down here.

_____

_____

_____

_____

You may have found several places where you think this happened. I assume you agree that one occasion was his deceit by silence and lying. The more glaring example of his dishonesty was his decision to report on Tom Bedachek's record that he had performed the therapeutic procedure when he had not. His deceitfulness and dishonesty are not applicable only in the health professional and patient relationship; intentional lying causes harm by undermining trust and misleading the other in ways that diminishes their right to autonomy. He has ignored the duty to do no harm. The principle of veracity is supportive of the duty to be truthful too. No circumstance excuses him from these important principles of ethical decision making. Making himself look more responsible than he was does not justify his lying.

Entering false statements on a medical record also is illegal. He is committing *legal fraud* because the home health care agency will be paid for treatment it did not perform. This act could cost him his professional career and lead to criminal sanctions. What are some of the reasons this breach of professional responsibility is viewed as so serious by society as a whole?

If you are reasoning about this as a utilitarian, you are on the path to legitimating his course of action on the basis of the overall good consequences you may believe will result. Within professional ethics, however, the ethical principles not to harm and truth telling (veracity) in regards to the patient take on the strength of duties. They are vital as means to honoring that in the role of professional the patient's interests take priority. A caring response requires unequivocally that the decisions be patient-centered. Therefore, to the extent that Matt understands his role as a health professional, he cannot justify withholding key information or making false statements in the record without understanding that he is engaged in wrongdoing.

 SUMMARY

As a student, your role as a moral agent includes that you are not protected from ethical dilemmas and that you must participate in deciding how to arrive at a caring response in a specific situation.

During your formative years as a student, you have an opportunity to refine your ethics skills, although at times they make you uncomfortable.

Step 4: Explore the Practical Alternatives

Yet another step in ethical decision making is to seek the viable alternatives and find the one that most fully approximates or achieves a caring response.

One of the reasons health professionals enjoy working with students is that students often provide creative approaches to old problems. Professionals who have been facing similar issues for years get bogged down in habit or become discouraged because attempted solutions have not been successful in the past. (How many times have you heard, "We've tried that before, and it didn't work?")

Your unwillingness to offer suggestions is not a morally neutral act. Sheer robustness, arrogance, or ill-placed criticisms are not welcome. At the same time, as a student, you are a moral agent whose scope extends to your readiness to voice your thoughtful opinion when you are invited to do so and to taking a posture of readiness to contribute such ideas rather than standing by passively and keeping your insights to yourself.

Although Matt has seriously breached the responsibilities consistent with his role as a moral agent, he can still offer suggestions from the perspective of what he observed in the Bedachek family. Of course, he also has a moral responsibility to contribute his thoughtful ideas regarding all the other situations he has had the opportunity to witness and participate in during his tenure in this clinical setting.

 SUMMARY

You have a moral duty to participate with others in seeking practical alternatives for patients faced with difficult ethical decisions. You have a right to receive support and guidance for this from your faculty in both the classroom and clinic.

Step 5: Complete the Action

The fifth step in ethical decision making is to act. Students' responsibilities include the four forms described in the following paragraphs.

Act Within the Limits of Competence and Self-Confidence

Always seek to balance your knowledge, skills, and abilities with the need for supervision. This helps ensure that the patient is the beneficiary at all times. With this overriding guideline in mind, the next three forms are simply logical complements.

Act According to Convictions

Some general protections for health professionals to honor their integrity and therefore avoid moral compromise were introduced in Chapter 1. Similar protections should apply to students. For instance, during your student experience, you have a responsibility to make your convictions known so that you are never placed under pressure to participate in a procedure that undermines your religious or other deeply held convictions. Religious observances may pose another reason for you or your fellow students to want special consideration—for example, to participate in holiday traditions and rituals. Every professional educational program should have a formal or informal mechanism in place to ensure that you and your student colleagues are able to offer rationales for wishing to abstain and an appeals process in place for disagreements. Of course, you have the responsibility to inform your educational program administrators and supervisors in advance of any such situation so that patient care is never compromised. Whenever possible, there should be plenty of lead-in time for your request to be heard and considered in a timely manner.

Right Any Wrongdoing

Another dimension of living according to your convictions is to right any wrongs you yourself have done in regard to a patient or other situation within your student professional role. Matt should admit his wrongdoing to Madeline Notch right away. No one enjoys having to do damage control after wrongdoing, but Matt needs to engage in self-care that will serve him well in the future when he errs. There is no better investment than taking care of yourself by keeping your conscience clear. His admission will also ensure that Tom is spared any additional harm as a result of a missed dressing change. Tom's cognitive disability places him at risk of neglectful care of health complications. As the caregiver, Matt's duty is to honor the principle of nonmaleficence.

Reflection

Matt should admit his wrongdoing of lying about the wound dressing as soon as possible. If you were Matt, how would you go about correcting this serious error in ethical judgment?

_____

_____

_____

_____

You must begin to practice during your student years if you are going to be able to admit shortcomings and mistakes throughout your career. Nothing is more harmful to you professionally and personally than to get into the habit of "covering up" your mistakes or deceits. When approached thoughtfully, professors and supervisors almost always are forgiving of student missteps and stand ready to discuss and help prevent such breaches from happening again.

Address Others' Wrongdoing Constructively

As you recall in the story of the five students, the idea that academic integrity involves also holding colleagues accountable for their wrongdoing begins in the classroom. Here we remind you that it continues through your clinical education experiences as well.

This arduous moral task of addressing others' wrongdoing constructively is also a part of everyone's responsibility in the health care environment, including yourself and your fellow students. Quiet, diligent observation is a reliable guidepost in your assessment of wrongdoing by your fellow students or by professionals. As we have noted, a legitimate worry about expressing your concern arises because as a student you may be aware that you do not have full knowledge of the situation. In his study, Branch[3] noted that medical students tend to question their own moral judgment when faced with differing values expressed by authority figures. During many years of working with students in the health professions, we have found the same response to be true, generally speaking. In Chapter 5, Alexia Eliopoulos, who had completed her physical therapy preparation and was an employee, hesitated after talking to Ms. Carroll because she was warned that she "did not have all the facts." To make certainty more elusive, as a student you are not an actual employee of the institution in which you are placed and therefore are unfamiliar with its policies. You probably do not know the in-house mechanisms that employees use for resolving concerns and conflict, and even if you do, they may not apply to you.

In the end, these challenges should not keep you from addressing ethical wrongdoing. For instance, Matt knows with certainty that Ms. Notch acted wrongly in sending him to the Bedachek's home alone, no matter her rationale. Matt, however, did not challenge that act so that he also acted with poor judgment. Rather than the two of them maintaining a conspiracy of silence, he can help report his own wrongdoing in the context of acknowledging that she, too, was a partner in the way this situation unfolded.

Step 6: Evaluate the Process and Outcome

In the sixth and final step of ethical decision making, the moral agent steps back from the heat of action and goes over the process to think about what can be learned about a truly caring response, how it might be done better next time, or how it applies to other situations. Only through this conscious process will your own moral development be enhanced.[6] By now you are aware that a caring response in regard to present or future patients should ultimately drive your motivation at all times. If any action or inaction flew in the face of this basic core of your professional identity, that path should not be taken again.

Your reflection also should include an acknowledgment that you are "in it together" with your clinical faculty; their job is to guide you in ways that will encourage you, not discourage you. A study of 272 nursing students in a baccalaureate educational program showed that when clinical faculty as individuals were themselves "caring [toward students], gave encouragement and positive feedback, demonstrated . . . new procedures, encouraged critical thinking, clearly stated faculty expectation of students, and conducted pre- and post conferences,"[7] students learned the important dimensions of their clinical role more effectively. If on reflection you are experiencing that type of treatment, you will want to model your own behavior toward others in your work situation in the future on how you yourself were treated.

Given the situation in which Matt finds himself, he certainly owes it to himself to reflect on what happened and why. He also has a moral responsibility to future patients not to let this negligence and the deceit that followed happen again. He has a moral responsibility to himself to regain his self-respect by gaining more insight into the incident.

 SUMMARY

If you reflect back over steps 1 through 6, you will see that a student's moral agency applies at every step of ethical decision making.

Strategies for Success as a Moral Agent

The student role has more vitality and enjoyment built into it than risks and ethical challenges. The opportunity to apply your ethical knowledge and skills in real-life situations will help your confidence grow and experience deepen. The most difficult situations are those that involve the report of wrongdoing, one's own or that of others. We invite you to continue to search for ways to address them when they do occur. A few notes on strategies for such disquieting student moments are offered here.

Most educational programs have well-developed institutional policies and procedures to protect students who follow the processes designed for reporting concerns. Freely use channels within your institution set up for students in your professional program. You should be made familiar with them before going into your clinical education experiences. If you do not receive this orientation and you run into trouble, your clinical supervisor, fieldwork staff, and academic advisor are obvious sources of information and support. It is also most helpful to reflect before reporting apparent problems. A well-reasoned concern is a well-respected one because it shows your ability to self-assess and evaluate.

An essential rule of thumb is to honor the confidentiality of everyone involved, reporting only information that is relevant to the situation and containing the report to documented evidence. Understandably, if you report on an error in judgment you made, you may be asked to justify how it happened and work with your supervisor or others to rectify it.

Summary

In summary, there are special ethical challenges during your student years that involve both the peculiarities of the student-supervisor or student-professor relationship and the limits of your own knowledge and experience. From the time you enter your professional program, you are a student-professional and are bound to certain duties and guiding professional values. It is the mutual task of students, classroom faculty, and clinical supervisors working together to ensure that students trust their developing competencies and abilities, understand their role as moral agents, and act appropriately to help ensure that a caring response consistent with the demands of professional responsibility are exercised. In fact, the purpose of this book is to help you think clearly about a wide variety of ethical situations before you are faced with the more weighty responsibilities associated with professional practice after completion of your studies.

Questions for Thought and Discussion

1. This morning, Andrea, a student working in the outpatient clinic, notices two men sitting in the waiting area. She recognizes one as her dad's business partner, Mr. Brown, and greets him. She recalls that in a recent visit she made to her parents' home for dinner her father had expressed concern about Mr. Brown's failing health, which has begun to interfere with his earnings. Mr. Brown and the other man are chatting amiably, despite that they make a striking contrast—the silver-haired Mr. Brown and the seamy young man with a torn leather jacket. She remembers her dad's admiration for Mr. Brown's ability to "cross classes" and have friends in all walks of life. She goes to hang up her coat and when she returns to the waiting area the other man has disappeared and Mr. Brown is sitting alone.

   Andrea is somewhat shy about her assignment to take Mr. Brown's clinical history. Mr. Brown seems relaxed about it, however, and even a little bemused as she earnestly questions him and checks off the answers on her sheet. She leads him to the dressing room where he will undress for his tests. While heading back to her desk she notices that something had fallen from his pocket just before he entered the dressing room. She rushes back and picks up the packet. Inside the brown bag are a syringe and a small plastic bag of white powder. On the outside of the bag, written in a smudged scrawl on a piece of white tape, it says, "Brown, $450." She feels panic rising up in her chest and hopes beyond hope that her suspicion is unfounded.

   If you were in Andrea's situation, what do you believe you should do or not do? Does her role as a student professional dictate what she should do in regard to sharing this information with her father? Her supervisor? The police? That is, would it make any difference if she had met Mr. Brown on the street when her terrible discovery had been made?

   Discuss the steps you would take in arriving at your decision, emphasizing the professional moral duties, rights, and character traits that will help to inform and guide your decision and the special challenges you face as a student professional in this setting.

2. You have learned in your preclinical professional education that use of a certain procedure has been discontinued almost everywhere because of a dangerously high incidence rate of harmful side effects. You observe it being performed regularly in the setting where you are currently assigned, a place with a good reputation (apparently well deserved, generally speaking). In fact, as you observe patients' responses to the procedure, you become convinced yourself of good reasons not to use it. Now you have only 1 week left in this rotation and raise your concern with your supervisor. She responds, "Actually, we know that, and we don't like it either. Our health plan, however, does not allow us to use the newer procedure because it is four times as expensive as this one."

   Do you have a moral responsibility to recommend this site be discontinued for students? Why or why not? Do you have a moral responsibility to do anything in this situation? If yes, what?

3. You overhear a fellow student say to another colleague, "I just pretended to treat her. She was sleeping and will never know the difference. It's such a drag to treat someone who is so out of it." This student has cheated a patient out of her treatment. Is this different from cheating on a classroom test? Is so, why is it? If you observed a classmate cheating, should your response to it be different than if you learned that a patient was not treated? In each case, what should you do?

4. Your friend who is serving in the same clinical setting with you stops you in the hallway to ask you what he should do. His wife has called, crying, saying she feels really sick and would like him to come home right away. He has already missed several days because his uncle died and he also had a bout of the flu. The supervisor spoke with your friend this morning about how they would have to try to make up for some of the absences by providing special opportunities for him to cover areas he has missed. In fact, she told him that she has arranged for him to assist in an evaluation that starts at noon and will take about 4 hours, but from which he will benefit tremendously. He cannot get home and back in time for the beginning of the procedure.

   How should you respond? Why?

   What do you think he should do? Why?

REFERENCES

1. Purtilo, R., Haddad, A., 2005. Respect for yourself as a student. In: *Health professional and patient interaction*, 7ᵗʰ ed. WB Saunders, Philadelphia, PA, pp. 61–79.
2. Doherty, R., Purtilo, R., 2009. *Case study adapted from on-line self study; Unit 1, ethical foundations in the health professions.* MGH Institute of Health Professions, Boston, MA.
3. Branch, W.T. Jr., 2000. Supporting the moral development of medical students. *J Gen Intern Med* 15 (7), 503–508.
4. Arnold, R.M., Fello, M., 2000. Hospice and home care. In: Sugarman, J. (Ed.), *20 Common problems—Ethics in primary care.* McGraw Hill, New York, pp. 118–128.
5. Garcia, T., 2006. Ethics in home care. *Home Health Care Manage Pract* 18, 133–137.
6. Bankert, E.G., 2002. Care and traditional ethics: Enhancing the development of moral reasoning among nurses. *Int J Human Caring* 6 (1), 25–33.
7. Brewer, M.K., 2002. Being encouraged and discouraged: Baccalaureate nursing students' experiences of effective and ineffective clinical faculty teaching behaviors. *Int J Human Caring* 6 (1), 46–49.

7

Surviving Professional Life Ethically

Objectives

The reader should be able to:

- Describe what "a caring response" entails when the object of care is you.
- Discuss the place of self respect in your ability to survive professional life ethically.
- Evaluate the phrase "you owe it to yourself" from the standpoints of a duty to be good to yourself, aspirations for yourself, and responsibility to yourself as a caregiver.
- Describe what a personal values system is and its relationship to caring for yourself.
- Evaluate your own personal values system.
- Identify two types of threats to personal values encountered in the health professions and some strategies for meeting them ethically.
- Describe the idea of a reflection group and its function in helping to maintain personal integrity.

New terms and ideas you will encounter in this chapter

self care	responsibilities to	cooperation with
self respect	yourself	wrongdoing
personal values	exemplar	principle of material
system	conscience	cooperation
duties to yourself	conscientious	reflection group
aspirations	objection	

Topics in this chapter introduced in earlier chapters

Topic	Introduced in chapter
Personal morality	1
Integrity	1
Moral repugnance	1
A caring response	2
Responsibility = accountability + responsiveness	2
Moral distress	3
Emotions	3
Ethical dilemma	3
Intent	3
Moral agency	3
Duties	4
Beneficence	4
Six-step process	5

Introduction

You have come a long way in thinking about the ethical dimensions of professional practice in a general way, and in Chapter 6, you focused on them in relation to your role as a student. This chapter gives you an opportunity to think about the essential task of *self care* as you assume your professional role and throughout your professional life. Use of the six-step process for self care issues, many of which have ethics problems embedded in them, will illustrate ways for you to take care of yourself in your professional role. We believe it is extremely important that you honor your deep personal values and needs because as a professional you are always expected to think about others. How can you also take care of yourself in ways that prepare you to flourish in your professional role in all kinds of situations you will encounter? Janice K.'s story helps to focus this discussion.

 The Story of Janice K., Her Personal Values, and the Policies of Her Workplace

Janice K. is a dietician employed by a community health clinic affiliated with a large multihospital health plan. Part of the mission of the clinic is to provide nutritional counseling and services for people in an underserved area of her community. She loves working in this setting and believes that her professional responsibility includes helping to ensure that people in such areas have the same access to health care benefits as everyone else. Until now, she has told many of her friends and family how delighted she is to have found this position in a town where she can be close to her family. But recently everything has changed. Janice is distressed because she has learned that the health plan has designated her clinic as a site where abortion counseling and services will be added to its family planning programs. Janice has strong religious convictions that abortion is murder and that this practice should be stopped by whatever means possible. In her words, "Whenever an abortion is performed, two patients, mother and child, are harmed and the latter is murdered. This is against any interpretation of professional ethics that I can imagine. It's against life."

She realizes that her personal morality is bumping up against society's legal acceptance of abortion procedures that are carried out in medically competent settings. But this is no comfort. She is anxious, has been experiencing sleeplessness, and is also feeling vulnerable and angry about this turn of events, just when everything seemed to be falling into place.

This story could lead to many interesting and important ethical discussions, but in this chapter, we focus on the prime importance of your personal values and needs as foundational wellsprings of survival in your professional career. Many of your values have a moral component, comprising your personal morality. You have had some opportunities to think about your personal morality already in the course of studying this text. In Chapter 1, you were introduced to the ideas of personal morality and integrity and some ways that society tries to protect these in professionals. In Chapter 6, your integrity was raised again in regard to areas where you must exercise your moral agency as a student. So far, every story in this text has posed an ethical problem to you as you try to put yourself into the shoes of the person who is the moral agent searching for a caring response. Now you have an opportunity to step back and focus on yourself.

In Janice's situation, her beliefs and the values that inform those beliefs are powerful forces that guide her thinking about her duties and what kind of character traits she should strive to develop so that she can flourish as a human in any situation, including her workplace. That is the challenge each of us faces. The next section turns the lens from your quest for a caring response solely focused on the well-being of the patient to considering what you can to do act in a way that takes good care of yourself too. Is there a way to think about a caring response to yourself that honors your own values and needs, even in your role as a professional? We think yes.

The Goal: A Caring Response

At the center of finding a caring response to yourself is the development of deep *self respect*. Respect comes from a Latin root that means to hold something or someone in high regard. Respect for the dignity of individuals is an overriding virtue in professional ethics. But respect is almost always understood as referring to the deference one pays to another person, particularly the patient. Where in professional ethics is there encouragement to cultivate and incorporate respect for oneself?

Traditionally, very little about self respect has been found in the professional ethics literature. It has taken an understanding of modern moral psychology to bring it together with respect for others. An American moral philosopher, John Rawls, relied heavily on psychology to help clarify the relationship of respect for self and respect for others.[1] As adults, he notes, one source of self respect is the awareness that we are contributing to society's well-being. Professionals have an opportunity for almost daily feedback about how their contributions to patients' lives are helping society. This feeds the idea that their own needs also deserve to be respected. And so unlike other analyses that make respect solely a virtue about how to respond to others, Rawls interprets the development of self respect as an engine that can drive our daily activities towards human flourishing. True self respect allows us to flourish as selves and, in turn, allows us to have high regard for the societal tasks we assume to do our part in supporting human flourishing for others as well.

Your understanding of self respect as a wellspring that nourishes your professional obligation to respect others will result in your recognition that a lack of self respect will undermine your ability to enjoy deep job satisfaction.[2] A recent study highlights that health professionals who find meaning in their professional activities also have a strong connection with their deep values and moral orientation and strive to live according to them.[3] Their self respect partially is tied up with having basic values from which to draw and is reinforced by acting according to those values.

In short, the often overlooked attention to building self respect is an extremely important dimension of exercising a caring response toward yourself.

The Six-Step Process in Self Care

The six-step process of ethical decision making can be applied to challenges that threaten to pit your care of yourself against other loyalties and duties that you face in your professional role. It sounds contradictory to put yourself ahead of others when Chapter 2 focused so intensely on the focus of your care being with the patient first and foremost. Now we have an opportunity to examine further what happens when and if your personal beliefs, convictions, needs, or limitations counsel you to put yourself first and how to be sure that in these instances you do not unduly compromise your professional responsibility to take the patient's interests deeply into account.

Step 1: Gather Relevant Information

In all situations that involve questions of decisions about self care in your professional role, a key piece of information is that there are many barriers to acting in your own best interest. You will be faced with ample opportunities to compromise your own care in your professional role. The situation Janice faces presents an ethical challenge regarding how to live out personal values based on her religious convictions in an institutional environment. She believes that to go along with the clinic's proposed new practice threatens to compromise her spiritual and psychological well-being. Understandably, she is distressed about how to exercise self care. But there are other common types of situations too. For instance, one challenge arises when the workplace is short staffed. Many professionals decide to stay overtime or work on their usual days off to help fill a gap of patient needs that otherwise will go unmet, even though they know that their duties to their families or others are short-changed. Harder still to justify for many is that they simply need a break from the workplace pressures even though patients and colleagues will suffer. In a previous chapter, you met the young professional who wanted to go to a church supper on Friday evening to socialize with her new rural neighbors and in rushing through her patient care situation felt she had made a serious mistake. Although in this instance we would agree, the problem is that for many young professionals like her this one unfortunate situation may undermine her self-confidence in the basic idea that she does need to make decisions that serve her well personally over the long haul of her demanding workplace responsibilities.

We may seem to be overstressing health professionals' tendency to compromise self care, but the professional literature supports the seriousness of the tension professionals experience. The stresses sometimes arise out of the culture of the professions themselves. This is illustrated in a study of physical therapists who incurred work-related musculoskeletal disorders. The investigators found that the therapists' need to continue behaviors they believed best expressed care for the patients, together with their desire to appear knowledgeable and skilled in their ability to remain injury free, sometimes worked against their recovery from injury. These therapists had to leave the profession because of disturbing symptoms associated with their injury, a loss for them, their patients, and the clinical environment of health care.[4] A part of the terrible irony of this situation is that the American Physical Therapy Association at that time was a sponsor of Decade, an international, multidisciplinary initiative to improve health-related quality of life for people with musculoskeletal disorders. Members of this and other professions often have been unable to "practice what they preach," with high prices to pay for it. As health professionals, we must reflect on our own needs and values and begin early in our careers to analyze the influence that they have on our practice.

Information Gained from Identifying Your Personal Values

A *personal values system* is the set of values you have reflected on and chosen that will help you lead a good life. Usually people adopt personal values that partially overlap with societal values and that are in harmony with

PERSONAL VALUES SYSTEM

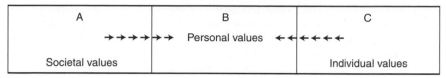

Figure 7-1. Personal values system. (From Purtilo, R., Haddad A., 2002. *Health professional and patient interaction*, 6th ed. Philadelphia: WB Saunders Company, p. 3.)

them.[5] Amy Haddad and Ruth Purtilo have represented and explained values in more detail according to the following scheme:

In Figure 7-1, area *A* represents values developed by society. Many times we accept these values because we want to live peacefully and harmoniously in society. Examples include obedience to traffic laws or other laws, adherence to etiquette, and willingness to pay taxes. Area *C* represents individual values that are important to you simply because you value them individually. You receive personal benefits from them. Many people cherish time to relax with a good book or pursue a hobby or sport. Having time alone "doing nothing" can be restorative and relaxing. The area of overlap, area *B*, represents values that you have internalized so that they not only are shared by other people in society but also are perceived as your own values. The motivations for accepting them are that leading a good life includes not only living harmoniously in society but also experiencing personal satisfactions and self-fulfillment. For many, some of these values include friendship, economic independence, and the realization of certain character traits such as fairness or courage. Most people integrate these three into a lifestyle and personal values system, drawing at times on all three areas: *A*, *B*, and *C*. Many values are moral values, and in this case, you can readily discern their relation to the personal, group, and societal moralities presented in Chapter 1.

Reflection
Name some personal values that help to give meaning and enjoyment to your life. Include at least one that you would identify as a moral value, such as honesty or justice.

_____

_____

_____

_____

As you study to become a professional, you will also incorporate some professional values into your personal values system. That process has already begun, and it is highly probable that values introduced into your professional preparation will help to make your career choice fitting within the context of your life. In terms of your professional activities, most of them will be moral values. The upshot is that while we are emphasizing self care in this chapter, the integrity that allows you to go forward with clarity and job satisfaction will require that your professional values be taken deeply into account in every decision you make.

 SUMMARY

> Your personal values system gives you the foundation for decisions that support self care. When faced with an ethical issue that involves how to honor yourself, it allows you to act on your own convictions in a meaningful way that best protects your moral integrity as a person. Your professional values must be included in this deliberation for you to maintain professional integrity.

Step 2: Identify the Type of Ethical Problem

It is easy to see that Janice is experiencing moral distress. She appears to like the clinic and her job, and until now, she has had no reason to be concerned about its practices or policies. Now her emotional alarm system has gone off, signaling that something is wrong. She is anxious, experiencing sleeplessness, and also feeling vulnerable and angry. We can assume with some certainty that Janice is convinced she is doing harm to herself by participating in a system that allows abortion. From that standpoint, it would make sense for her to withdraw from this institution altogether and apply her skills elsewhere. However, this inclination comes into conflict with some other considerations that constitute an ethical dilemma. She is concerned that if she withdraws completely, she is doing nothing to try to stop this procedure from being offered, thereby, in her words, allowing "both mother and child to be harmed." And she believes in the services to the socially marginalized population that she can help to provide, knowing that many of her colleagues are reticent to work at this site that they consider to be in a "dangerous" part of town. If she leaves, she believes the clinic will have a hard time finding a qualified replacement for her. Is that serving her personal values better than staying and working from within the system (Figure 7-2)?

In other types of conflicts regarding self care, such as a whether to give up one's day off because of a short-staffed workplace or to take a much needed "personal mental health" day of rest, the ethical problem may

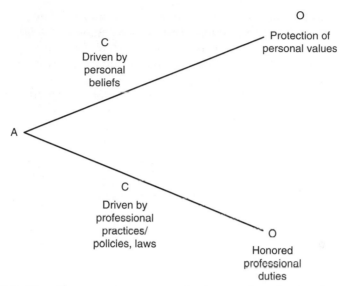

Figure 7-2. The dilemma when personal values and professional expectations conflict.

present its own set of considerations. We briefly address each of these in step 3 but focus our attention on Janice's situation.

Step 3: Use Ethics Theories or Approaches to Analyze the Problem

Janice may gain valuable insight into the course of action that will best help her come to a quiet place in her own conscience by engaging in deep deliberation about any duties she has to herself in this situation.

How is one to interpret the odd phrase, "You owe it to yourself?" Does this mean that you have a duty to be good to yourself? We believe yes.

The Duty of Self Care

In Chapter 2, we included care as a duty in our deliberation about the meaning of a caring response. It is usually interpreted as a duty of caring for others, but it applies equally to oneself. In Chapter 4, duties were placed under the usual umbrella of expectations of moral conduct between individuals. Duties usually describe commitments that individuals make to other people or groups to act in certain ways that are believed to uphold the moral life. Therefore, it is unusual to talk about *duties to yourself.* One philosopher among others who made a compelling case to do so is W. D. Ross, a 20th century British moral philosopher influential in developing the idea of moral obligation who included the duty of self care and a commitment to improving yourself among his list of duties. He believed that the duty of beneficence (doing good toward others) and doing good toward yourself arise because each of us should produce as much good as possible. Only in honoring the claims on your own health and welfare and in responding to claims from others can a complete picture of the overall good being produced be expressed. In other words, Ross treated self care as a duty in that it brings about good generally, but, of course, you are the major beneficiary![6] His (rule) utilitarian weighing of benefits depended on everyone keeping these duties or rules. We can expect Janice to find a way forward in her dilemma that allows her to honor her duty to be faithful to her religious beliefs while weighing the various alternatives she has open to her. Her moral distress will continue to keep her feelings and emotions alive as she works her way through the challenge she faces.

Reflection

Can you think of some examples in your everyday life when you were not being "good" to yourself, even harming yourself? What are reasons you chose to cheat yourself this way?

_____

_____

_____

_____

The idea of a duty to oneself seldom is reflected in ethics codes of the professions, probably because of the "other directedness" of the professions' orientation. The closest we have come to finding one that emphasizes being good to yourself is the American Nurses Association Code of Ethics for Nurses that states, "the nurse owes the same duties to self as others, including the responsibility to preserve integrity and safety, to maintain competence *and to continue personal and professional growth.*"[7] Others do emphasize the duty to remain competent and continue to develop professionally too, but almost always those duties are cast into the context of your professional duties to patients and societies.

Aspirations of Self Care

Another way to think about self care is that it is an aspiration worth achieving. An *aspiration* is an ideal standard of excellence toward which you strive; when you have attained that standard, you have gained a better quality of life. Therefore, even if you do not agree that taking good care of yourself has the full force of a duty, you can embrace it as something worth cultivating. We believe that anytime you realize such an aspiration, you do owe it to yourself to reward the accomplishment. For example, when you have aspired to lose weight or make a high grade in a course and you achieve it, you owe it to yourself to acknowledge your success by going out to buy a new pair of jeans or taking time from studying to read a novel. Similarly, in the realm of the moral life, you may aspire to be courageous, to go the second mile, or to set an example of high moral character for others. Has there been a time recently when you experienced this kind of self-satisfaction (Figure 7-3)? The primary reward in this case is in seeing the good you are capable of bringing about and knowing you have made a stride in developing a high moral character. You owe it to yourself to stop to enjoy the good it has done for others. You owe it to yourself to be aware that next time it will be easier.

 SUMMARY

> Reinforcing in yourself the good that comes about by honoring your duty of self-improvement or aspiring to be good to yourself will help you prepare for healthfulness and a chance to flourish throughout your professional career.

Responsibilities of Self Care

A third way of conceptualizing what it means to include a caring response to yourself among your professional tasks is to think of *responsibilities to yourself*. As you recall from Chapter 2, responsibility includes accountability but also has the root idea of responsiveness embedded in it. Responsiveness will guide you toward being kind and gentle with yourself as you face difficulties. Health professionals can be extremely demanding of themselves, believing they must grin and bear it quietly. Janice's sleepless nights and

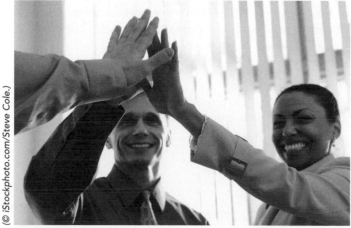

(© iStockphoto.com/Steve Cole.)

Figure 7-3. Celebrating personal achievement.

agitation do not have to prevail, wearing down her spirit and body. In this regard, responsiveness to her personal values is a sign for her to pay attention to what they hold for her and a rich way to understand how self care fits into her moral life as a professional. Only in this way will she be able to improve herself professionally and personally and learn more about how her professional role provides an opportunity for self-fulfillment.

Remaining competent professionally. Professionals are not able to achieve fulfillment in work if they fall behind in the knowledge and skills of their profession. Society recognizes this benefit when it imposes requirements to ensure that they continue to maintain a high level of professional competence by taking continuing education courses and demonstrating proficiency in other ways. Sometimes relicensure or recertification examinations are required after a number of years. Almost all states require clinicians to demonstrate that they have taken steps to engage in lifelong learning professionally. One goal of these requirements is to safeguard your patients, but for most people, the idea of being competent on the job is closely related to their feelings of accomplishment and satisfaction too. Many professional and licensing organizations ask clinicians to reflect on a professional development plan. Professional reflection can help guide individuals in thinking about linking their personal and career goals. In that case, your self-improvement in professional areas involves consideration of both your patients' and your own well-being. Recall Ross's observation that we should bring about as much good overall as we can, including more good for ourselves!

Improving yourself personally. Beyond improvement in professional areas, responsibilities of self care include the development of personal health habits, skills, and interests. Do you have hobbies or other interests? A well-rounded person always makes a better professional insofar as he or she has relief from the demanding routine of professional work. One of the best safeguards against becoming bored or burned out is to have outside compelling interests that require concentrated attention and provide delight. It is not an accident that many application forms for programs of study or jobs include a question about your interests, hobbies, and personal skills unrelated to work.

Reflection

What are some ways you enjoy spending your time outside of your work and study? List them in order of priority.

_____

_____

_____

_____

Being an exemplar. Many persons in society, as well as professionals, believe that professionals have a responsibility to be exemplars of a healthy lifestyle. An *exemplar* is someone who demonstrates a quality to an unusually high degree, therefore becoming an example to others. No one can argue with the fact that a healthy lifestyle is a plus in terms of being able to live a high quality of life. But the exemplar idea goes further. For example, a dietician who is obese because of poor dietary habits, a physically unfit physical therapist, a respiratory therapist who smokes cigarettes, a social worker or psychologist who does not attend to personal emotional problems, or a nurse who consistently gets too little sleep or abuses prescription medications would be soundly criticized on the basis of being a health professional who should "know better." The health professional does know better, strictly from a knowledge perspective, about the deleterious effects of obesity, unfitness, mental stress, driving oneself, and other abuses or neglects of the body and mind. But what do you think? How are health and health behaviors linked?

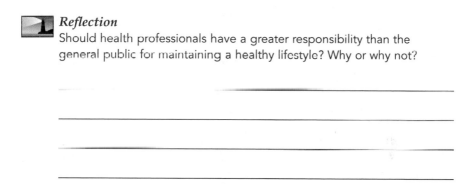

Reflection

Should health professionals have a greater responsibility than the general public for maintaining a healthy lifestyle? Why or why not?

_____

_____

_____

_____

We find it unconvincing that personal excellence in health matters related to their field is a special responsibility of health professionals. Rather, sometimes people who choose a health profession have it as a component of their own personal values system to be fit, maintain healthful eating and sleeping patterns, and take steps to remain in good physical and mental health. In this regard, a health professional may experience a sense of personal responsibility to continue to improve his or her own healthfulness.

Step 4: Explore the Practical Alternatives

Let's return specifically to the story of Janice, whose challenge is to be caring of herself around the ethical dilemma she faces. We will assume that she has taken her duties to herself into account, is committed to living up to her highest aspirations, and accepts the importance of living responsibly. In other words, she is trying to decide what to do that will be consistent with self care. She has been talking with her religious advisors, friends, and colleagues about her values and convictions, all of whom were well aware of her position. They have different ideas about what her response should be. Among the alternative courses of actions suggested to her are the following:

1. Distribute antiabortion pamphlets around the clinic.
2. Talk with patients in the clinic to get their opinion and be guided by their responses to this proposed new service.
3. Quit working in this clinic and find another job.
4. Pray about this turn of events.
5. Call some groups to come and picket the clinic in protest.
6. Talk with her direct supervisor to understand more about the new service and express her concern.
7. Go directly to the top administration of the health plan (of which the clinic is one unit) and try to persuade those in authority not to include this service.
8. Tolerate the situation; it is a pluralistic, diverse society, and some people who could not receive it elsewhere will want to take advantage of the abortion service.
9. Go about her work diligently and not get involved in taking care of any of the abortion patients.

Earlier in this chapter, we posed the question to you, "What do you believe she should do?" You might examine your own response now in light of the alternatives Janice has identified. Given that she is experiencing moral distress and has an ethical dilemma involving not only her own sense of duties, aspirations, and responsibilities to herself but also those associated with being a professional and an employee of an institution, she understands that the whole range of options deserve her discerning judgment. She also is well aware that this clinic has other values she agrees with such as providing quality care to underserved populations. She needs a starting place of deliberation and a decision to act once these alternatives each have been considered thoroughly.

Let Your Conscience Be Your Guide

It is a pretty sure bet that Janice is struggling with what it entails to let her conscience be her guide. How many times have you heard that phrase when you were about to do something that others had some doubt about? What is a *conscience* anyway? The Oxford English Dictionary describes it as "The internal acknowledgment or recognition of the moral quality of one's motives and actions, the sense of right and wrong as regarding things for which one is responsible."[8] This is the starting point of deliberation that Janice has chosen, and her alternatives all reflect some measure of the work she has done to examine her own conscience. Already her first reaction has been refined by going through a reflective process of ethical decision making. All of her proposed activities indicate her objection to the proposed service, and on that basis, she can be said to be a conscientious objector. However, conscientious objection as a concept has a more specific meaning.

Conscientious objection. *Conscientious objection* is an act of resistance or defiance against existing practices, policies, laws, and other expectations that others in that person's position have agreed to. The objector asks to be an exception. The root idea came from the military in which otherwise eligible inductees refuse to serve on the basis of religious or other deeply held objections to war. The burden of proof is on the objector; many democratic nations have allowed alternative service if the person's reasons are accepted as legitimate. Of the alternatives Janice has identified, the one that most closely resembles conscientious objection is number 9. To implement this alternative allows her to practice her skills in a setting that has some other benefits to patients and herself, but it will require that she work with the administration of the clinic for their acceptance of the grounds of her objection for one subset of patients. In Chapter 1, you encountered the legal concept of moral repugnance designed to protect objectors on religious or other grounds from having to participate in the procedure of abortion. Whether or not her involvement as a dietician will be seen as participation in abortion as a procedure is up to the administration to decide.

Conscientious objection has arisen in situations other than abortion in the health care setting. Some include the participation by pharmacists, nurses, or others in capital punishment via lethal injection, work on religious holidays or, in some cultures, on the Sabbath, touching dead bodies, or conducting a physical examination on the opposite gender. Increasingly, health care institutions are recognizing the wisdom of developing policies to spell out the conditions when conscientious objection will be honored.

Common themes in such policies are that a conscientious objection is a legitimate position for a person to take but will **not** be honored if:

- the abstention is discriminatory against a patient or class of patients (e.g., Muslims, gay men);
- the degree of negative patient impact is too great (e.g., emergency care is compromised, the timing is deleterious to serious patient needs, no substitute is available); or
- the cumulative burden on other employees is too great.

The benefit of Janice's workplace having this type of policy is that as she considers her alternatives she can go into the situation knowing that she will be treated equitably with other employees and will have an idea of how the institution will be "listening" as she states her case. At the same time, patients who are anticipating or have undergone an abortion and who have nutritional needs that require the dietician's expertise must be given the same high quality of care as all other patients. Therefore, if she asks for abstention from treating these patients (or working with health professionals more directly involved in the abortion procedure) and another dietician is not found to care for the patient, Janice will be required to place the patient's needs above her own conscientious objection.

One part of the distress Janice is feeling is that at times all of us find ourselves in a situation where we believe there is wrongdoing but are not in complete control to stop it. Furthermore, sometimes opportunities for achieving a good end and avoiding other greater wrongdoing can depend on "cooperating" with wrongdoing in some fashion. A way to think about the justification for *cooperation with wrongdoing* is embodied in the *principle of material cooperation.* You will note that the scholars who have developed this moral principle depend on the relationship of our intent and the ensuing conduct we choose in such dilemmas. They take seriously the truth we posited in our introduction to ethical problems in Chapter 3: an ethical dilemma entails acknowledging that sometimes harm is one effect of achieving something more morally compelling, although the goal is to minimize the harm. At the same time, one must never directly intend the harm.

The principle of material cooperation. The following guidelines are offered in the principle of material cooperation:

- Cooperation with wrongdoing is easier to justify if the wrongdoing will happen with or without one's personal cooperation.
- Cooperation cannot be directly intended by oneself. The cooperation is occasioned solely by one's position as a member of a group, such as employment in an institution where there is wrongdoing.
- The more remote the personal cooperation the better.
- The benefit that is attained by the degree and type of cooperation one tolerates must greatly outweigh the wrongdoing that results from other alternatives that attempt to block the wrongdoing.

In a specific situation, this general set of guidelines for when one might justify cooperating with wrongdoing to some extent has to be submitted to further interpretation.

Reflection

From this point of view, what, if any, of Janice's alternatives would include some cooperation with the institution but might be justified as she weighs her various professional duties and responsibilities?

_____

_____

_____

_____

We believe that all of the alternatives, except number 3, require her to reckon with the fact that she is choosing to stay within an institution where she believes wrongdoing will be taking place. Each of these alternatives is her attempt to integrate her personal and professional values without leaving the institution completely. In this decision, she joins eons of others over the ages who have chosen to remain within the system as moral change agents rather than absenting themselves completely. The other benefits or harms that each of her alternatives will engender must be part of her ethical decision making process.

Step 5: Complete the Action

Janice, along with anyone else faced with affronts to personal values, must have the courage to take whatever steps are necessary once a full deliberation is completed. Courage is self care in its starkest, most challenging form. Tantamount for her to consider at this point of action is that if she wishes to continue as a professional she will need to ensure that her act, based on her personal values, does not detrimentally impact the individual care she is providing to patients assigned to her. The goal of a caring response to the patient cannot be compromised in her professional role, no matter what her caring response to herself prompts her to do. Moreover, some of Janice's alternatives will not be welcomed by her institution or many of her colleagues. It follows that she must be prepared to accept the employment consequences of her action, if they are judged by the institution or existing laws to be unacceptable, and the possible disdain from some colleagues with whom she has enjoyed a comfortable relationship.

In the next chapter of this book, we examine the institutional setting in more detail with insights that complement those that in this chapter have focused primarily on you, the individual, faced with situations that threaten deep personal values and convictions.

Step 6: Evaluate the Process and Outcome

Janice's process and eventual decision will give her an opportunity to engage other colleagues in what she went through. They, too, will thereby have an opportunity to reflect on their own personal values and how and when such values may present moral distress or an ethical dilemma. We highly recommend that your place of employment have a mechanism that allows you to gain the insights of others when faced with, or looking back on, a difficult ethical decision. We have found that such a mechanism, which we call *a reflection group*, is extremely helpful for ensuring self care and a high-quality well-working professional environment (Figure 7-4).

Whether the group is designed to assist in your discernment around decisions you are about to make or in looking back on what happened, it brings the collective wisdom of the group to bear on what can otherwise be an extremely lonely journey.

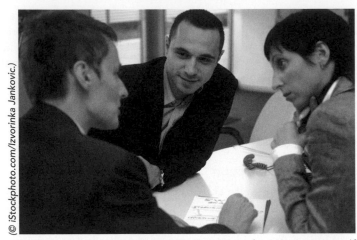

(© iStockphoto.com/Izvorinka Jankovic.)

Figures 7-4. A reflection group is one mechanism for maintaining self respect while meeting professional obligations.

Because in this chapter we have not revealed the actual decision Janice makes, we focus on her prospective action and assume that the members of the reflection group are drawing on their past reflections from previous dilemmas involving their personal values. As you recall, that is the function of step 6, to learn from previous experience and prepare for the next encounter. We affirm the use of the reflection group for prospective action and retrospective analysis because full preparation is the best antidote to having to do damage control later. We also presume that they will meet after Janice has acted to help her in her analysis of what happened and what is to be learned from it.

> Preparation in advance is self care at its best, and sharing your values with your group will give everyone a chance to be supportive within the confines of their own value system.

Additional alternatives to the ones Janice identified may open up if she engages in discussion, and her colleagues also can help her anticipate some of the things she will need to take into account to be sure she is making a decision consistent with a deeply caring response to herself. All kinds of discussion might come up in a group of colleagues when taking care of oneself is included in the deliberation. We conclude this chapter with speculation about a couple of topics that are likely to be included in what we will call "Janice's reflection group."

Opportunities for Self Care in Any Situation

At least two major areas present opportunities for professionals to examine and further strengthen their personal value system.

Responding to "Bad" Laws, Policies, and Regulations

Janice is an example of how a person can experience a threat to personal values by virtue of what he or she perceives as a bad law resulting in bad institutional policy or practices. Bad laws, policies, or regulations come in many forms. They might be poorly stated, therefore providing poor guidance, or worse, they seem to be morally wrong in their emphasis. Someone in Janice's reflection group might suggest that they read the play, *The Dark at the Top of the Stairs*, by the great American playwright William Inge, because it is a fine illustration of how individuals sometimes are unwilling or unable to interact with the "powers that be" who make and revise policies. The setting for the play is the home of the Rubin Flood family in a small Oklahoma town, where he, his wife Cora, and their two children are living. It takes place in the 1920s, during a prosperous time for this area because of an oil boom. What we see of the Flood's house is the living room, but there is a flight of stairs at one side, and at the top of it is a second floor landing. Some of the most vital activities in the play, the moments that set direction for the rest of it, are played out on that landing, but the Flood family never integrates those activities into the process of resolving the small sorrows, tragedies, and missed opportunities that finally threaten their integrity as individuals and as a family.[9]

Policies that cause consternation because they appear to challenge personal values sometimes can be effectively addressed and changed. It need not include an ethical dilemma. Janice's reflection group may take the opportunity to discuss policies or practices that affect their personal health that they feel are hindering them from effective self care. For example, concern about the personal effects of fatigue, including its deleterious effects on good patient care, has appeared in the professional literature.[10] Still relatively lacking are studies that show the price professionals pay for not being able always to remain comfortably within the boundaries of their own religious or other beliefs. One recent survey of more than 2000 practicing US physicians from all specialties revealed that many ". . . do not consider themselves obligated to disclose information about or refer patients for legal but morally controversial medical procedures." However, the investigators did not ask their subjects about the price the latter felt they paid for following their conscience.[11] In addition, the moral residue that accompanies situations of moral distress such as the one Janice is facing is an occasion for suffering. Rushton observes that health professionals "sorely are lacking in self-compassion, renewal and the cultivation of resilience" to address their suffering and "when suffering is unresolved and remains in the unconscious, it will likely reappear when similar experiences of suffering occur, or may manifest itself as inappropriate or disproportionate responses to other situations."[12] Janice's reflection group can be one resource to begin the discussion of how to support each other in their suffering.

Reflection

Can you think of a health care policy you would write that would strengthen one or more of your personal values in your work setting? If so, jot it down before going on so that you can think about it as you read further.

_____

_____

_____

_____

Janice's reflection group should examine their perceptions of whether their professional roles require them to get involved in policy. For example, if Janice tells the group that her role as a dietician does not include trying to change policies other than those directly related to dietetics, she will feel more vulnerable and may believe that her only option is to leave the workplace. At the same time, if she discerns that a part of her role generally is to question policies in her workplace, she will feel more empowered to act within the system. In the latter case, she can prepare to objectively present her ideas to the people who are involved in making and revising the family planning policies, understanding that her beliefs and convictions may not prevail in the final outcome. At the very least, she has gone into the discussion with the intent to stop a practice that she thinks is morally wrong. By being willing to speak her mind within the system, she may also have an opportunity to hear the arguments on the other side and learn the reasons why other people are supporting them even if she is not persuaded to support them herself.

Maintaining Vigilance

Janice's reflection group will identify some policies and practices in their institution that they can rely on. But they also will benefit by reflecting on how no general safeguards can identify the actual content of each individual health professional's values and beliefs. In the end, it is up to each of them in the group to be vigilant. Vigilance means continual alertness and watchfulness. The same goes for you. You and you alone are the only one who can maintain the vigilance necessary to treat your personal integrity with the care it deserves. Sometimes conflicting values come into play when you are trying to protect your sense of personal integrity in your professional role, just as you surely face them in your other roles. For instance, the religious values that led to Janice's position about abortion may come into conflict with values that have led her to become a professional or to take this job in the first place. Her values and beliefs may also prohibit her use of violence and confrontation as forms of resistance.

Does Janice's predicament have anything to do with her responsibility for self-improvement? The answer is yes because every challenge to her personal values system provides an opportunity not only to act in accord with her beliefs but also to respond optimally. We continually reflect on our values and gain new insights as situations arise. As we change, so do our values at times. For one thing, Janice may incorporate new insights and receive counsel from the group that will modify her decision from what she thought she would do when she first encountered the challenge or how she will respond differently next time. If she is alert to the details of other past challenges to her personal integrity and uses them wisely as a teacher to help guide her in what she should do in each new situation, she will have taken advantage of a grand opportunity for improving her odds in the direction of her hoped for results. Over time, Janice's (and our) practiced attention to what works best will better prepare us not only for moral leadership in our professions but also for all of life's difficult choices.

 SUMMARY

A reflection group is one mechanism for assessing prospective and recent decisions involving self care in the professional role. By sharing concerns and exercising personal vigilance, all professionals can become better equipped to respond more effectively, efficiently, and caringly with each new situation, remaining true to a caring response to ourselves.

Janice and others in her reflection group will benefit from the knowledge and insights they share that were prompted by her situation. They may decide to make a statement for themselves or others to help tie themselves to the mast of resolve regarding self care.

Summary

A focus on the well-being of others often is the sole emphasis in health care ethics. Chapter 6 and this chapter propose that to survive ethically throughout professional preparation and your entire career requires self-awareness, experiences (and reflection on them), a commitment to living according to your personal values system, vigilance in maintaining personal integrity, and strategies for fulfilling responsibilities to yourself. Overall, we hope we have met our goal for this chapter, namely to highlight that not all self care is preparation for the most challenging ethical moments with the highest stakes. Acting out of a position of self respect, taking good care of yourself generally, and being kind and gentle with yourself will prepare you for confident ethical decision making and a fulfilling professional career. Self care is one of the greatest gifts you can give yourself. In Chapter 8, you will have an opportunity to further examine how colleagues and the institutional mechanisms for support and accountability in health care also are relevant to your survival ethically.

Questions for Thought and Discussion

1. Melissa Y. is a therapist who works in a chronic pain clinic that includes some inpatient beds. She has become distressed in the last month because she is increasingly convinced that one of her longtime nurse colleagues is "siphoning off" some of the narcotic medications intended for the patients. Her personal values and her professional sensitivity dictate that she pursue the issue. If you were Melissa, how would you proceed? With whom? Why?

2. Some of the physicians who participated in the Nazi medical experiments testified that their activities did not run counter to their personal values. When asked how this could be, they stated that they were simply "doing their job." Discuss the limits of using an individual's personal conscience, convictions, or understanding of his or her professional role as the ultimate standard of moral judgment. What, if any, higher standard is there? What types of checks and balances do you want to have in place to minimize wrongdoing in an institution or society?

3. "Some days it would be better if I just stayed in bed," Bob thought. He started out the day by oversleeping, thereby missing his first patient appointment. When he went out for lunch with Bill, his colleague at work, his car was rear-ended at a stoplight. Now he is treating a patient who has just been diagnosed as having lung cancer. Bob expresses his sympathy regarding this bad news. The patient retorts, "You shouldn't sympathize. It's people like you who are part of the problem! You preach about health, but you smoke like a chimney. If you can't be a better example than this to common folks like us, you should get out of the health care field and leave it to someone who knows how to take care of his own health." Bob, who has been fighting the cigarette habit, suddenly feels guilty. He wonders if his smoking really is that bad of an example for his patients. He wants to respond to the patient but cannot think of what to say regarding this indictment. Can you help him make an appropriate response? Why do you think your idea is an appropriate remark? Is the patient right?

REFERENCES

1. Rawls, J., 1999. *A theory of justice*, 2nd ed. Harvard University Press, Cambridge, MA.
2. Purtilo, R., 2005. New respect for respect in ethics education. In: Purtilo, R.B., Jensen, G.M., Royeen, C.B. (Eds.), *Educating for moral action: A sourcebook in health and rehabilitation ethics*. F.A. Davis Co, Philadelphia, PA, pp. 1–10.
3. Green, B.H., 2006. The meaning of caring in five experienced physical therapists. *Physiother Theory Pract* 22 (4), 175–187.
4. Cromie, J.E., Robertson, V.J., Best, M.O., 2002. Work-related musculoskeletal disorders and the profession of physical therapy. *Phys Ther* 82 (5), 459–472.
5. Purtilo, R., Haddad, A., 2005. Respect. The difference it makes. In: *Health professional and patient interaction*, 7th ed. WB Saunders Company, Philadelphia, PA, pp. 3–14.
6. Ross, W.D., 1930. *The right and the good*. Clarendon Press, Oxford, England, pp. 26–27.
7. American Nurses Association, 2001. *Code of ethics for nurses with interpretive statements*. ANA, Washington, DC.
8. CD-Rom version 3.1, 2004. *Oxford English Dictionary*. Oxford University Press, Oxford, England.
9. Inge, W., 1968. The dark at the top of the stairs. In: *Four plays*. Grove Press, New York, pp. 223–304.
10. Gaba, D.M., Stevens, S.K., 2002. Fatigue among clinicians and the safety of patients. *N Engl J Med* 347 (16), 1249–1255.
11. Curline, F.A., Lawrence, R.E., Chaine, M.H., et al., 2007. Religion, conscience, and controversial clinical practices. *N Engl J Med* 356, 593–600, quote 593.
12. Rushton, C.H., 2008. Caregiver suffering. In: Pinch, W.E., Haddad, A.M. (Eds.), *Nursing and health care ethics: A legacy and a vision*. American Nurses Association, Chicago, quotes 300 and 294, respectively.

8

Living Ethically Within Health Care Organizations

Objectives

The reader should be able to:

- List several areas of health care addressed by organization ethics.
- Define the term mission statement and the role of a mission statement in an organization.
- Describe what policies are and what they are designed to accomplish within health care and other organizations.
- Identify how the utilitarian approach to organizational arrangements such as policies and practices serves everyone well and conditions under which serious shortcomings may arise from relying solely on this approach.
- Describe several ethical principles that are useful in the analysis of organization ethics problems.
- Identify three rights of professional employees in health care organizations.
- Name some virtues of organizations and why they are important in today's evolving health care system.
- Name some business and management challenges in organizations that warrant ethical reflection.

New terms and ideas you will encounter in this chapter

organization ethics	stakeholders	principle of
mission statement	cost effectiveness	participation
policy	organization ethics	principle of efficiency
conflict of interest	committee	

Topics in this chapter introduced in earlier chapters

Topic	Introduced in chapter
Values and duties	1
Courage	1
Moral agent	3
Moral distress	3
Ethical dilemma	3
Locus of authority problem	3
Virtue	4
Prima facie and absolute duties	4
Utilitarian theory	4
Principles approach	4
Beneficence	4
Nonmaleficence	4
Justice	4
Autonomy	4
The six-step process of ethical decision making	5
Aspirations	7

Introduction

So far, we have focused on the individuals and the ethical challenges they face in their professional role and work environment. In this chapter, we turn more directly to the organizational dimensions of health care. Another critical area of ethical reflection in health care is *organization ethics*. Organization ethics pays attention to the values, character traits, rights, and duties expressed in:

Mission statements

Policies and other administrative arrangements

Business priorities

Organization ethics cuts a wide swath across your professional life. The field addresses issues in organizational structures that deliver health care, those that regulate health professionals or health care practices, professional associations, businesses that provide health care equipment or material for procedures, pharmaceutical companies, and those involved in remuneration for professional services. Subsets of organization ethics are business ethics, management ethics, administrative ethics, and legislative ethics, to name some. Each addresses the conditions under which an organization's and society's moral expectations can be reconciled. They focus on the larger societal and bureaucratic organization of modern health care; therefore, their goals are not limited solely to the ethical goals of individual health professionals. Institutional policies and actions affect patient care, so a lens must be placed on health care organizations and professionals. For instance, a business goal of increasing the profit margin each year is legitimate for a business enterprise. Business ethics addresses the conditions required for that profit margin to be gained, with adherence to high ethical standards set by its consumers of their products or services, society, and the organizations themselves. Robert Hall[1] notes that health care organizations have ethical problems that in many ways are similar to good business management anywhere, but because of the special place the professions have in society, these organizational structures must be styled to fit the type of role its employees and "clients" play. As a participant in various health care organizations, your challenge is to assess whether the rights, values, and duties by which they abide affect your ability to offer a caring response to patients when measured against the standard of your professional values and duties. To illustrate one version of how the ethical challenges of working within an organization affects health professionals, consider the following story.

 The Story of Simon Kapinsky and the Subcommittee to Implement a Green Health Plan

The Chief Executive Officer (CEO) of StarServices, Inc, a for-profit major health plan, has asked Simon Kapinsky, a senior member of the professional staff in one of the plan's units, to chair the ethics subcommittee of the health plan's greening advisory council. The advisory council recently was formed to set new policy and practices for StarServices, Inc, to operate as a "green health plan" in regard to the services it offers. On review of the material from the CEO, Simon learns that the Board of Trustees of the health plan signed a contract 2 years ago to build or remodel all of its treatment (not research) units according to concepts of ecologic architectural design. Simon is aware that the flagship hospital in the health plan (where he is employed) already has undergone major renovation, but he was not fully aware of the scope of the project. In the proposal, the greening of the health plan is being financed one fourth by StarServices, Inc, one half by bonds in the city where the major institutions of the health plan are located, and one fourth by Green International, a private architectural firm whose purpose is to showcase ecologic architecture in public buildings. Green International claims that the new health plan structures will become the showcase for eco-friendly medical facilities in the next 50 years. The estimated overall cost is $36 million, but Green International emphasizes that much of that cost will be recovered by offsetting operating costs and also by the amount of business this eco-friendly model project will generate. When Simon returns the material to the CEO, the latter emphasizes, "With the flagship hospital in the health plan already renovated, StarServices, Inc, is positioned to move ahead substantially toward its strategic goal of becoming the greenest health plan in the world. Welcome to the leadership

SUMMARY

Like codes and oaths for health professionals, mission statements are organizations' public statements designed to declare to all the type of organization it is, including its core ethical values and ideals.

Policies and Administrative Practices as Information

A *policy* is a statement designed to establish formal and informal guidelines for practice within an organization. Obviously, policies should be consistent with the values of the organization. They also should be specific expressions of how the ideals in the mission statement can be carried out by the people in the organization and those the organization hopes to attract or serve. If policies are to be followed, they must also be clear, practical, flexible, and consistent with the values of the people or groups to whom they apply.

Currently, policies in health care reflect both traditional health care ethics and business ethics. One group whose mission was to deliver high-quality patient care once commented, "No money, no mission." This is probably the perspective from which the CEO of StarServices, Inc, was responding to Simon's query about the approach the organization was taking to meet their goal of going green. The goals of the organization often are not fully met simply by focusing on the model of a single patient and health professional. As you can imagine, the picture is not always rosy because an organization's policy may come directly into conflict with professional ethics standards. In fact, it is often at the level of policy that goals for individual patients' well-being or justice among groups come into direct conflict with business interests. Recently, one of the authors conducted a workshop in a private health care facility that had adopted a "no AIDS patients" policy because of the high costs of services for many such patients. The health professionals were distressed because the facility was in the process of building a new multimillion dollar reception area and surrounding gardens with the hope of its beauty being the draw to "beat out the competition." This decision by the trustees of the facility was interpreted by the professionals as being a triumph of profits over patients, and still they agreed that the patient load was down because of increased competition in their geographic area.

SUMMARY

Few health professionals today are in situations where they can ignore organization policies. Still, professional values must guide their own decisions.

The Realm-Individual Process-Decision Making (RIPS) model of ethical decision making developed by three physical therapists maintains that partially because of the changes in the health care system, all ethical issues that involve patient care now also have business or administrative and larger societal dimensions. The three realms of ethics (individual, institutional [i.e., organizational], and societal) always are present.[2] Glaser,[3] who has a similar scheme of the three realms, portrays it well (Figure 8-1).

Step 2: Identify the Type of Ethical Problem

Simon and his colleagues on the ethics subcommittee of the greening advisory council are experiencing moral distress. Their guts tell them that something is wrong in the whole approach StarServices, Inc, is taking in its pursuit of an otherwise laudable goal of becoming "the greenest health care plan in America."

They also feel the pinch of an ethical dilemma. On the one hand, they recognize that they have a duty of loyalty to the goals of their employing health care organization, StarServices, Inc. Honoring its goals is an expression of these employees' willingness to acknowledge that being an employee provides the context for them to make a living while honoring their professional commitments. At the same time, they know that they have a responsibility to assess whether their loyalty is ethically supportable in the current challenge they face. They were placed in a consultative role and asked to make recommendations to help ensure that the health care plan

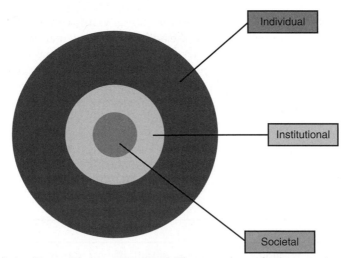

Figure 8-1. *(From Glaser, J.W., 2005.* Three realms of ethics: an integrating map of ethics for the future. In Purtilo, R.B., Jensen, G.M., Royeen, C.B., (Eds.), *Educating for moral action: a sourcebook in health and rehabilitation ethics.* F.A. Davis, Philadelphia, PA, P. 120.)

succeeds in its worthwhile project, but their dilemma is in feeling that this project's success may be at the cost of compromising a caring response to patient groups using the facility. They began their task enthusiastically and earnestly and had a reasonable expectation that their concerns would be heard. Simon is on the horns of a dilemma with two right courses of action facing him, one pointing to his loyalty to the organization, the other, more compelling, to his loyalty to the well-being of patients. The subcommittee is facing the possibility that they are involved in a serious conflict of interest situation. A *conflict of interest* situation occurs for professionals when they incur interests that significantly threaten their professional duties and commitments.[4]

Simon and the subcommittee also have a locus of authority problem. Although aware that their role ultimately was advisory, they believed that they brought an essential ethical perspective and area of expertise to this business enterprise. In fact, they were appointed to do so. Their positions as leading professionals in this organization should have given them the say-so to have their questions taken seriously by the administrators and advisory council. In fact, their concerns were based on thoughtful ethical reasoning, which caused them to take seriously their moral agency as guardians of patients' well-being. They believed they were on solid ground regarding their assumption that this health care organization should protect quality care for patients above all other priorities.

One important lesson the subcommittee members are learning is that there are many *stakeholders* in the type of project they have been pulled into, with different and sometimes conflicting values and priorities. A stakeholder is a person, group, or other entity that has a deep and compelling interest in a situation that it wants to protect. Because there are ethical issues involved, the stakeholders all are moral agents with their part to play in arriving at ethically acceptable courses of action. Two major stakeholders are the professionals and the administration or management. In order of priority, some common loyalties that cause ethical conflict between health professionals and the top level administration of a health care organization are listed subsequently.

Where Do Health Professionals' Priorities Lay?	Where Do the Organization's Priorities Lay?
High-Quality Patient Care	Fiscal Viability
• Other professionals, teammates	• Employee protection
• Patient satisfaction	• Being competitive in the marketplace
• Workplace effectiveness and efficiency	• Patient/consumer safety and satisfaction
• Societal expectations/laws upheld	• Laws, regulations upheld
• Professional values	• Community support
• Self-fulfillment	• Institutional efficiency

Reflection

In examining these two sets of loyalties, where, if any place, do you see complementary interests where the administration of StarServices, Inc, and the ethics subcommittee of professionals are likely to find common ground for discussion and eventual agreement? List them here.

_____

_____

_____

_____

Why have you chosen these? Describe in a sentence or two before going on.

_____

_____

_____

Step 3: Use Ethics Theories or Approaches to Analyze the Problem

Several ethical approaches can be considered when an administrative proposal is being assessed. Unfortunately, it appears that Simon and the concerns of his subcommittee are being ignored, but we do not know that for a certainty because he did submit meeting minutes and a copy of their questions to both the health plan administrators and the chair of the greening advisory council. All we know is that the subcommittee has been disbanded without a chance to discuss their concerns. At any rate, it is important for you to walk through the approaches that the combined group of administrators and professionals could use to discern what finally should be done.

Utilitarian Reasoning in Organization Ethics

Utilitarian reasoning is the usual approach to a potential structural change in an organization. Understandably, from the administrative and business standpoint, an ethically supportable policy or procedure is one that brings about the best outcomes overall based on a utilitarian value system designed to provide the greatest good for the greatest number. It follows that from an organizational standpoint, considerations of individual autonomy may be submerged in favor of such utilitarian considerations as efficiency of operations and economic stability. Simply stated, the organization that fulfills its function of providing a worthwhile service efficiently usually is believed to justify the means used to attain that end so long as the net result is a greater balance of benefits to humanity than would be realized if the organization did not exist.

The idea of *cost effectiveness* often is cited as the appropriate goal of health plans. A definition of cost effectiveness is that the greatest quality of care possible is provided at the lowest price. No one can argue with that underlying utilitarian ideal. The administrative arrangements, however, may succumb to the serious criticism that such efficiency can best be achieved through cutting costs by means that actually compromise high-quality care.[5]

Taking these general considerations into account, the combined group can profitably discuss the question of whether StarServices, Inc's proposed course of action appears to encourage practices that will do more good than harm overall. No one will argue against the idea that a green organization is a benefit to the community, and from a market competition and community support standpoint, it stands to benefit the organization greatly. The burden of proof on the organization is to show that the goal of high-quality patient care is protected and encouraged so that the subcommittee will be convinced that their patient-centered concerns are unfounded.

The criticism often leveled at pure utilitarian thinking generally applies to the current situation under discussion. The policy or procedure that works as a general touchstone cannot provide the optimal solution to every situation. It may be inappropriate or inadequate to handle specific problems faced by the organization and its constituents. Therefore, the utilitarian equation merely provides boundaries. We all find ourselves breaking general guidelines when overriding them is ethically justified—for example, parking in a no parking zone to assist at the scene of an accident. That is, of course, why there is a prima facie, but not an absolute duty, to honor organizational arrangements based solely on utilitarian reasoning. What may be best for most people most of the time may not be best in a specific situation. It is from this level of concern about whether a caring response to individual or groups of patients will be compromised that the addition of several principles helps to enrich and fill out the ethics subcommittee's ethical analysis.

Principles Approach in Organization Ethics

From a principles approach, several ethical principles can further delineate values and duties to which this particular organization must answer.

The principle of beneficence is one key. Although utilitarianism emphasizes overall good consequences that are brought about by a course of action, beneficence requires the moral agents to delineate the type of good that the act itself is. For instance, consider specific benefits that may be a part of the combined group's discernment about the next step. If a proposed course of action allows some members of the organization to be exemplars in terms of improving patient satisfaction while increasing employee morale and demonstrating good stewardship of environmental or other resources, these specific benefits can be heralded apart from the overall good consequences.

The principle of nonmaleficence demonstrates the flipside of beneficence. The administration that creates moral distress by silencing the voice of concern brought by thoughtful professionals such as the ethics subcommittee is harming its employees and risking a decrease in professional staff morale more widely. Moreover, as StarServices, Inc, looks toward implementing their ideal of a green health care organization, the combined group of administrators and subcommittee members must work together to minimize any harm that would ensue through new policies, practices, or resource priorities that compromise the professionals' ability to bring about a caring response because of cuts in goods or services.

The philosopher John Rawls, to whom you were introduced in the previous chapter, holds that the principle of justice is a fundamental virtue of institutions. His position is that if an organization is fair in its assignment of rights and duties and makes provision for a fair distribution of its resources, then all individuals in those institutions will be able to live more moral lives.[6] If the administration of StarServices, Inc, can show that its proposed course of action will continue to honor the distribution of patient care resources based on patient-centered considerations of need (rather than on market and other business benefits), a major concern of the ethics subcommittee can be laid to rest as far as justice is concerned.

The principle of respect also is relevant. All stakeholders in this situation deserve respect. The interests of administrators and trustees counsel toward a green organization because it shows respect to the larger community through saving and protecting natural resources and by being accountable regarding health-related environmental concerns. They are aware that health care institutions are among the highest waste-producing and toxin-producing entities and are committed to demonstrating a viable alternative.[7] The professionals' goal of showing respect for the patients through their search for a caring response creates a reasonable expectation that their workplace conditions will support that search. This is a strong argument in the subcommittee's favor that whatever changes are made in patient care services, they do not compromise the professionals' duties of a care-centered workplace.

SUMMARY

Utilitarian reasoning almost always must be used to determine the best possible balance or benefits over burdens when organizational policies and procedures are being implemented. At the same time, principle approaches involving the dictates of beneficence, nonmaleficence, justice, and respect considerations refine the ethical analysis in a specific situation to guide decision makers.

Step 4: Explore the Practical Alternatives

The institution has taken the alternative of outsourcing the task originally assigned to Simon's ethics subcommittee. This leaves the ethics subcommittee to consider their practical alternatives now that they have learned their request for a discussion of their questions has not been honored and they have been disbanded. They are disappointed, of course, and some are angry. Before making their request, they did do considerable work on the project. They identified duties, relevant principles, and virtues they believe should govern any future recommendations from the standpoint of their professional role as moral agents. They took into account that "the bottom line" of money does matter in organizations and that administrative decisions always must keep "the big picture" in focus, weighing the costs of one priority against another and honoring the importance of efficiency within the organization as a whole. Although they judged that a utilitarian approach is not alone a sufficient basis for ethical analysis, they agree that it is one critical aspect of ethical concern when it comes to an organization's general positions, policies, and practices. But they also have reckoned with the moral rights and reasonable expectations with which they undertook the responsibility of trying to help address a major change in the character, public image, and internal practices of StarServices, Inc, including their right to relevant policies that will enable them to complete their subcommittee tasks according to high ethical professional standards. In all of this, they moved forward initially with the assumption that the top administration and trustees want to foster an environment consistent with the high moral and service standards of patient-centered health care. Now they have convened again to decide the course to take because, formally, their function as a subcommittee is completed and their request for clarification and discussion before advancing a proposal has not been honored.

 Reflection
List some practical alternatives Simon and the ethics subcommittee have open to them.

_____

_____

_____

_____

Surely one course of action would be to do nothing more. However, no one in the group wants to just let the matter drop. Would you? Why or why not?

_____

_____

_____

_____

We see the following alternatives.

- The subcommittee can urgently request that their work be extended and make a recommendation without the benefit of having had their serious questions addressed. Some suggest that many changes can be made without any alteration in the number or kind of services offered through the health plan.
- Simon may continue to communicate privately with the CEO and chairperson of the greening advisory council about the ethical reasoning that informed the subcommittee's concerns.
- If the health plan has an *organization ethics committee* designed to examine the larger organization's ethical problems that arise, they could request a consultation with that group to get further insight and advice.[8]
- The members could ignore the top administration but begin to discuss their concerns with colleagues at their own levels of organizational seniority and responsibility, hoping for a "bubble up effect" that will get the attention of the top administration before policies are set in stone.
- They could link arms with advocacy groups in the community to put external pressure on the administration to be responsive to any patient care concerns the changes may raise.

Steps 5 and 6: Complete the Action and Evaluate the Process and Outcome

We do not know which of these alternatives the subcommittee will pursue. We believe that the first three are the most viable as the next steps before the subcommittee considers taking this issue outside the organizational structure. The group must have the courage to take whatever steps the members decide on, individually or as a collective moral voice, once they have discerned what each of the alternatives might achieve. Short of this, their time, energies, and collective best judgment surely will give way to other priorities. Health professionals who are forced to provide care in a changing environment where policies and practices seem at odds with the demands of their moral roles experience a feeling of loss of control, stress, discontent, and disheartenment.[9] The ethics subcommittee's goal to help set direction that upholds the organization's high ethical standards of patient care may be thwarted if they lag in their efforts now.

As with all important ethical challenges, their willingness to reconvene as a "reflection group" (see Chapter 7) to evaluate the process and outcome of their experience will strengthen them for future leadership efforts within their organizations. Moreover, they can find ways to share their successes with other staff and health professions groups attempting to deal with similar challenges regarding the increasingly rich mix of priorities that health plans are facing.

Educating for Moral Agency Within Organizations

Taken as an educational opportunity, there are at least two areas of their ethics subcommittee experience that may make good professional staff seminars in their workplace or at meetings of their professional organizations. We conclude this chapter with introducing them here.

Living with the Business Aspects of Health Care

Health care organizations are businesses, but not only businesses. Bodenheimer and Grumbach[10] maintain that the following three major forces drive the organization of health care in the United States and, to some degree, in all economically developed nations: (1) the biomedical model, (2) financial incentives, and (3) professionalism. The service of health care is expressed through the biomedical and clinical skills of the professionals, the financial grounding through financial incentives, and the particular ethical standards through professionalism. Still, the financial incentives often are targeted in the literature as creating the biggest challenge to the professionals. In other words, the challenge for health professionals is the requirement of living with the "business" of health care but not letting it govern all the values and priorities of practice.

Business language often conjures up negative images of greedy health care institutions driven by profit at all costs. Such organizations do exist and, of course, create ethical dilemmas for any health care professional who works in them because they fail to meet reasonable expectations of patients and society. Not all health care institutions, however, are driven solely by a monetary bottom line. Many health care organizations are distinguished by their vision, mission, and sensitivity to the implications of each when making decisions about the business. The business functions of any organization are designed to help meet the appropriate goals of that organization, whatever those goals may be. An examination of the priorities of an organization outlined on page 165 of this chapter highlight why some major themes in business ethics are honesty in advertising, transparency in dealings with partners and clients, fairness in the treatment of employees or others, criteria for quality control of the product or service, the meaning of fiscal accountability from the standpoint of taking everyone's legitimate interests into account, and the duty of respect for others in all the organization's interactions.

 Reflection
Specify some ways a health care organization such as a hospital, nursing home, home health agency, or health maintenance organization (HMO) would have to gear its business goals, policies, and practices to meet high ethical standards of patient care.

_____

_____

_____

_____

To survive ethically within the organization where you work, you will need to identify the business realities and critique them. Although it goes beyond the parameters of this book to fully address the business dimensions of your practice, the next generation of health professionals, to which you will belong, will be forced to be more cognizant of them. One of the most interesting challenges for you is that the organizational structures in which you may find yourself are much more diverse than even a few years ago. For example, in addition to the more familiar settings of hospitals, clinics, rehabilitation centers, or hospice, you may be working aboard a cruise ship, in a school system, in the military, at a children's camp, at a nursing home, or with a sports team. In each instance, your professional values must be honored and the business aspects of the workplace understood.

┌───┐
| SUMMARY |
├───┤
| Both a firm grounding in professional ethics and astute awareness of the |
| business dimensions of health care are necessary for a full picture of eth- |
| ical problems in today's health care organizations. Organizations should |
| be shaped by patient-centered health care arrangements. |
└───┘

Rights of Professionals in Organizations

The ultimate administrative decisions in most organizations are made by those in powerful positions within the structure, although today multilevel input sometimes is invited. The greening advisory council and its ethics subcommittee are examples of StarServices, Inc's mechanisms to invite multilevel input. In other words, more and more people from all echelons of an organization hierarchy are currently becoming involved in administrative decisions.

The Right to Participate

This stance is consistent with the idea that everyone in an organization has a basic moral right to become involved in appropriate ways. The moral *principle of participation* is seldom included in lists of ethical principles applicable to health care ethics but is often cited in social ethics and political treatises on democratic societies. It arises partly from the more familiar principle of autonomy because it supports the idea that you, in your role as a professional, have a right to help determine aspects of your workplace that directly affect your well-being. Your involvement in organizational arrangements and review of practices or policies are the only way you can ensure that you will not be forced to sacrifice important personal and professional values to overriding organization values such as efficiency. Workplace efficiency can be applauded when it is brought in line with the professional values of faithfulness to patients' and professionals' rights and prevention of harm to anyone. But only by participation of concerned professionals is that outcome assured. Simon and his colleagues were offered— and took—the opportunity to participate in making sure patient-centered care was not compromised. Their right to participation was welcomed and then apparently taken away.

A good place for you to start exercising your right of participation at the organizational level is in your own place of employment or your professional association. Part of the ability to be involved in policy is to be able to ascertain where organizational arrangements are being made and revised. Pertinent questions include:
1. What are the names of groups responsible for making organizational arrangements and setting policies and practices? To whom, exactly, does each report?

2. Who sits on the organization's various committees, and what are their qualifications?
3. What must I do to be nominated for or appointed to a group?
4. To whom must I speak to learn more about a group and express my interest?

The Right to Employment Protections and Guidance

It is your right to assume that your organization will have a range of policies and other administrative arrangements that give clear direction for your professional practice. Depending on the nature of your patient population and the services offered through the organization, you should be able to find the following types of policies or guidelines related to patient care:

- Informed consent policy;
- Withholding and withdrawing life-sustaining treatment policy;
- Assisted suicide and abortion policies;
- Advance directive policy;
- Surrogate decision making, health care agents, durable power of attorney for health care, and guardianship process policies;
- Do not resuscitate (DNR) policy;
- Confidentiality and privacy policy;
- Organ donation and procurement policy;
- Human experimentation regulations (policies and procedures);
- Conflicts of interest policy (including patient care and research policies);
- Patient admission, discharge, and transfer policy;
- Impaired providers policy (including reporting procedures for impaired providers and medical errors);
- Conscientious objection policy and procedures;
- Reproductive technology policies; and
- Grievance procedures.

Reflection
Can you think of other policies, procedures, or guidelines that would pertain to your professional responsibilities?

_____

_____

_____

_____

The Right to a Virtuous Organization

As you recall, virtue theory turns the lens on a situation to examine the type of person one ought to be. Philosophers, economists, and others maintain that institutions and other organizations do have character traits or virtues. They also acknowledge the power of organizational structures to affect the lives of individuals in our highly bureaucratized society. You have a right to be assured that your workplace administration shows sincere and intense commitment to creating a humane or "virtuous" organization. Because most organizations are governed by a small number of people who have the final say over what will happen to everyone, this commitment must begin with the individuals who have the most power and authority. The traits of health care organizations are one important focus of serious reflection today, and we invite you to participate in this exciting dimension of your professional career.[11]

You already have learned that efficiency is one virtue of organizations because they are designed to meet multiple needs and render multiple services. The *principle of efficiency* can provide a moral basis for conduct that benefits all. From a social standpoint, many would say that a "good" or "well-run" organization is an efficient one. From the standpoint of your tasks within a health care organization, however, you would benefit from institutions and systems that reflect others virtues too.

For example, you have also already learned earlier in this chapter that a commitment to justice in the organization's assignment of benefits and burdens is a virtue that organizations can strive to meet.

Can you imagine what a courageous organization would be like and what type of policies and administrative guidelines you would find there? What about a compassionate or merciful institution? You can help to construct policies, practices, and other arrangements that allow your workplace to exhibit a commitment to organizational virtue.

Summary

Undermining the ethical goal of virtuous organizations is their capacity to fragment lives, alienate individuals from their values and connectedness, and marginalize already oppressed groups. Organizations have a moral obligation to help prevent such destructive conditions from occurring.

We have seen some challenges at work in the StarServices, Inc, health plan. Because so many people spend more time each week in the organizations of work, government, education, health care, and religion than they do in their own homes, all organizations must assume an influential role in helping to foster high moral standards.

This chapter takes you, the moral agent, out of the clinic or other immediate work environment and into the committee room and administrator's offices. As the complexity of the health professions and health care environment continues to grow, so do the necessity and opportunity for becoming involved in the development of mission statements, policies, and administrative and business practices. Such involvement should enable you to maintain professional standards and a high level of ethical practice. The six-step process of ethical decision making can guide you in your role in this situation. Despite the help that the organization policies, practices, and environment can provide, they are not an automatic guarantee of high-quality patient care or fair practices toward employees, patients, or others. You still must apply skillful ethical reasoning about ethical problems as they present themselves.

Questions for Thought and Discussion

1. Can you describe an employment situation in which you can imagine quitting in protest over an ethically unacceptable policy of the organization? What is it? List the pros and cons of quitting. Now list some changes that would allow you, in good faith, to continue in the organization.

2. Eudora Cathay has been a unit clerk at the same community hospital for 2 years. The position of unit clerk is a demanding one that involves answering the phone, relaying messages, coordinating laboratory personnel in their rounds, responding to physicians' requests, and making sure that patients are in the right places at the right times. Eudora's striking appearance is enhanced by her African dress style. Some of the more conservative members of the staff, particularly physicians and administrators, have been disturbed by her style of dress. Others find it attractive and an interesting change from the wall-to-wall white uniforms everywhere in the hospital. The dress policy does not require unit clerks to wear a uniform and stipulates only that they be neat and well groomed (which she is) and dressed "appropriately" (which is controversial). Someone in an administrative position asked Eudora to dress more conservatively. She refused on the grounds that she was neat and well groomed and any further demands were an invasion of her privacy. She was fired for her refusal to comply, amidst rampant rumors of racism. Discuss her situation in light of good organizational policy. Should there be a dress code? Is there anything ethically relevant about how employees dress? Why or why not?

References

1. Hall, R.T., 2000. *An introduction to healthcare organizational ethics.* Oxford University Press, New York.
2. Swisher, L.L., Arslanian, L.E., Davis, C.M., 2005. The realm-individual process-situation (RIPS) model of ethical decision making. *HPA Resource* 5 (3), 1, 3, 8.
3. Glaser, J.W., 2005. Three realms of ethics: An integrative map of ethics for the future. In: Purtilo, R.B., Jensen, G.M., Royeen, C.B. (Eds.), *Educating for moral action: A sourcebook in health and rehabilitation ethics.* F.A. Davis, Philadelphia, PA, pp. 169–184.
4. Gabard, D., Martin, W.W., 2003. *Honesty and conflicts of interest: Physical therapy ethics.* F.A. Davis, Philadelphia, PA, pp. 142–158, definition p. 143.
5. Casilino, L., Gillies, R.R., Shortell, S.M., et al., 2003. External incentives, information technology and organized processes to improve health care quality for patients with chronic diseases. *JAMA* 289, pp. 434–441.
6. Rawls, J., 1991. *A theory of justice*, 2nd ed. Harvard University Press, Cambridge, MA.
7. Pierce, J., Jameton, A., 2004. *The ethics of environmentally responsible health care.* Oxford University Press, New York, pp. 43–60.
8. American Society of Bioethics and Humanities, 2009. Part 3: Organization ethics. In: *Core competencies for health care ethics consultation.* American Society of Bioethics and Humanities, Glenview, IL, pp. 12–15.
9. Blau, R., Bolus, S., Carolan, T., et al., 2002. The experience of providing physical therapy in a changing health care environment. *Physical Ther* 82 (7), 648–657.
10. Bodenheimer, T.S., Grumbach, K., 2002. *Understanding health policy: A clinical approach*, 3rd ed. McGraw-Hill, New York, pp. 62–65.
11. Lawrence, D., 2003. *From chaos to care: The promise of team-based medicine.* Da Capo Press, Cambridge, MA.

9

Living Ethically as a Member of the Health Care Team

Objectives

The reader should be able to:

- Describe some major areas of professional life that present ethical challenges as a member of a health care team.
- List five guidelines that are useful in assessing whether a prospective place of employment supports teamwork that is ethically and clinically of the highest quality.
- Discuss several reasonable expectations a health professional can have of professional peers.
- Define peer review and assess its usefulness as a mechanism to maintain the high moral standards of a profession.
- List several types of impairment that health professionals may experience that create ethical challenges for the whole team.
- Discuss some general guidelines on how to gather relevant information regarding an alleged incident of incompetent or unethical professional conduct.
- Outline the appropriate steps to be taken in a whistle-blowing situation.
- Develop several alternative strategies for dealing with a colleague who is engaging in incompetent or unethical conduct and describe probable outcomes of taking each line of action.

New terms and ideas you will encounter in this chapter

health care team	peer review	impairment
dual relationship	whistle blowers/whistle	
supererogatory	blowing	
peer evaluation		

Topics in this chapter introduced in earlier chapters

Topic	Introduced in chapter
Ethical dilemma	3
Faithfulness or fidelity	4
Beneficence	4
Justice or fairness	4
Nonmaleficence	4
Deontology	4
Utilitarianism	4
Ethical reasoning	4
Six-step process of ethical decision making	5
Self care as a responsibility	7

Introduction

This chapter launches a new focus. Up until now, you have been considering your moral agency role as an individual student or professional. But you are a moral agent in respect to other roles you assume, too, one of the most interesting being as a member of a *health care team*. A health care team is a group of professionals, sometimes with adjunct staff to assist, that becomes the unit of decision making. A team is designed to meet the same ethical goals of a caring response as individual professionals so that members of a team, working together, will accomplish collectively what individual professionals aim to do. You have already seen some examples of professionals working together to provide optimally competent care to patients. Now you will observe them as they also participate in other team activities, demonstrating that the search for a caring response to them can be as important for good patient care as is your commitment to finding a caring response toward a patient. Usually, the two focuses of your care are completely compatible with your ultimate goal of doing what is best for each patient. In fact, team-oriented care was designed to enhance the effectiveness of this goal. Occasionally, however, problems arise within teamwork that threaten to compromise the patient's good, the team's effectiveness, or both. You have an opportunity here to examine both some strengths and challenges in teamwork. The story of Maureen Sitler and Daniela Green is one example of how conflict or questions arise about the ethically right thing to do.

 The Story of Maureen Sitler and Daniela Green

> Maureen Sitler is the chief respiratory therapist in the respiratory intensive care unit (ICU) of a large university hospital. Two staff therapists are in the unit with her.

Maureen has been on vacation during the last 2 weeks and arrives home late Sunday night. When she reports to work on Monday morning, she finds a note on her desk saying that Karen, one of the two staff therapists, has had to leave town to be with her mother, who has had a serious heart attack. Karen writes that she will be gone at least this week and maybe next.

The other therapist, Tom Morgane, arrives and brings Maureen up to date on the activities. He assures her that, as usual, the patient load soared immediately after she left and that the unit has been buzzing ever since.

They sort through the current patient load and are relieved that no new patients have come in over the weekend. They decide that between them they can just manage for the day. Suddenly, Maureen feels weary, as if she had never been on vacation.

She is writing names of the patients on the schedule board in the office when a unit clerk brings a note to her detailing four patients in other parts of the hospital who need therapy. The note is from the hospital's other respiratory therapy department chief, the one who serves the general inpatient population. Often the two directors make such requests of each other when their own loads are especially heavy. Maureen's first impulse is to refuse to accept any more patients, but she takes the note to her desk.

The first patient is an 81-year-old widow with inhalation burns. She accidentally started a fire that gutted her kitchen when a kitchen towel caught on fire. The second referral is a 3-year-old child with congenital lung and bronchial deformities. Another repair of the bronchial tubes had been performed. The third patient is a 31-year-old woman with severe asthma.

Maureen lays out the three referral sheets in front of her without bothering to read the fourth and studies the schedule again. At most, they can accept only one more patient today. She decides to call the other chief therapist, Sandra Haynes, to ask her judgment regarding the relative urgency of these patients.

She is dialing, tapping idly with her forefinger on the one referral she has not yet read, when the name Daniela Green leaps off the page at her. She picks up the referral and reads it. Her heart begins to pound in her throat. She slams down the receiver and runs to the treatment area where Tom is working. "This can't be our Dannie!" she exclaims. Tom puts a hand on her shoulder, "I'm sorry. I forgot to tell you with so much else to catch up on. As you can see, she was hospitalized with severe pneumonia while you were gone. We should find a way to fit her in."

Maureen feels sick to her stomach. Daniela Green is the head nurse in the oncology unit. Daniela and Maureen often have the same patients, so more often than not, they find themselves on the same health care teams, whether it be in the oncology or respiratory ICU units or as members of the rehabilitation team. Daniela recently gave an excellent in-service workshop for the physical therapy, occupational therapy, and respiratory therapy departments. On a number of occasions, Maureen and Daniela have attended plays and other social events together. Two years ago, they initiated a drive to find support for improving, or as they put it, "humanizing," the environment of the waiting areas throughout the therapy areas. On several occasions, Maureen has called on Daniela as a "sympathetic ear" and has found her insightful and understanding. During her vacation, Maureen had been thinking that she should take the time to cultivate this budding friendship, knowing that it could take root and deepen.

Maureen's first reaction is to squeeze Daniela into the treatment schedule, no matter what. But something stops her. How can she be fair to all the patients on the list, she thinks, and still respond to the additional loyalties of kinship she feels toward her teammate Daniela?

You will have an opportunity to reflect on this story throughout the chapter because it highlights several strengths and types of ethical challenges that you could face—and probably will face—in your role as a team member. The first thing we will consider is the importance of providing support to and accepting support from each other as teammates.

The Goal: A Caring Response

No one who works in the health care setting day in and day out escapes moments of self-doubt, anger, or utter frustration. As you read in Chapters 6, 7, and 8, a great deal is expected of you in regard to taking good care of yourself as a student or professional and in getting along in the organizational structures of health care. Even so, at times, your involvement in the human suffering of illness and disease is intense, the responsibilities arduous, and the challenges monumental. The wear and tear of taxing schedules, patients whose problems seem overwhelming, or a day in which everything that could go wrong does can discourage even the most competent, optimistic person.

Being a member of a health care team is one of the most fundamental facts of life in today's health care system, and when the team is working well together, it is one of the most certain hedges against being worn down by the challenges of your work (Figure 9-1).

Maureen Sitler's situation illustrates well how understandable (and how wonderful) it is to develop friendships in the workplace. It is not surprising, considering that you will spend some of the best (and if not the best, at least the most) hours of your life in workplace settings. Friendships, a love relationship, and business partnerships with people you will meet first as a team member are all within the realm of possibility.

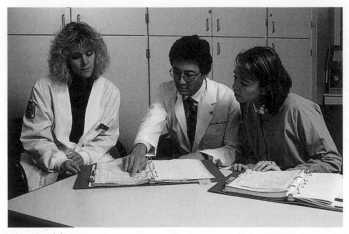

Figure 9-1. Health care team. (From Christensen, B.L., 2005. *Foundations of adult health nursing*, 5th ed. Mosby, St Louis)

Many institutions currently recognize the need for team support. In some institutions, there is an effort to hold departmental or interdepartmental meetings so that issues may be addressed in a nonthreatening, supportive setting. This type of arrangement usually improves and sustains good working relationships among team members and provides a refuge where individuals can receive needed support. They provide opportunities for deliberation, negotiation, and communication clarification to facilitate consensus building in complex situations. In any department, such arrangements can help to humanize the environment for workers and patients alike.[1] In this regard, it makes sense to think of teamwork as the institution's acknowledgment of such stresses and the implementation of actual mechanisms to address them as its caring response to the situation.

In the previous chapter, we suggested some ways to "check out" the health care environment when applying for a new position in a health care setting. Wisdom counsels that in your fact finding, you inquire whether there is a support network among team members as well. To make an assessment, the following suggestions may help:

1. Inquire of your future employer whether there are team meetings or other sessions to freely discuss everyday stresses on the team.
2. Ask some of the team members you will be working with what they find to be the most stressful aspects of their work in that environment.
3. Ask them how each, as an individual, deals with the stresses of his or her role on the team and whether the environment as a whole is supportive or divisive.
4. Make a mental note of potential teammates who appear to be likely sources of support for stress or if no one appears to be potentially supportive.

5. Perhaps most important, try to ascertain whether it will be possible to help try to decrease or eliminate sources of team stress and who will help accept responsibility for fostering such change.

 Reflection

What other questions or concerns would you address when applying for a position and trying to assess how well key team members seem to work together? List them here.

_____

_____

_____

_____

Fortunately, it is highly probable that you will find a supportive net of team members in your work setting. Once you are employed, or if you already are, you can help create a greater support network among team members by being attentive to the blahs and blues that a colleague seems to be experiencing, by risking sharing your own "doubts or discouragements" with people you judge to be trustworthy to help you through them, and by making suggestions regarding the need for mechanisms designed to work through problems as a team. As Maureen's situation implies, friendships may take root in the shared experiences, concerns, and time spent with other members of the health care team. A friend you meet in a work situation may become the key figure in building a supportive network, and as friends, the two of you can provide support to each other and others. The joy of discovering and cultivating such a friendship is among the most rewarding of the many fringe benefits of a health professional's career.

The ethical components guiding close, convivial working relationships are similar to those in the health professional–patient relationship.[2] Team members also should be recipients of caring responses from you and others. Some ways to achieve these responses include telling the truth, honoring confidences, acting with compassion, and respecting the dignity of your colleagues.[3]

 Reflection

Because you are a moral agent with the responsibilities associated with it, what do you think you should be able to reasonably expect from your fellow teammates? Name some things that would indicate that you are the beneficiary of their respect and care.

_____

_____

_____

_____

From our own experience, we have developed a list of reasonable expectations regarding team relationships—things we believe one should be able to count on based on the ethical principle of fidelity to each other. These expectations are:

1. Collegial trust and the shared goal of a caring response.
2. Substantive assistance from teammates regarding questions about good patient care or other matters of professional judgment.
3. A willingness by all teammates to carry a fair share of the workload.
4. Sympathetic understanding regarding work-related stresses.
5. An environment conducive to a high level of functioning and one that fosters work satisfaction for everyone involved, not just some members of the team.
6. A commitment by everyone to respect differences in values, contributions of other team members, and embrace each person's unique gifts.
7. Encouragement to develop both professionally and personally within the work environment.

As you think of other things you would expect and want to help protect and encourage, be bold in making suggestions to those with whom you work. Sometimes a well-placed word can help to increase everyone's imagination about how the team can work together more effectively.

 SUMMARY

Good teamwork is based on respect. You can expect respect from others and also must show respect to them.

With the background established thus far in this chapter, turn to the six-step process of ethical decision making to learn how it also applies to team issues.

The Six-Step Process and Team Decisions

We take Maureen's situation, with its potential for favoritism toward Daniela, to give you an opportunity to apply the process of ethical decision making introduced in Chapter 5. So far, you have applied it to situations involving health professionals' decisions regarding direct patient care and organizational dimensions of your work. At the same time, interprofessional issues also will arise among team members, and those issues lend themselves to analysis and (hopefully) resolution by use of the same process. Some ethical considerations you have not yet encountered must be taken into account in a team peer relationship. The last part of this chapter focuses on the challenges of peer review and the duty to report unacceptable conduct of a teammate.

Step 1: Gather Relevant Information

Maureen has to gather all the relevant information about the patients on the waiting list that she would be morally obligated to do in any event. However, right away you can see that her discovery of Daniela as one of her potential patients complicates the situation in at least two ways: she has to decide whether her loyalty to her team member should have any bearing on her choice, and she has to reckon with the fact that the two of them are now in a "dual role" with each other (i.e., as colleagues and also as professional-patient) if Daniela becomes her patient.

Team Loyalty as Relevant Information

We surmise that because Daniela is Maureen's colleague this factor alone is influencing Maureen's ethical reasoning. No one would question how important it is to provide support to professional peers, and now here is a peer with a need to which Maureen is able to respond. It takes little imagination to understand why Maureen's emotional response is to immediately accept her as one of the patients. It would be easy to give Daniela the VIP ("very important person") treatment, slipping her in ahead of the others in the busy schedule, regardless of whether she will benefit the most. We do not know exactly why Tom urges Maureen to "fit her in." His statement may be based on something he knows about her physical situation relative to the others on the list. More likely, he is responding to the same urgings that Maureen is experiencing. He might also be imagining the backlash among their other teammates and professional colleagues throughout the institution if word gets out that Daniela was not given high priority knowing that teams have a shared responsibility for their decisions and outcomes.[4] Maureen probably is well aware of these relevant "facts" of the situation.

The Ethical Challenge of Dual Roles

The two women are not only teammates but also enjoy a warm personal relationship. In other words, they are in a relationship both as peers and as friends. Now they are plunged into a third type of relationship: they are about to encounter each other as therapist and patient in a health professional–patient relationship. Within health care settings, this type of situation is referred to in the literature and ethical guidelines as a *dual relationship*.

The situation of a dual relationship is always one occasion for careful reflection about appropriate boundaries in the professional setting.[4] As Maureen tries to sort out her priorities in her role as a health professional, who will be treating the patient, Daniela, she becomes strikingly aware that she and Daniela are in a new psychological dynamic with each other. The health professional–patient relationship has ethical parameters that do not pertain to their relationship either as professional peers or as friends. In her professional role, if Maureen's favorable bias toward Daniela becomes an occasion for allowing an uncaring response to the other patients on the list, she will have acted unethically. Although Daniela may accept this situation with equanimity and understanding, anyone who has been very ill knows that it is difficult not to want attention immediately. The favoritism one would automatically hope for and reasonably expect from a friend is not alone sufficient reason for Daniela to receive top priority treatment as a patient.

 SUMMARY

Loyalties to one's teammates and the situation of dual roles create occasions for ethical discernment.

Steps 2 and 3: Identify the Type of Ethical Problem and Use Ethics Theories or Approaches to Analyze It

Maureen, the moral agent in this situation, is faced with an ethical problem.

We judge that she has an ethical dilemma. Why? First, other things being equal, she would be justified in responding positively to her professional colleague. It is morally appropriate for members of the team to pay due respect to each other. As you recall, earlier in this chapter we suggested a list of what you can "reasonably expect" from teammates in terms of their support. Our list was based on our own experience and the principle of faithfulness (fidelity), knowing that if a team does not stay together in its shared goal of providing good patient care, it will fail in meeting that goal. Therefore, it is not at all morally questionable that Maureen would be invested in the well-being of her colleague.

Maureen also has the duty to search for the most caring response to any one of the patients on that list, and Daniela is one. This peels off all the layers of other concerns and leaves the core of the patient–health professional relationship. If she believes any or all of those other patients have a more pressing need for her services than Daniela, Maureen cannot honor both her fidelity to her teammate and her duty of beneficence that is at the ethical core of her professional role.

In this type of dilemma, the conflicting principles of fidelity to her peers and beneficence to the patients on the list summarize her ethical quandary. However, her moral agency carries with it the power to allow harm or less than optimal benefit to ensue for the patients in relatively greater need if she is swayed by criteria inappropriate to a health professional's decision.

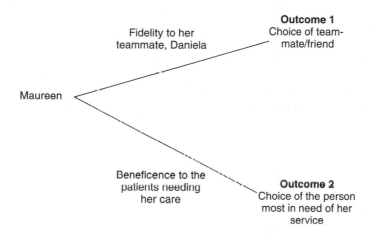

Given that these principles are markers to moral duties that Maureen is working with, one can conclude that she is sorting this out according to the framework a deontologist would use. As straightforward as this appears, Maureen may also be acutely aware that the consequences of not accepting Daniela, whatever the assessment of her relevant need, will be deleterious to the morale of the rest of the team. Therefore, she will have to further weigh in those utilitarian considerations before making her final decision.

 Reflection

Having analyzed the situation this far, what more would you want to know to decide whether her duties or utilitarian considerations should govern her decision?

_____

_____

_____

_____

What character traits would you want Maureen to have when she is making this decision?

_____

_____

_____

_____

Step 4: Explore the Practical Alternatives

Several options are open to her, including:
1. Accept Daniela Green for treatment because they are friends.
2. Accept Daniela because she is well loved by many people in the hospital and to not give her priority will adversely affect the staff.
3. Not accept Daniela because showing favoritism in such instances sends
   the wrong message.
4. Not accept Daniela because she is in less immediate need of this particular health professional's services than the other three patients
   seem to be.
5. Choose randomly who among the four patients will be treated today
   (draw straws).
6. Accept the three other patients and treat Daniela after hours.
   Can you add others?
   Consider the first option. As we discussed earlier, all things being equal,
you would expect a friend or colleague to act favorably on your behalf and
would be prepared to do likewise. One display of friendship and colleague-
ship is this type of commitment. But Maureen's ethical dilemma reveals that
accepting Daniela for this reason oversimplifies the ethical problem she is
facing because it ignores the reality of conflicting commitments.

The second option entails a type of utilitarian reasoning. Again, we
speculated earlier that if Daniela is not accepted for treatment, the morale
of the whole hospital may be affected. The staff may think, "The same thing
could happen to me. Would my colleagues overlook me for someone else,
too?" Maureen might say, along this line of reasoning, "Particular loyalties
and justice aside, it just does not pay in the long run to accept for treatment
those who do not command the sympathies of the hospital the way that
Daniela does."

Practically speaking, this type of reasoning often underlies decisions. But
the moral point of view requires that the various duties experienced in the
health professional–patient relationships not be ignored so facilely. Accepting Daniela for the reason stated in the second option again oversimplifies
the ethical dilemma Maureen is facing.

The third option again emphasizes the difficulty of trying to proceed fairly or impartially when faced with a decision that involves someone the decision maker knows and cares about. Refusing Daniela treatment primarily because she and Maureen are teammates intuitively seems as unfair as automatically giving her top priority because of it. And so, acting on the third option is not a morally adequate decision either. In contrast, Maureen's idea of telephoning her respiratory therapist colleague, who may know the other patients, is a good plan. The other therapist might provide insight and more balanced judgments regarding unfair biases Maureen would introduce by having such a vested interest in her friend's welfare.

We know the ethical priority in regard to Maureen's dilemma is the health professional–patient relationship rather than her relationship with another team member.[5] Why? Because Daniela is in this situation due to her clinical condition and her need for Maureen in this instance specifically is the need that a patient experiences in relation to a health professional. Moreover, neither of them would want to allow suspicion that because they are both health professionals they had fallen suspect to a depersonalizing aspect of health professions practice—namely, the health professionals' propensities to cover for, show favoritism toward, and link arms with other health professionals.[6] Any appearance that this is happening must be avoided. Therefore, whether the bonds of friendship are generally more binding than the health professional–patient relationship may be an extremely interesting question, but the governing framework for this situation (and Maureen's position of moral agency in it) must be the health professional–patient relationship.

The fourth option comes much closer than the previous three to a decision that takes the following important ethical considerations into account:
1. The health professional–patient relationship as the proper relationship governing the decision;
2. The principle of distributive justice that helps to guide allocation of scarce resources (in this case, Maureen's energies and time); and
3. Acknowledgment that the relative degree of clinical need is the appropriate criterion by which all four patients should be compared.

More detailed discussion regarding the criteria on which to base distributive justice decisions in health care are postponed until Chapter 15. Here it is sufficient to point out that the degree of clinical need combined with Maureen's potential to be of benefit in each case is a reliable guide for the type of decision Maureen must make.[7] Because patients' needs differ, Maureen does not have to resort to other criteria of selection (the fifth option).

If Maureen accepts this type of ethical reasoning regarding the proper moral criteria for determining who should be accepted for treatment, it should in no way diminish her desire to expend her best energies for Daniela. The sixth option would enable her to do just that. By accepting the others on the basis of their greater clinical need, she would meet the requirements of fairness to the other patients, who would receive treatment instead, but this does not prevent Maureen from taking an extra step to help her colleague. Philosophers call Maureen's conduct *supererogatory*, a type of morally praiseworthy conduct that goes beyond duty.[8] The problem for Maureen (and anyone who falls back on this solution), of course, is that although it might make her feel better about this particular situation, it cannot be used as a general practice to always "fix" conflicts involving how to deal with scarce resources.

 Reflection

If you listed additional options, this is a good time to take a few minutes and analyze each.

_____

_____

_____

_____

Step 5: Complete the Action

If Maureen decides not to show any favoritism toward her colleague, we have helped her move in the direction of getting her priorities in order so that however much she may wish she did not face a dilemma, at least she knows why she will set priorities as she does.

Step 6: Evaluate the Process and Outcome

Once Maureen has made her decision and acted on it, she would be wise to reflect on it with other members of the team. Hopefully, her action will have been such that a desire to give preferential treatment to a friend or close colleague will have been successfully weighed against the demands of her moral role as a professional; this is worth sharing with the other members of the team so that all of them will be better able to face a similar situation in the future with more confidence.

⊙ SUMMARY

Loyalty of professional colleagues is laudable in itself but does not preclude the moral necessity of honoring the tenets of ethical practice as a professional.

Peer Evaluation Issues

A second category of ethical challenge in team membership arises around the concept of *peer evaluation*. The basic idea is that a professional is asked to evaluate the performance or other aspects of a colleague who is in a similar professional position. Increasingly, members of professional organizations, educational institutions, and treatment facilities are asked to evaluate the quality of their colleagues' work and moral character.[9]

The standards against which the evaluation is judged may be set by your professional organization or immediate workplace or may be imposed by governmental or other agencies and you may find it mandatory to participate in them. Two varieties of peer evaluation are peer review and whistle blowing.

Peer Review

Peer review is designed primarily to ensure that high standards of professional practice are upheld in your workplace. It may be a resource that the administration uses when salary increases, honors, promotions, or other work-related distinctions are being determined. Letters of recommendation you write for a colleague who is applying for a new job is a form of peer review that will be used by the prospective employer. Therefore, although the main emphasis in peer review is on its value as a procedure to ensure that standards and practices remain of high quality in the health professions, it also functions secondarily as a personal profile of a person's progress (or lack of it) in attaining professional stature. Peer review documents taken together often generate data that then become a basis for comparisons among similarly situated colleagues.

With this understanding of peer review, let us go back to Maureen Sitler, whom you met at the outset of this chapter. But now, the focus will be on her relationship with her colleague, Tom Morgane. Maureen and Tom have not told anyone at work that they are in love and are planning to be married in autumn. They are both in their early 30s and wish to remain at their current place of employment because of the benefits they have built up by staying there and their favorable opportunities for advancement and also because they enjoy the part of the country where they live.

Although both are about the same age, Maureen has worked longer as a respiratory therapist, and everyone agrees that she is exceptionally well qualified as director of the respiratory therapy unit in the ICU. She has written several articles, engaged in clinical studies, and learned some difficult diagnostic techniques through special training.

News has just come out that Sandra Haynes, the other chief respiratory therapist, has decided to take a position elsewhere. The hospital administration has decided to merge Maureen's and Sandra's departments into one large unit, and a nationwide search will be conducted to find the best person to be the director. There are two in-house candidates within the institution itself. Maureen is one, and the other is a woman who has been in the other department about as long as Maureen has been in the ICU and who also seems well qualified.

After the first extensive search is made, four people are still in the running. Both Maureen and the other woman are among them. As part of the administration's attempt to make an informed choice, they now ask several people to submit peer evaluations of Maureen and the other candidate. Tom is among those asked to make this peer evaluation of each of the two candidates.

Maureen and Tom are elated at the possibility that Maureen may be appointed director of the new department. Tom believes that Maureen is well qualified, but he also knows that she very much wants the position. They both are aware that her substantial increase in salary would be helpful for them financially and may even enable them to put a down payment on a house.

Reflection

Should he write a letter of recommendation for his future wife? Why or why not?

_____

_____

_____

_____

The following paragraphs share our line of thinking. See if you agree and why or why not.

Tom may think that whatever he says is not going to make a difference anyway. But that is an avoidance of assuming the responsibility he has been asked to assume. From a moral standpoint, he should try to work out a method of acting responsibly by writing the assessment. At the same time, anyone who finds out about his "other" relationship with Maureen will certainly cast doubt on his objectivity and, likely, his intentions.

Because the primary purpose of peer review is to help maintain the standards of professional practice, he must do some soul searching to assure himself that the high esteem he has for Maureen professionally really is based on the high quality of her work and her skills. If he can give a positive response to that issue, he should go ahead, letting the administration know, however, that he and Maureen are engaged to be married. He should document his statement with examples of her work and try especially hard to recall areas where he believes she can continue to grow. Disclosing that he has a vested interest as a friend or fiancé will allow the person reading his letter to take into consideration the bias he may introduce. Hopefully, the person reading the review will know that it is difficult enough to comment on one's peers and that an additional emotional challenge is introduced by their intimate personal relationship.

Even when the added component of friendship or a love relationship is not present, peer review by team members can be an emotionally taxing situation. Essentially you are being asked to engage in a process of affirming or discrediting your fellow team members in relation to their professional quality and skills. Why is it so difficult? In the first place, all health professionals have some doubt about their own judgments from time to time, simply because the nature of professional practice is fraught with ambiguities. As a result, it is not surprising if you are hesitant to pass negative judgment on someone else's activities, knowing well that everyone has an Achilles' heel. Second, there is the fear that if you are too rough on colleagues, the tables may one day be turned on you. Finally, sometimes loyalty to one's profession acts as a deterrent to saying anything negative about one of its members. Whatever the source of the difficulty, the health professional who assumes this responsibility with an honest, fair, and compassionate approach can help to uphold the high standards of professional practice. In the end, this approach benefits the peer, the patients, and the professions themselves.

An advantage of peer review as a mechanism is that this practice usually involves obtaining the considered opinions of several people. When it can be done without compromising confidentiality, this practice helps to mitigate biases that might arise from having only a superior conduct the review on his or her own. The person who reads the reviews (i.e., the administrator, search committee chairperson, or other) looks for areas of congruence among the several reviewers. If one evaluation is radically out of line with the others, further clarification may be sought.

 SUMMARY

The aim of peer review is to uphold the high standards of professional practice. Your participation in such a process is one of your professional responsibilities.

Blowing the Whistle on Unethical or Incompetent Teammates

A serious team-related ethical challenge of another type arises when there is evidence that a team member is engaging in unethical or incompetent behavior. When such a person is reported, the person or persons making the report are called *whistle blowers*, and their action is called *whistle blowing*.

Currently, professional organizations, and government licensing and disciplinary boards, are acknowledging that unethical and incompetent behavior does occur by health professionals, clinical investigators, and health care administrators. The bases of such behaviors include *impairments* from severe substance abuse, the apparent inability to exercise sound professional judgment, severe depression, paranoia or other mental disorders, or breaches of professional integrity through sexual abuse of patients, theft from patients or institutions, chronic lying, fee splitting, and practicing without a license or under other false pretenses. You need not watch soap operas to know that health professionals include all types of people.

To make matters more complicated, usually the knowledge of harm to patients or colleagues gradually comes to the attention of colleagues, and often in a form that creates many questions about the legitimacy of the rumor, the mental stability of the person in question, or other troubling factors. Consider the following examples. A rumor is circulating that Ms. Werthheimer, a nursing unit clerk, accused Patient A of threatening to kill her by poisoning her food, and she claims to have reported him to the CIA. Mr. Grabowski, a surgical technician, is said to have reported to work after an unexplained absence of 3 days with the smell of whisky on his breath and contaminated the surgical suite by not scrubbing in properly. Money has been reported missing from patients' homes after Mrs. Waltham has made a home visit to them. The mother of a young boy accuses Alan DeJong of sexually abusing him during a recent treatment. An old woman claims that Dr. Sakabuto tried to suffocate her with a pillow during the night. Word is out that Mr. Fried forged his papers and is not a graduate of an approved school.

Dramatic examples of wrongdoing often hit the newspapers. At the same time, more common problems arise that are not as dramatic but that potentially are just as dangerous to patients. For instance, take the case of a health professional who has family problems and copes by excessive lack of sleep or abuse of over-the-counter or prescription medications.

These rumors are about teammates one works with, side by side, consults with, and has shared lunch or coffee with for months or years. Even the person who seems rather strange or is considered a loner is more easily dismissed as a curiosity than viewed as an enemy among the ranks. Unfortunately, rumors are more easily believed as carrying a kernel of truth when the person is disliked or suspected in the first place. But, even so, in almost all cases, this type of rumor is first met with disbelief by most people. Indeed, to base one's judgment solely on such a report would be morally indefensible behavior.

What should guide you in your attempt to arrive at a caring response when faced with hearsay information? As in most such situations, the information should not be totally denied or ignored, but a final judgment about the person should never be made on this tenuous ground. The process of gathering relevant information must be taken especially seriously. The characteristics of the person who makes the complaint should be taken into consideration, but he or she should never be dismissed as senile, crazy, irrational, or otherwise unable to report accurately what has happened. At the very least, the person making the complaint should be asked directly for details. A further step is to ask whether he or she is willing to put the complaint into writing. Although this in itself does not render the alleged offender guilty, it is a sign that the person observing the conduct is willing to describe his or her perceptions of the situation in writing and probably would be willing to defend it before a grievance committee or in a court of law if necessary. Hesitance to report a peer in cases of a serious offense often comes from fear of reprisal from the alleged offender or fear of stigma (e.g., in cases of rape).

So long as safety is not an immediate concern, it is wise to hold your judgment in abeyance as long as the report remains at the level of one report by one person, especially if the person is not willing to document the incident in writing. If a pattern of alleged abuses or mistakes emerges, it definitely must be followed up immediately. Almost all institutions currently have appropriate processes for reporting suspicious or outright improper conduct. These processes are designed to protect the rights of everyone involved, to provide due process under the law, and should be followed rigorously.

The moral decision to blow the whistle on a fellow team member can be among the most agonizing in your career as a health professional.[10] From a psychological viewpoint, there is tremendous potential for your own ego, beliefs, and hopes to take a battering. The loss of an errant colleague also can signal the loss of a friend or the loss of your belief in ideals you thought were shared ideals. Understandably, it is a comfort to believe that you will not be faced with such a dilemma, especially if the offender is a close friend. But to hope for such good fortune does not excuse you from trying to prepare for it. Your moral character is always tested. It takes a full dose of courage, patience, and fortitude; a striving toward justice; much compassion; and a capacity for sympathetic involvement to know when and how to proceed with incriminating evidence when a colleague or friend is implicated.

 Reflection

Before reading ahead, list some courses of action you could take if you increasingly believed that your colleague was seriously addicted to alcohol.

1. _____

2. _____

3. _____

4. _____

One alternative in some situations is to stave off a developing problem before a real offense is committed. Often, the breaking point between a professional's attempt to maintain self-esteem or professional responsibilities and total resignation to the destructive forces at work within is the realization that colleagues have turned their backs. Most people know when they are in trouble. At the point of greatest need and alienation, a direct contact coming from someone who cares enough to confront the problem tactfully often can provide courage for one to seek help and can be the thin thread back to more sound functioning. Morag Coate, a British writer quoted in Kay Jamison's book *Night Falls Fast: Understanding Suicide*, was contemplating suicide but decided not to take her life when she became convinced that her doctor cared. She wrote afterward, "Because the doctors cared, and because one of them still believed in me when I believed in nothing, I have survived to tell the tale."[11] It makes no difference whether it is a patient or teammate who loses the will to go on because of whatever serious problem he or she is facing. You, the one link, may be sufficient for the person who is spinning out of control to get her or his bearings.

Whenever possible, you should act to affirm such a person as someone in a struggle and offer your support. This may include recommending that the person not continue to practice, at least until he or she is on more solid footing. The motivation for risking yourself enough to reach out to a fellow team member in distress often arises from a sense that it could be you in a similar situation and that, in some fundamental regard, we all are in the game together. Many years ago, the poet John Donne captured our interdependence in this famous phrase:

> "No man is an island, entire of itself; every man is a piece of the continent, a part of the main; if a clod be washed away by the sea, Europe is the less . . . any man's death diminishes me, because I am involved in mankind; and therefore never send to know for whom the bell tolls; it tolls for thee."[12]

Second possible alternative is to do nothing. The shortcoming of this position is that once you have identified the potential problem, doing nothing also is a course of action. When harm to others or the teammate's self is likely to ensue, your neglect has become complicity. The professional disciplinary committees of most states and the codes of ethics of most professions now count this type of inaction as an offense as serious as committing wrongdoing yourself. Chapters 6 and 7 addressed this situation briefly in the discussion of your moral agency as a student and as a professional.

 Reflection

If you have not already done so, check the code of ethics of your chosen profession to see if it includes a statement of responsibility to report unethical or incompetent colleagues. Write a few notes about how it would and would not help you.

_____

_____

_____

_____

A third course is to act decisively to remove the teammate from a position in which he or she can do further harm. This is the appropriate course of action once the relevant information has been gathered and analyzed and is persuasive. A secure rule of thumb is to keep the information as contained as possible using the usual channels of communication and institutional or other disciplinary mechanisms designed for this purpose. It is extremely important to honor the alleged violator's privacy, respect, and legal rights, no matter how grievous a "crime" you may think the person has committed.

Unquestionably, there are some difficult judgment calls involved in actually taking the final step of whistle blowing. Some checkpoints include:

- If possible, you should communicate to the person that you have reached the point where you plan to call attention to his or her alleged violation of ethical, competency, or legal standards.
- Decide whether to talk to anyone else before you act, knowing that sometimes there is strength in numbers and also that your own perceptions may be skewed.
- Give careful attention to whether you have exhausted the other possibilities that may allow you to take a less radical step and still be responsible in your role as a moral agent.

Should you be faced with a whistleblowing situation, your ability to strike a balance between your sensitivity to the human situation and a commitment to proceed will require courage. The attention you have given to it here will serve you well.

As always, any opportunity you have to help prevent such situations is time extremely well spent. Short of that, if your institution has developed guidelines about unethical or incompetent conduct, use them as aids. If not, you and your teammates can contribute greatly to the constructive functioning of the institution by helping to develop policies that will implement whistle-blowing procedures with the following goals. Guidelines should:

- encourage thorough documentation;
- ensure due process judiciously;
- provide as much support all around as possible; and
- require that the institution persevere to the completion of the review and take action consistent with the findings.

Completion probably will involve the role of several others, such as administrators, regulatory board members, risk managers, or designated people in professional associations. The actual personnel and processes vary. Your job in seeing the issue to completion is to work diligently within prescribed professional and other organizational mechanisms.

 SUMMARY

Whistle blowing may involve reporting impaired, unethical, or incompetent colleagues. In addition to the rights listed in Chapter 8, you also have a right to expect guidelines that ensure protection of all parties involved while the appropriate bodies follow up on your report and that the investigation will be accompanied by appropriate action.

It is in the heat of challenging situations regarding peer evaluation that certain character traits disposing you to be thoughtful also will help you to know whether and how to proceed. An acute sensitivity to the various people affected combined with the courage to act and the desire to act compassionately is an essential moral tool in such situations.

Summary

This chapter focuses on several sources of support professionals have and can offer as members of a health care team. You have a right to expect support from your teammates and from your institution. The challenge of remaining ethical in peer evaluation situations was discussed, as were serious challenges that arise when a colleague is engaging in unethical or illegal behavior. In the latter situation, the person may be ill, extremely stressed, addicted, or devious. Whatever the cause, your motive for whistle blowing or other considered action should always be to protect patients, clients, or even society from the harm such a person may cause. Your moral agency positions you so that you can do no less than that.

Questions for Thought and Discussion

1. You and Uri enjoy a good working relationship as members of a health care team, although you do not know much about his personal life outside of the work situation. You notice that during the past few days he has become increasingly irritable toward you. You wonder if it is something you have said or done that is making him angry.
   a. What steps, if any, should you take to address this issue?
   b. Would it make any difference in how you proceed if it appears that his attitude is interfering with the quality of his work? Why?

c. How will you handle it when another member of the team expresses her worry about his behavior and asks if you have noted anything disturbing about him in recent weeks?

2. You are asked to give a job recommendation for your friend Arthur. You have worked closely with Arthur for more than a year on the same health care team and feel qualified to provide such a recommendation. Arthur is an energetic, fun-loving person, and you enjoy his friendship. His manner with patients is sometimes disturbing to you, however. He seems careless at times, almost to the point of negligence. Quite honestly, you would have to recommend him with qualification for the position to which he is applying.
   a. Why would you agree or refuse to provide a recommendation?
   b. Do you have a responsibility to your colleague to tell him that you are giving him a "qualified" recommendation? Why or why not?
   c. Do you have a responsibility to tell the party requesting the recommendation that you and Arthur are friends? Explain your position.

3. Dr. Roland Heisler is a senior physician on the health care team in the unit where Ms. Barbara McKenzie is the head night nurse. At about 7:00 PM, he is admitted to the unit as a patient with chest pain and is seen by a colleague, Dr. John Phillips. Several hours later, Dr. Heisler calls Barbara McKenzie into his room and asks her for a sleeping pill. She says that Dr. Phillips did not order a sleeping pill, reportedly because the patient said he did not need one. Dr. Heisler says that now he needs one. She puts in a call to Dr. Phillips, but he does not return it. Dr. Heisler is getting more and more aggravated and threatens to "go get one from the supply room" himself. Should she give it to him from the large supply of sleeping pills in her supply room? Defend why or why not, drawing on the duties, rights, and role issues discussed in your study of ethics so far.

4. You are told by a young patient, whose complications from childbirth required her to remain hospitalized on the obstetrics ward, that Dr. Redmarck, a medical resident assigned to her case, is acting "inappropriately" toward her. She says she is scared, and she looks it. When you ask what she means, she says, "Twice this week he has stopped in during the late evening and has asked to examine my breasts. At first I didn't think anything about it, but then I started thinking that it didn't have anything to do with my condition. . . . He pulls the covers way back, and lifts up my gown. The way he looks at me and touches me down there. There's something strange. I dread seeing him." What steps would you take in response to this information?

References

1. Purtilo, R., Haddad, A., 2007. Self-respect through nurturing yourself. In: *Health professional and patient interaction*, 7th ed. WB Saunders, Philadelphia, PA, pp. 73–79.
2. Purtilo, R., 2000. Thirty-first Mary McMillan lecture: A time to harvest, a time to sow: Ethics for a shifting landscape. *Physical Ther* 80, 1112–1119.
3. Clark, P.G., Cott, C., Drinka, T.J., 2007. Theory and practice in interprofessional ethics: A framework for understanding ethical issues in healthcare teams. *J Interprofessional Care* 21 (6), 591–603.
4. Purtilo, R., Haddad, A., 2007. Professional boundaries guided by respect. In: *Health professional and patient interaction*, 7th ed. WB Saunders, Philadelphia, PA, pp. 213–225.
5. Purtilo, R., 2004. Professional-patient relationship: Ethical issues. In: Post, S. (Ed.), *Encyclopedia of bioethics*, 3rd ed. vol. 4. Macmillan, New York, pp. 2150–2157.
6. Ashley, B., O'Rourke, K., 1997. The health care profession. Section 4.1. Professions: Depersonalizing trends. In: *Health care ethics: A theological analysis*, 4th ed. Georgetown University Press, Washington, DC, pp. 69–71.
7. Sugarman, J., 2000. Conflicts of interest and obligation. In: *20 Common problems: Ethics in primary care*. McGraw-Hill, New York, pp. 98–99.
8. Beauchamp, T.L., Childress, J., 2009. The continuum from obligation to supererogation. In: *Principles of biomedical ethics,* 6th ed. Oxford University Press, New York, pp. 47–52.
9. Purtilo, R., 2004. Teams-health care. In: Post, S. (Ed.), *Encyclopedia of bioethics*, 3rd ed. vol. 5. Macmillan, New York, pp. 2495–2497.
10. Purtilo, R., 1994. Interdisciplinary health care teams and health care reform. *J Law Med Ethics* 22 (2), 121–126.
11. Jamison, K., 1999. *Night falls fast: Understanding suicide.* Knopf, New York, p. 255.
12. Donne, J., 1624. *Mediation XVII.* In: *Devotions upon emergent occasions and several steps in my sickness.* A.M, Thomas Jones, London.

Ethical Dimensions of the Professional-Patient Relationship

10

Why Honor Confidentiality?

Objectives

The reader should be able to:
- Define the terms confidentiality and confidential information.
- Identify the relationship of a patient's legal right to privacy with his or her reasonable expectations regarding confidential information.
- Describe the concept of "need to know" as it relates to maintaining confidentiality.
- Discuss the ethical norms involved in keeping and breaking professional confidences.
- Name five general legal exceptions to the professional standard of practice that confidences should not be broken.
- Consider practical options that a professional can take when faced with the possibility of breaking a confidence.
- Discuss some important aspects of documentation that affect confidentiality.
- Compare ethical issues of confidentiality traditionally conceived with those that have arisen because of computerized medical records and patient care information systems.
- Describe the key ethical strengths and challenges of the recent US federal regulations related to privacy considerations (Health Insurance Portability and Accountability Act of 1996).

New terms and ideas you will encounter in this chapter

trust	the medical record	Health Information
confidentiality	Health Insurance	Technology for
confidential information	Portability and	Economic and
right to privacy	Accountability	Clinical Health Act
need to know	Act of 1996	of 2009 (HITECH
patient care information	(HIPAA)	Act)
systems (PCIS)	protected health	health record databases
health information	information	panel of laboratory tests
managers		

Topics in this chapter introduced in earlier chapters

Topic	Introduced in chapter
Hippocratic oath	1
Character traits or virtues	2
Codes of ethics	2
Ethical dilemma	3
Beneficence	4
Nonmaleficence	4
Fidelity	4
Autonomy	4

Introduction

In this chapter and the next several chapters, you will have an opportunity to think about specific ways in which patients learn to put their *trust* in you. You already have met some patients through the stories that have been presented to help focus your thinking. The idea of *confidentiality* in health care has ancient roots as a basic building block of trust between health professionals and patients. For instance, the Hippocratic Oath, written in the fourth century BC, says,

> *"And whatsoever I shall see or hear in the course of my profession, as well as outside my profession...if it be what should not be published abroad, I will never divulge, holding such things to be holy secrets."*[1]

And so confidentiality is a splendid place to begin this focus on basic components of trust building. The story of Twyla Roberts, an occupational therapist, and Mary Louis, a patient, helps set the stage for reflection on confidentiality.

🐚 The Story of Twyla Roberts and Mary Louis

Twyla Roberts works as an occupational therapist for Marion Home Care Agency. Her patients are primarily elders, but she also occasionally treats children. All of Twyla's visits are performed in the home setting. She evaluates and treats throughout the community, and the agency is interconnected with two of the area hospitals and several outpatient clinics. The organizations are well connected electronically in one patient care information system. This arrangement allows Twyla to enter her patient information into the hospital's database and also to receive instant, thorough information on any activity her patients may have in the larger health care system. This electronic record also contains the patient health history and treatment activity. She refers to it many times each day and enters her own data each evening.

Thus, the clinical record of her patient, Mary Louis, is in "the system," and her progress after a fall is narrated. Mary has just been discharged from the hospital after a fall at home. She was seen by a surgeon, several nurses, a physical therapist, an occupational therapist, and when she was preparing for discharge, a social worker. She is now referred to the home care agency for a home safety evaluation and for ongoing therapy to regain function of her right hand, which was injured in the fall.

Twyla has been taught to document all relevant information about a patient; therefore, she is surprised about her own reluctance to record a conversation that occurred with Mary today. During their treatment session, Mary blurts out that the reason for her injury was not a fall. She has fallen in the past; however, this time her injury was the result of a domestic dispute. Mary's husband, who has middle-stage Alzheimer's disease, has been showing more signs of agitation. He became confused one evening, and a struggle ensued. Mary tried her best, but she was neither able to effectively reorient her husband nor manage his aggressive behavior. The incident ended abruptly when Mary's husband pushed her down the stairs. Despite her disorientation at the time, no one asked specifics regarding how she fell and so in the ambulance she told them she tripped rather than revealing the truth.

She says to Twyla, "I probably shouldn't have told you about this either. Now my secret is out. Please don't tell anyone. I am actually ashamed for my husband, you know. I don't want anybody to know about this. I am really afraid it might affect his ability to stay home. If my daughter finds out, she will surely have him sent to a nursing home. I know he is getting worse, but I would just die if we could not be together. Promise me you won't say anything!" Twyla does not promise, but neither does she tell Mary that her secret is not safe. Instead, she tries to talk with her about the importance of seeking respite care and of getting more assistance for her husband. But Mary says once again, "Please don't tell anyone."

Tywla completes her treatment and goes to the computer. She opens Mary's record and notes that the social worker, Michael White, was concerned about the home situation. He found Mary's husband to be quite irritable during hospital visits and so interviewed Mary several times without her husband but did not elicit any evidence that would classify him as a safety risk. Twyla realizes that if she documents this conversation, Mary's secret will be out for everyone on the patient information system to read. Suddenly, she realizes that Mary has shared information with her that she really wishes she did not have. Now Twyla wishes, too, that when Mary started talking about it she would have stopped her and said she could not promise to keep it confidential. But she did not. Still, she fears that if she does not document their conversation, she could regret it later.

1 *Reflection*

What should Twyla do next? Why? What should she ultimately do in regard to this situation? Why?

_____

_____

_____

_____

Many dimensions of Twyla's ethical quandary are identical to questions that have made confidentiality a compelling issue over the centuries. At the same time, because she lives in an era of computerized data entry, storage, and retrieval of patient information, her situation also is highly contemporary.

The Goal: A Caring Response

In light of all you have learned about Twyla and Mary, you know that her ethical goal of finding a caring response requires her to address both traditional and contemporary dimensions of confidentiality and the specific type of confidential information that this patient has shared. She needs to be clear about what confidentiality is and its appropriate use and limits. She needs to understand the related concept of privacy and to be savvy about new challenges regarding the use of computerized networks designed to manage information about patients.

Identifying Confidential Information

The most commonly accepted idea of *confidential information* in the professions is that it is information about a patient or client that is harmful, shameful, or embarrassing. Does it necessarily have to come directly from that person? No. Information that is furnished by the patient directly, or comes to you in writing or through electronic data, or even from a third party, might count as confidential.

Who is to be the judge of whether information is harmful, shameful, or embarrassing? The person himself or herself is the best judge, but any time you think a patient has a reasonable expectation that sensitive information will not be spread, it is best to err on the side of treating it as confidential. Of course, as Figure 10-1 illustrates, it is possible to go to extremes so that the best interests of the patient are lost in the process. A good general rule regarding potentially confidential information is to treat caution as a virtue.

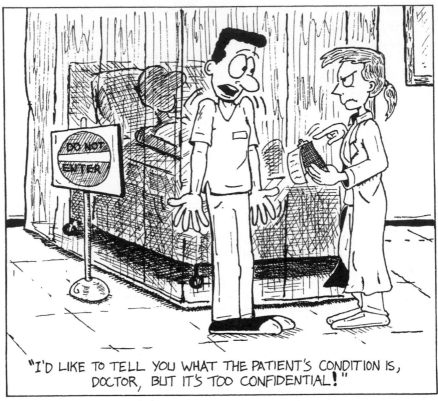

Figure 10-1.

Confidentiality and Privacy

Sometimes the notion of confidential information is discussed within the framework of the constitutional *right to privacy*.[2] This framework is not incorrect because the right to privacy means that there are aspects of a person's being into which no one else should intrude. We return to this idea of privacy later. At the same time, confidential information creates a situation a little different than privacy, taken alone.

Patients who share private information have chosen to relinquish their privacy because they have a reasonable expectation that sensitive information will be shared with certain people to further their welfare but with no one else.[3] The patient thinks, "I may have to tell you something very private, perhaps something I'm ashamed of, because I think you need to know it to plan what is best for me. But I do not want or expect you to spread the word around." There is an implicit understanding in the relationship that you, the professional, can perform your professional responsibilities only with accurate information from and about the patient. Patients and family caregivers trust that health professionals have the competency to maintain professionalism in communicating information necessary for health care delivery.

When you have confidential information from patients, they have a right to expect that you will honor your professional promise of confidentiality.

 SUMMARY

Confidentiality is one of the most basic principles in health care practice, and it is the most long-standing ethical dictum in health care codes of ethics. Confidentiality is the practice of keeping harmful, shameful, or embarrassing patient information within proper bounds. The right to privacy gives legal standing to this ethical principle.

Reflection
Go to the code of ethics or other guidelines of your profession and write down what it says about confidentiality.

_____

_____

_____

_____

Confidentiality, Secrets, and the "Need to Know"

Developmental theorists tell us that concern about confidentiality begins when a child first experiences a desire to keep or tell secrets. Secrets manifest a developing sense of self as separate from others, and the desire to share secrets is an expression of reaching out for intimate relationships with others. How secrets are handled in those early stages of development can have long-lasting effects on an individual's sense of security, self-esteem, and success at developing intimacy.[4] The power of a secret, or of being in a position to tell a secret, is nowhere conveyed more clearly than when a 2-year-old child has a secret pertaining to someone's birthday present! When was the last time that you had a secret that was so potent it was difficult, maybe impossible, to keep?

It is not considered a breach of confidentiality if you share "secret" information with other health professionals involved in the patient's care as long as the information has relevance to their role in the case. In fact, to share it is deemed essential for arriving at a caring response because up-to-date, thorough information is the structure on which high-quality health care delivery to a patient depends.[5] Some information comes from your clinical evaluation of the patient's condition; the rest has to come from the patient.

A reliable general test for who among team members should be given certain types of information is the *"need to know"* test. Need-to-know information is necessary for one to adequately perform one's specific job responsibilities. Does he or she need this information to help provide the most caring response to the patient? Sharing of clinical information must occur so that the health care system can effectively care for a patient. Information that passes the need-to-know test must be distinguished from that which a teammate might be interested to know and especially from information that has no bearing on the teammate's ability to offer optimum care.

 SUMMARY

Taken together, the immediate aims of confidentiality are to:
1. Facilitate the sharing of sensitive information with the goal of helping the patient.
2. Exclude unauthorized people from such information.
3. Discern need-to-know information from mere interest when deciding what to share.

 Reflection

Susan is a nurse who works in the orthopedic department of a large urban hospital. Her son's girlfriend was admitted to the medical department of the same hospital for treatment of a staph infection in her right ankle. Susan's son asks his mom to "look in the computer and find out what is going on with his girlfriend." What should Susan do?

_____

_____

_____

_____

If you answered that Susan should not access her son's girlfriend's record, you are correct. Susan is not a health professional on the team caring for this woman, so she does not have a "need to know" the details. She could go to visit the girlfriend in the hospital and offer her support; however, accessing her medical record would be a breach of confidentiality. Any information about a patient should never be passed along to someone not involved in the care of a patient. All patients have a right to privacy.

What if Susan worked in that department and was the nurse assigned to take care of her son's girlfriend? In this case, Susan would have a "need to know." If she was assigned to care for the girlfriend, she would need to access the medical record for relevant clinical details. Susan may choose to recuse herself from the case and seek an alternative patient assignment given that she knows the girlfriend; however, this decision would depend on other factors such as the needs of other patients on the unit and staffing.

Her need to know still would not warrant her sharing the information with her son.

Keeping Confidences

In Chapters 2 and 4, you were introduced to the ideas of caring and the character traits that a health professional should cultivate. Keeping secret information that flows from patient to health professional is not valued as an end in itself but rather as an instrument that serves trust. And the ultimate value that both the keeping of confidences and the subsequent building of trust points to is human dignity.

SUMMARY
Keep confidences
to
Build trust into the relationship
to
Maintain patients' dignity

To decrease trust is to cause harm. Understandably, when there are no conflicts, the health professional will be motivated to keep the confidences entrusted to him or her because it has long been understood that a trusting health professional–patient relationship must be built. Confidentiality serves as one cornerstone for that solid foundation. However, conflicts often arise in regard to keeping patient confidences, and health professionals must decide how to best balance these competing interests. This is reflected in a number of codes of ethics. Many contain statements similar to this one from the American Medical Association (AMA) Principles of Medical Ethics:

> *"A physician shall respect the rights of patients, of colleagues and of other health professionals, and shall safeguard patient confidences within the constraints of the law."[6]*

In such statements, the conflict is presented as one in which the health professional's duty to benefit and refrain from harming patients by keeping their secret is pitted against a duty to prevent harm to the patients themselves, to someone else, or to society.

Breaking Confidences

Although as you have seen previously, the importance of confidentiality is recognized in both law and professional practice, in certain cases, the most caring response requires breaching the patient's confidence.[7] Historically, such cases involved preventing harm to others, such as carriers of contagious diseases who wished to keep the condition a secret. The person does not have the prerogative of keeping the secret by requiring the professional to keep silent about the condition.

Legal exceptions to the standard of practice that confidences must be kept, except with the patient's consent or at the patient's request to break it, include the following[8]:

- An emergency in which keeping the confidence will harm the patient.
- The patient is incompetent or incapacitated, and a third party needs to be informed to be a surrogate decision maker for the patient.
- Third parties are at serious risk for harm (e.g., sexually transmitted diseases, child or other abuse).
- Request for commitment or hospitalization of a psychiatrically ill patient.
- A serious risk that many others may be harmed (a terrorist threat).

A good general rule of thumb is that you must not share confidential information unless it is required by the law or authorized by the patient personally. The presumption is that health professionals try to minimize the number of exceptions. Most patients do not know about the limits of confidentiality. It is a good practice to advise them before rather than after they have divulged sensitive information.

In conclusion, breaking confidences always entails at least one harm. Two questions we always ask when faced with such a decision are:

1. When is the harm of threatening the fragile trust in the relationship outweighed by the benefit?
2. How can the amount of harm be kept to a minimum when it becomes ethically appropriate to break a confidence?

The burden of proof is always on the health professional to minimize the harm.

The Six-Step Process in Confidentiality Situations

With the previous description of what confidentiality is and when it may legally or ethically be breached, let us return to the story of Twyla Roberts and Mary Louis to see how confidentiality works in everyday practice.

Step 1: Gather Relevant Information

One aspect of Twyla's concern arises from the nature of Mary's comments. She always assumes that patients are telling the truth (until she has had it proven to the contrary). If so, she may want to talk to her more about her knowledge of the event because to do so will help her understand the situation better. Was this the first time such an event occurred? Does Mary feel unsafe in her home? Is Mary's daughter involved in the care of her parents? How well is the spouse's dementia condition being managed? Increasingly adults with dementia are receiving care in the community sector. What resources are available to Mary? To her spouse? How will Mary's role as a caregiver be impacted by her new injuries? Who are the other stakeholders in this case?

Another avenue of discussion Twyla may wish to pursue is why Mary does not want "anyone" to know. She has blurted out some reasons. Often spouses of patients with Alzheimer's disease withhold information on the basis of detailed moral, social, and psychological considerations that involve deep emotional investment. Family dynamics are often complex, and dissenting opinions regarding care plans can negatively impact the quality of life for couples.[9]

Steps 2 and 3: Identify the Type of Ethical Problem and the Ethics Approach to Analyze It

Twyla knows that, despite these caring responses, in the end it boils down to whether she should document their conversation in Mary's medical record, knowing that by doing so she is opening this information to others.

 Reflection
What kind of ethical problem does Twyla have? Is it moral distress? An ethical dilemma? Take a minute to jot down your response before proceeding.

_____

_____

_____

_____

In some instances of confidentiality, moral distress may face the moral agent. However, Twyla has not been prohibited from documenting the conversation. She is experiencing such distress from her belief that she should document the conversation but knows it may cause harm to Mary. At the very least, it will shake Mary's trust in her. She cannot achieve both the outcome of keeping the confidence and the one of doing her duty to document relevant information. She is facing a classical version of an ethical dilemma.

 Reflection
From the standpoint of a health professional's goal of arriving at a caring response, name three ethical principles that will help guide your thinking about your conduct in regard to keeping confidences.

Principles:

1. _____

2. _____

3. _____

Name some character traits that will help you in these challenging situations.

Character Traits

1. _____

2. _____

3. _____

If you answered with the principles of beneficence, nonmaleficence, or fidelity and the right to autonomy, you are grasping the ethical principles or elements that support confidentiality. A key character trait is trustworthiness (i.e., your part of the bargain if you are asking the patient to trust you). Other traits include kindness, compassion, and courage to break confidences when it is ethically or legally necessary to do so.

Step 4: Explore the Practical Alternatives

What options does Twyla have in trying to discern what to do?

One way that Twyla can handle this situation is to keep the confidence by sharing it with another health professional on the team who would have a good reason to learn about this information. Often a health professional's inability to assess whether a person outside the immediate health care team should be given information leads the professional to discuss it with a trusted colleague first. For Twyla, one person seems to be the obvious choice: the social worker who treated Mary at the hospital. Part of the motive of this discussion among professionals would be to clarify whether Mary has spoken to anyone else and also to confirm how she should proceed.

Often, an additional outcome of this type of in-house discussion is to determine whether further action on behalf of the patient should be taken. Social workers are well trained in the policies and procedures that relate to elder abuse and neglect. By collaborating with the social worker, Twyla expands her knowledge and maximizes resources. If Mary remains unwilling to self report or talk with professionals or family regarding her circumstance, Twyla will be in the type of situation that the AMA (and many other) codes have in mind when they suggest that breaking the confidence may "become necessary in order to protect the welfare of the individual." In Mary's case, the social worker may agree wholeheartedly that Mary's comments warrant documentation and follow up. He may suggest that Twyla again recommend that Mary make an appointment to follow up for caregiver support. The suggestion could be put in such a way as to assure her that it is Twyla's concern for Mary and her spouse that prompts the suggestion. It may be exactly what Mary needs.

Another option for Twyla would be to say nothing but still make note of the conversation on the patient's record.

Do you think this is a good idea? We do not. It breaks the confidence of the patient without taking any further direct action to let her know what she has decided to do and why. Although it may relieve the health professional's anxiety, at least momentarily, in this case, it probably will serve little useful moral purpose in regard to helping Mary. In some cases, Twyla may see this as her only alternative, but she has not yet tried to go back to Mary to warn her of what she has determined she must do.

If Twyla goes directly back to Mary and reveals to her in a supportive way that the conversation was deeply troubling, Mary quite possibly could gain better insight into the seriousness of her comments. Mary may be suffering from mental stress and caregiver fatigue, two common outcomes of spousal care giving in long-term, serious conditions.[10] Twyla can be a help in referring Mary to someone who can assist her and her husband. But at least she will know that in choosing to proceed as she did (in telling her about his serious condition), Twyla did not take this plight lightly. She used her ethical reasoning.

Step 5: Complete the Action

This case, like many we discuss, does not admit of simple answers. It would seem, however, that given all the aspects of her role as a moral agent, Twyla should go back to Mary immediately to discuss her concern. She also should let her know that she is compelled to at least document the conversation because it is information highly relevant to her own care, and a part of her moral duty to document such exchanges.

Step 6: Evaluate the Process and Outcome

Obviously, any caring professional would be concerned about the consequences of overriding a patient's wishes in a situation where the latter thought she could count on the professional to keep a "deep, dark secret." Whatever Twyla decides to do, she will benefit by taking time to review her actions and motives each step of the way.

Confidentiality, Records, and Patient Care Information Systems

Another aspect of confidentiality raised in this story is the process of information sharing and record keeping that goes on within the health care (and other institutional) systems. For example, Mary's report of abuse, if documented, will remain in her permanent electronic record. The issue of how far this information should and can go takes on greater importance when one considers modern, computerized systems of record keeping called *patient care information systems (PCIS)*. Virtually all major health care institutions and agencies currently use computerized data sheets that enable easy entry, storage, and retrieval of almost any information. This aspect of the patient's care has become so sophisticated that a group of professionals called *health information managers* are key members of the health care team. Their primary role is that they "are responsible for designing and maintaining the system that facilitates the collection, use and dissemination of health and medical information."[11] Depending on what is requested and the policies of the health care plan at her institution, the information regarding Mary's self report may be released to insurance agencies, other care providers, people conducting research, or state agencies. In short, Mary's and her husband's living situation is in danger of changing because of information documented in her record. Twyla must be aware that if she records their discussion, Mary's husband may get stuck with a stigmatizing profile.

Although ethics as expressed in the codes of ethics of most health professions requires that information about patients be kept confidential unless some strongly overriding argument for disclosure exists, the realities of modern health care make this difficult. As noted previously, these medical records are accessible to many different people and agencies, for many different reasons, and computerized data systems compound the problem. Thus, any information that may impair the patient's ability to function freely and confidently in society must be more carefully weighed than ever before it is recorded in the medical record.

The Medical Record

The medical record is an extremely useful document for health professionals. Medical records can be found in both paper and electronic form. Records are systematic accounts of a patient's encounter with a health provider. They serve as a repository of information. They are generated by and contributed to by many providers in various health delivery settings. An electronic health record (EHR) is an electronic record of patient health information. Not unlike the paper record, EHRs often include patient demographics, progress notes, problems, medications, relevant social history, medical history, vital signs, laboratory data, and diagnostic reports. Regardless of the type of medical record used, information about the patient that is true and is relevant to his or her health care ought to be recorded there. At the same time, harm can be done if faulty, erroneous, speculative, or vague information is included because it can be duplicated and spread to several locations in both paper and electronic medical records.

One example of this is the story of a middle-aged woman who was hospitalized at a university hospital where many invasive and dangerous procedures were carried out to evaluate a problem of incipient renal failure. Several doctors were writing the orders for these tests, and she judged that none of them bothered to explain fully what was being done or why, even though she signed consent forms. She became fearful, then hysterical, claiming that she could trust none of her doctors and that they were trying to kill her. She left the hospital against medical advice, and the medical intern writing her case summary included "acute paranoid-type behavior" as one of the notations. Thus, her subsequent encounters with health professionals were strongly influenced by this incorrect "diagnosis."

In this case, the patient was harmed by information in the record that was untrue. True information also can be harmful to a patient when not treated respectfully. For example, a 62-year-old man hospitalized after a stroke was lying in bed and overheard two health professionals outside his room discussing how he had suffered his stroke while "getting it on" with his wife. He was embarrassed and angry and refused to accept their treatment attempts after that. It made him distrustful of all the other health professionals involved in his care because he was sure that such gossip was not limited to the two whose conversation he had overheard. The information was written as part of his admitting history and physical: "The patient suddenly lost the function of his right arm and leg while having intercourse with his wife." Sexual activity or habits are often relevant to medical care (e.g., in the case of sexually transmitted disease or sexual dysfunction); in such cases, information should not be fodder for idle gossip in hospital corridors.

As you return to the story of Twyla and Mary presented at the beginning of this chapter, it is important to recognize the great power of the information about your patients or others. Three guidelines are applicable:
1. Questionable information should be clearly labeled as questionable.
2. True information that is not relevant should not be recorded.
3. All information should be handled among health professionals with regard for the privacy and dignity of patients.

Information recorded in the medical record can be of great help or harm to the patient. For this reason, the medical record needs to be treated with a great deal of respect. Health information managers and others involved with medical record information are usually highly aware of the power of these documents. They function as the gatekeepers for the records and rightfully take great pains to keep the records in order and to make sure that they are available to those professionals who need them and who have a right to see them. Conversely, they also need to be careful that the records are not abused or released to unauthorized persons. Sugarman notes:

> *"The increasing use of electronic medical records and the creation of computerized databases, while clearly beneficial for many aspects of patient care, raise important questions regarding privacy and confidentiality. The easy retrieval and transmission of such records make them tempting targets for those interested in unauthorized access."*[12]

Electronic communications are discussed further in Chapter 11; however, it is important to remember that confidentiality applies to all information communicated regarding the patient, whether in verbal conversation, handwritten documentation, or electronic communication.

 Reflection

Have you ever seen this disclaimer on the end of an e-mail or fax?

"The information transmitted in this email is intended only for the person or entity to which it is addressed and may contain confidential and/or privileged material. Any review, retransmission, dissemination or other use of or taking of any action in reliance upon this information by persons or entities other than the intended recipient is prohibited. If you receive this email in error, please contact the sender and delete the material from any computer."

Why do you think that it is there? How does it relate to confidentiality?

_____

_____

_____

_____

In the end, everyone is responsible for the confidentiality of patient information. Whether it be professional colleagues engaging in a conversation in the corridor, those handling the management of formal records, or the individual health professional properly disposing of work sheets and notes, taking care to log off the computer after use, and being vigilant in the use of fax or copy machines. The technology of health care information is only as effective as the professionals and others who use the devices allow it to be.

SUMMARY

Confidentiality finally comes down to each professional being vigilant about the flow of patient information, guided by the goal of using information to help the patient.

Patient Privacy: Health Insurance Portability and Accountability Act of 1996

Concerns about the collection, storage, and use of sensitive information have led to much discussion by patients and the public in recent years, so that the notion of private information increasingly has been mentioned as relevant to considerations of confidentiality. In 1996, the United States passed regulations under the *Health Insurance Portability and Accountability Act (HIPAA)*, which imposed considerable new constraints on the use and disclosure of a patient's personal and clinical information. These regulations went into effect in April 2003 and continue to govern patient privacy as related to health care communications. A major goal of HIPAA is to ensure that an individual's health information is properly protected while allowing the flow of information needed to promote high-quality care.

This set of regulations, called the New Federal Medical-Privacy Rule,[13] took 5 years to go into effect. The basic intent is to control the use or disclosure of *"protected health information."* One area that this rule strongly affects is the handling of information for purposes of research. It also has been interpreted to mean that information about patients (including family members) cannot be released.

> *"The rule concerns all 'individually identifiable' health information created or maintained by covered entity, defined broadly as information about physical or mental health that either identifies an individual person or with respect to which there is a reasonable basis to believe the information can be used to identify the person."[14]*

A "covered entity" is defined as a health plan, data processing company, health care professional, or hospital.

The Health Information Technology for Economic and Clinical Health Act

The Health Information Technology for Economic and Clinical Health Act (HITECH Act), which was Title XIII of the American Recovery and Reinvestment Act of 2009, was signed into law in February 2009. Parts of this act expanded and strengthened the privacy laws that protect patient health information originally outlined under HIPAA. The HITECH Act provides additional provisions regarding privacy and security breaches, reporting of breaches, accounting of disclosures, restrictions of disclosures for sales and marketing purposes, and monetary penalties associated with HIPAA violations.[15] The act also designates funding to modernize the health care system by promoting and expanding the adoption of health information technology by 2014. This expands the federal government's effort to establish a national electronic patient records system by 2014 and provides for comprehensive records privacy and security standards. One of the challenges facing the United States national adoption of electronic medical records is ensuring the privacy of electronically accessed information. It is essential that both patients and a variety of health professionals participate in these policy discussions so that important ethical issues can be contemplated and decisions regarding *health record databases* and their approved usage can be articulated nationally and globally.[16] You will learn more about professional citizenship and moral advocacy in Section V of this text, which looks at ethical dimensions of the social context of health care.

As you can see, you are entering the health professions at a time when these new legal parameters about what can and cannot be shared will continue to be a source of discussion, revision, and refinement, hopefully so that the intent of preventing undue invasion of a patient's privacy can be balanced against the legitimate incursions into privacy that have served patients' interests well over the centuries. In other words, the notion of privacy as a conceptual core for information that needs to be taken into account for patient care is an appropriate move. The details of how this will be best accomplished continue to unfold.[17]

Summary

Keeping confidences is a general ethical guideline that the health professional can rely on to maintain trust and to foster dignity in the health professional–patient relationship. Sometimes, however, the interests of another person or society or even the best interests of the patient advise against keeping the confidence.

Current computerized methods of record keeping and information sharing raise additional, difficult ethical questions related to confidentiality. As a health professional, you must rely on sound clinical reasoning regarding the various moral obligations of professional practice, the rights of all involved, and the character traits that enable you to maintain a relationship of trust to arrive at a decision that is the most consistent with the goal of a caring response.

Questions for Thought and Discussion

1. Sonia is a nurse practitioner student completing her final clinical in an outpatient primary care setting. She is caring for Lea, a 42-year-old woman who visited the office last week for ongoing fatigue and

generalized weakness. Sonia conducted several blood tests on Lea (called a *panel of laboratory tests*) and told her she would get back to her with the results. Sonia's supervisor concurred with the laboratory tests Sonia requested but also added a human chorionic gonadotropin (hCG) test to the panel to rule out pregnancy as the cause of her symptoms. Sonia accessed the laboratory work via the computerized system and found all of Lea's laboratory test results were negative with the exception of elevated hCG levels. Sonia picks up the phone and dials Lea's number to inform her of the results. As she prepares to leave a message, she hesitates.

Why do you think Sonia hesitated?

What should Sonia say? Defend your response using ethical principles that support confidentiality.

2. The story of Mr. Shaw provides a good basis for thinking about some of the things you have just learned.

Ann von Essen is a health professional, and David Shaw is a patient in the hospital where she works. He has been referred to her for discharge planning.

Mr. Shaw is a pleasant man, 42 years old, whose family often is at his side during visiting hours. He was admitted to the hospital with numerous fractures and a contusion after an automobile accident in which his car "skidded out of control and hit a tree." He has no memory of the accident, but the person traveling behind him reported the scene.

The arrangement for his discharge is going smoothly. During one of Ann von Essen's visits, however, Mr. Shaw's mother, a wiry old woman of about 80 years, follows her down the corridor. At the elevator, Mrs. Shaw says, "I wish you'd tell sonny not to drive. It's those epileptic fits he has, you know. He's had 'em since he was a kid. Lordy, I'm scared to death he's going to kill himself and someone else too." Ann is at a loss about what to say. She thanks Mrs. Shaw and jumps on the elevator. She goes down the elevator for one flight, gets off, and runs back up the stairs to the nurses' desk. She logs on to the computer to review Mr. Shaw's medical record and finds nothing about any type of seizures. Put yourself in the place of Ann von Essen. Do you have confidential information? What should you do? Why?

Let us assume that in the state in which you work the law requires that people suffering from epileptic seizures be reported to the Department of Public Health, which in turn reports them to the Department of Motor Vehicles.

a. What do you think is the morally "right" action to take regarding Mr. Shaw once you have become the recipient of the information about his possible problem?

b. What duties and rights inform your decision about what to do?

c. Suppose you believe that it is morally right for the Department of Motor Vehicles to be advised of this situation. The obvious course of action is for you to inform the physician, the physician to report to the Department of Public Health, and the Department of Public Health to report to the Department of Motor Vehicles. If any of the usual links in this process are broken by failure to communicate the information, do you have a responsibility to make sure the Department of Motor Vehicles has actually received this information? Defend your position regarding how far you believe you and anyone else in your profession should go in pursuing this matter.

REFERENCES

1. Hippocrates, 1923. The Oath. In: Jones, W.H.S. (Trans.), *Hippocrates I*. The Loeb Classic Library. Harvard University Press, Cambridge, MA, pp. 299–301.
2. *Griswold v. Connecticut*, 1965. 381 U.S. 479. 85 S Ct. 1678.
3. Beauchamp, T.L., Childress, J., 2009. Professional-patient relationships. In: *Principles of biomedical ethics*, 5th ed. Oxford University Press, New York, pp. 288–331.
4. Winslade, W., 2004. Confidentiality. In: Post, S. (Ed.), *Encyclopedia of bioethics*, 3rd ed, vol. 4. Macmillan, New York, pp. 494–503.
5. Milton, C.L., 2009. Information sharing: Transparency, nursing ethics, and practice implications with electronic medical records. *Nurs Sci Q* 22 (3), 214–219.
6. American Medical Association, 2002. *Code of medical ethics*. The Association, Chicago, IL.
7. McHale, J.V., 2009. Patient confidentiality and mental health. *Br J Nurs* 18 (5), 944–945.
8. Gutheil, T.G., Appelbaum, P.S., 1988. Confidentiality and privilege. In: *Clinical handbook of psychiatry and the law*. McGraw-Hill, New York, pp. 2–29.
9. Tracy, C.S., Drummond, N., Ferris, L.E., et al., 2004. To tell or not to tell? Professional and lay perspectives on the disclosure of personal health information in community based dementia care. *Can J Aging* 23 (3), 203–215.
10. Blustein, J.T., 2004. The weight of shared lives: Truth telling and family caregiving. In: Levine, C., Murray, T.H. (Eds.), *The cultures of care giving: conflict and common ground among families, health professionals and policy makers*. The Johns Hopkins Press, Baltimore, MD, pp. 47–55.
11. Harman, L., 2001. *Ethical challenges in the management of health information*. Aspen Publishers, Inc, Gaithersburg, MD.
12. Sugarman, J., 2000. *20 Common problems. Ethics in primary care*. McGraw-Hill, New York, pp. 158–159.
13. U.S. Department of Health and Human Services, 2002. *Federal Register* 67, pp. 53182–53273.
14. Kulynych, J., Korn, D., 2002. The new federal medical privacy rule. *N Engl J Med* 347 (15), 1133–1134.
15. American Recovery and Reinvestment Act of 2009. One Hundred and Eleventh Congress of the United States, First Session, January 6, 2009. Available from: <http://frwebgate.access.gpo.gov/cgi-bin/getdoc.cgi?dbname=111_cong_bills&docid=f:h1enr.pdf> (accessed 8.10.09).

16. Milton, C.L., 2009. Information sharing: Transparency, nursing ethics, and practice implications with electronic medical records. *Nurs Sci Q* 22 (3), pp. 214–219.
17. Annas, G., 2003. HIPAA regulations—A new era of medical-record privacy? *N Engl J Med* 348 (15), 1486–1490.

11

Communication and Information Sharing

Objectives

The reader should be able to:
- Recognize the ethical relevance of communication in achieving a caring response.
- Identify six steps in the analysis of ethical problems encountered in healthcare communications.
- Understand the goals of healthcare communication.
- Describe why dignity is an essential component of ethical communications.
- Discuss the concept of shared decision making and its role in achieving a caring response.
- Identify several tools to aid in effective communication.
- Become familiar with national standards that relate to communication for safe and quality care.
- Reflect on how new technology can ethically impact health care communications.

New terms and ideas you will encounter in this chapter

nonverbal communication	dignity	patient rights and responsibilities
active listening	hope	health literacy
shared decision making	disclosure/ nondisclosure	hand offs
do not resuscitate		

Topics in this chapter introduced in earlier chapters

Topic	Introduced in chapter
Ethics committee	1
A caring response	2
Honesty and integrity	2
Patient rights and responsibilities	2
Moral distress	3
Deontology	4
Ethics of care	4
Narrative reasoning	4
Moral courage	4
Autonomy, beneficence, nonmaleficence, veracity	4
Six-step process	5
Responsibility	5
Team loyalty	9
Confidentiality	10
Trust	10

Introduction

Communication is an essential part of healthcare delivery. You have just read in the previous chapter about the importance of confidentiality. Confidence in another is a foundational aspect of the patient–health professional relationship. Confidentiality is about holding information. Communication is about sharing information. How information is shared in health care is vitally important. In this chapter, we turn to the ethical dimensions of sharing information in finding a caring response.

Consider the following scenario: Mary Beth is riding the train on her morning commute into work. She works as a recreational therapist in an inpatient mental health clinic. Sitting across from her is a young woman having a conversation on her cell phone. The young woman disregards her public surroundings, talking loudly throughout the call. Others on the train cannot help but overhear her as she talks openly in this shared space. Her conversation details a discussion she had last night with her mother about her sister's new husband. She elaborates how they suspect that the new husband has a serious problem with alcohol. She talks with detail of his drinking patterns and behaviors. She shares her concern regarding potential depression and abuse. Many individuals try to distance themselves from this young woman, but the train is full. They look away, reading their papers and listening to music. Mary Beth has neither with her. She closes her eyes and secretly hopes the young woman's cell phone will run out of battery life.

Reflection

Have you ever experienced such a situation? If so, what has been your reaction?

_____

_____

_____

_____

Is anything happening in this conversation that seems unethical? Why or why not?

_____

_____

_____

_____

This scenario highlights a social communication. It is a communication shared between two individuals through the long accepted mode of telephone technology. We believe the communication is not unethical but clearly demonstrates poor judgment and etiquette. The cell phone user may see the conversation as normal social discourse; however, it violates the privacy of both the people in the conversation and the commuters.

Reflection

What if the young woman talking on her cell phone was a health care provider sharing the story of a patient she treated? Would that be different? If so, how?

_____

_____

_____

_____

Communication

Communication is identified by many as a key foundational aspect of thera-peutic relationships.[1] Multiple research studies have shown that effective com-munication is an essential tool for the development of a successful treatment plan, improved patient knowledge, adherence to treatment regimes, and im-proved psychosocial and behavioral outcomes. Communication happens on many levels and in many ways. We do it so often that we often neglect to think of it or actualize its importance. Levetown helps highlights this well when she states "communication is the most common 'procedure' in medicine."[2] We communicate through spoken and written words and languages. We commu-nicate nonverbally. *Nonverbal communication* is expressed through body lan-guage, gestures, and mannerisms. We also communicate through various technologic means. Some of these are well established, such as telephones and pagers. Some are newer technologics, such as cellular phones and e-mail. Some are evolving technologies, such as blogs, video conferencing, text mes-sages, and social networking sites. Health professionals communicate directly with the patient him or herself and are also responsible for communicating effectively with other providers, family members, schools, interpreters, pay-ers, and other stakeholders to achieve the best care delivery. To do so, skilled communication is necessary.

The goal of this chapter is not to provide a comprehensive overview of communication in health care settings but rather to highlight how ethical problems may present surrounding such communications. Miscommunica-tions and poor communications often precipitate ethical problems. In the pages that follow, we hope that you will gain a broader understanding of the role of skilled communication in achieving a caring response.

The Purpose of Communication

A primary goal of health care communication is to achieve successful infor-mation transfer and exchange. It is a means of informing and advising our patients. But it is also about much more. It includes *active listening*. Active listening is used when a health professional listens to the patient's verbal and nonverbal communication. Active listening includes attention to cues in the conversation. It includes responding and validating to convey under-standing. Communication also includes educating, collaborating, coordi-nating, decision making, and partnering. Through communication, health care providers develop a relational dynamic with the patient, which when successful, serves to facilitate shared decision making. *Shared decision mak-ing* is the concept that decisions are made based on an underlying assump-tion of mutual respect and joint interest. Health professionals have both the opportunity and the duty to shape communications to hold respect in the relationship.

Shared Decision Making

Shared decision making values patient autonomy. Shared decision making is a process in which information is exchanged not *from* professional to patient but *between* professional and patient. Professionals sufficiently inform patients regarding the health options and best available evidence supporting those options, and patients share with providers their values, goals, and preferences.[3] In this way, decisions are better informed. The professional and patient then work together to arrive at the best decision option. In this model, because information is shared, the two partners can negotiate and commit to a collaborative agreement regarding health care decisions.[4]

 SUMMARY

Shared decision making is a tool for a caring response.

🥄 **The Story of Beth Tottle, Mrs. Uwilla, and Her Family**

Mrs. Uwilla is a 67-year-old woman from Haiti. She came to the United States to visit and assist her daughter and family with the birth of their second child. She is a widow and the mother of six children, two deceased, three living in Haiti, and one in the United States. Mrs. Uwilla is non-English speaking; her native language is a dialect of French Creole. Of modest means, Mrs. Uwilla supported herself caring for her grandchildren and other children in her rural Haitian village. A short while after arriving in the United States, Mrs. Uwilla collapsed on the sidewalk while walking with her daughter. She was taken to Mercy Trauma Center where it was determined that she sustained a severe subarachnoid hemorrhage from a ruptured cerebral aneurysm. She was admitted to the hospital and underwent a life-saving, emergent hemicraniectomy, a procedure in which the neurosurgeon removes a portion of the skull bone to allow for brain swelling. While in the intensive care unit (ICU), she underwent placement of a tracheostomy and a gastrostomy tube (G-tube). She was successfully taken off of mechanical ventilation but was unable to eat and continued to be fed via G-tube. Mrs. Uwilla was nonverbal and immobile and maintained a very low level of consciousness. Her tracheostomy was closed, but she remained minimally interactive and dependent in all activities of daily living.

Beth Tottle, the case manager assigned to care for Mrs. Uwilla, kept up to date regarding her clinical condition. It was her job to help coordinate a safe discharge plan for all patients on the neurosurgery unit. Mrs. Uwilla's daughter, Mica, delivered her new child and was able to visit her mother only sporadically as she was recovering from childbirth and had no other help at home.

Beth was helping to coordinate Mrs. Uwilla's care and asked Mica if anyone else could help. Mica told Beth that Mica's older brother Rene might be able to come to the United States to help. Rene had called the unit several times and kept up to date via phone calls. He is a religious man and was concerned for his mother. The doctors had told him it would take a few months for them to replace Mrs. Uwilla's skull bone and for the swelling to resolve. They have also told him that she may be able to receive rehabilitative care in the United States but that they would not know her options for sure until the case management team was able to do some searching.

After several phone conversations, Beth Tottle was able to convince Rene Uwilla to travel to the United States. He arrived 1 month into her hospitalization to assist the family in decision making regarding the next steps. He cried on seeing his mother in her hospital room. The day after he arrived, a family/team meeting was scheduled, during which Mrs. Uwilla's slow but steady progress to date was outlined. The resident physician told Mr. Uwilla that they need to make some decisions regarding her future care, most significantly her "code status." He states, "We are recommending your mom be made *do not resuscitate (DNR)*. This means if her heart stops, we won't restart it." The case manager and other members of the rehabilitative team also begin to educate Mr. Uwilla regarding the discharge planning process. Because Mrs. Uwilla is not a U.S. citizen and lacks health insurance, her options for rehabilitation are limited. They ask Mr. Uwilla to consider taking his mother back home to Haiti, although they realize that the care there will be suboptimal.

Mr. Uwilla is overwhelmed and angry and immediately responds to this by saying, "Now I see why it was so urgent to come here. You told me she would be rehabilitated here but now say that option is 'very limited.' Not only do you want me to get my mother out of here, you also want me to kill her. You see her as work—she is a human being! This is the woman who taught me to love. I can't be expected to immediately manage all of this. I am only one person." The team was caught off guard by his response, many of them looking to each other for assistance.

Reflection

What do you think led to Mr. Uwilla's response?

_____

_____

_____

_____

What are the communication needs of this family?

_____

_____

_____

_____

The Six-Step Process in Communication

Step 1: Gather Relevant Information

Beth Tottle's (and the care team's) duties of beneficence and veracity dictate that she must attempt to assess Mr. Uwilla's statement accurately. It is possible that Mr. Uwilla is asking the team this question because he wants them to reassure him that he does not have to face the uncertainty of his mother's recovery alone. It also is possible that he wants reassurance that he is part of the decision making process for his mom's care. Differences in power are quite prevalent in communication. These differences should be lessened in the shared decision making model; however, research shows that they continue to be prevalent in how professionals communicate with patients and families.[5]

It is important to be as sensitive as possible to the implicit, unspoken messages that are contained in language. This is true of all verbal communications between individuals. Here, Mr. Uwilla is expressing a nameless fear with the statement that the team wants him "to kill his mom." We know that he is a religious man and that there may be religious or spiritual beliefs associated with what he hears. He may have heard that in the United States individuals of an older age are not valued and perceive that the staff would like her to die. He is in a vulnerable situation at the moment. Often times, when DNR status is raised, it can be perceived as abandonment of the patient or family.

The health professionals must also acknowledge the fact that Mr. Uwilla and his family are from a Haitian culture. This is a different culture from that of the Western, predominately white care providers. Currently no one on the care team is of this cultural background. Beth herself knows very little from the Haitian point of view. She cannot help but wonder what illness or disability even means in the Uwilla's culture? This cultural point of view becomes ethically relevant information because it can serve to drive the decision making process.

Mr. Uwilla's anxiety is likely heightened by the feelings of helplessness and insecurity that arise when a loved one has an uncertain prognosis. Patients and family members are not the only ones who do not like uncertainty; health professionals often have difficulty with it as well. Uncertainty is a concept that implies limitations to knowledge of a particular outcome.[6] We often do not have adequate statistics to present a likely future course for patient conditions as seriously compromised as Mrs. Uwilla's. In neurosurgery, outcome after hemicraniectomy has been traditionally measured according to survival and level of disability; however, researchers and clinicians are now looking at measures of quality of life as well. Mr. Uwilla's real question may concern the extent of his mother's anticipated recovery. How will he know how much and when she will get better? Everyone has told him her recovery will be a long road. What does that mean? He may be asking beyond "What if her heart stops beating," to "Will you still care for her?" or "What is at the end of this tunnel?"

In summary, the first important step in Beth Tottle's assessment of this situation is to gather the relevant information by gaining a better understanding of what Mr. Uwilla heard, what he is asking, and what the sources of his discomfort are.

 Reflection

We have listed some types of information about the communication (or lack of it) we think are relevant. What other types of information would you want to have before proceeding in this situation?

Step 2: Identify the Type of Ethical Problem

This case provides an example of a poor communication that precipitates moral distress. Indeed, a central problem for Beth—and for the team of health professionals—specifically has to do with professional relationships and care planning. Nurses, therapists, chaplains, technologists, dietitians, pharmacists, social workers, and others may find themselves in the difficult position of being caught in the middle between the medical need for timely decision making and their own assessment of how a caring response consistent with the best interests of the patient can be realized. The structure of the health care system, as it has developed throughout history, has been characterized by hierarchical relationships. Currently, that model is being altered because more types of professionals serve as points of entry into the health care system and because of the greater sophistication of many team members. A well-coordinated team effort on behalf of the patient makes the most efficient use of resources, time, and energy and supports the patient's attitude of trust toward those entrusted with his or her care.

This story also highlights the impact of the context on ethical decision making. The role of the family caregiver (Mr. Uwilla) in this case is to protect hope. The role of the professional care providers (the team) is to predict hope. These roles are currently challenged by the clinical ambiguity, the possibility of a language or cultural barrier, and other factors.

Dignity as a Foundational Concept

As you will recall from previous chapters, respect for self and respect for persons are important character traits of health professionals. Haddock defines *dignity* as "the ability to feel important and valuable in relation to others, communicate this to others, and be treated as such by others."[7] This definition highlights the necessary regard for dignity in health professional and patient communications as it has shared meaning in the relational dynamic. Because communication is a relational dynamic, dignity can be considered as two values: other-regarding by respecting the dignity of others, and self-regarding by respecting one's own dignity.[8] You should recognize this concept from earlier chapters in which the concept of self care was introduced.

Reflection

Perhaps one of the best ways to recognize the importance of respect or dignity in communication is to reflect on a time when it was missing. Can you recall an interaction that you have had with someone in which you felt as though you were not treated with dignity?

How did that make you feel? How did it impact your autonomy or sense of control?

_____

_____

_____

_____

Communication: Hope and Disclosure

Hope. It has long been debated how to honor *hope* through discussion of *disclosure and nondisclosure*. Health professionals must balance how to best communicate clinical information as it relates to hope. Hope engenders the

Successful disclosure communications are both sensitive and concise. Underlying this bias toward greater disclosure of information is the conviction that if you convey the message that you still care and have the intention and ability to comfort, then it is possible to tell the truth and still help maintain the patient's trust and hope. Benevolence is expressed through honesty rather than played off against it.

Patient Rights and Responsibilities. An additional factor that supports direct disclosure of information to patients is the understanding of patient rights. It is believed that patients have a right to information about their conditions if they want this information. As introduced in Chapter 2, *patient rights and responsibilities* documents outline these patient (or consumer) protections. The goal of a patient's rights and responsibilities statement (Figure 11-1) is to strengthen consumer confidence that the health care system is fair and responsive to consumer needs; to affirm the importance of a strong relationship between patients and their providers; and to highlight the critical role that patients play in safeguarding their own health.[13] In such documents, there is an assumption that a patient has a right to the truth about his or her condition, and it is reasonable to believe that you, the health professional, do not have the prerogative of withholding it.

As a patient at Tingsboro Hospital, we want you to know your rights and responsibilities. We encourage you to communicate openly with your health care team and to advance your own health by being well informed regarding your care. Listed below are your rights and responsibilities.

Your Rights

- You have the right to receive accurate and understandable information to assist you in making an informed decision regarding your health care.
- You have the right to considerate and compassionate care that respects your culture, values, and beliefs. You have the right to this care regardless of your age, race, religion, sexual orientation, gender, or disability.
- You have the right to know that names of the health care providers involved in your care.
- You have the right to communicate with your providers in confidence and to have the confidentiality of your health information protected. You have a right to review and request copies of your medical records.
- You have the right to access emergency health services when and where the need arrives.
- You have the right to fully participate in all decisions regarding your health care, including the decision to refuse or discontinue treatment to the extent permitted by the law.
- You have the right to voice your concerns about the care you receive. This includes the right to a fair and efficient process for resolving differences with health plans, health care providers, and the institutions that serve them.

Figure 11-1. Patient's Rights and Responsibilities.

Continued

Your Responsibilities

- You are expected to provide to the best of your ability accurate and complete information regarding your identity, condition, past illnesses, medicines, and any other information that relates to your health.
- You are expected to ask questions when you do not understand, or believe that you cannot follow through with your treatment plan. You are responsible for your health outcomes if you do not follow the mutually agreed upon care plan.
- You are expected to treat all hospital staff, other patients, and visitors (and their property) with courtesy and respect.
- You are expected to keep appointments, be on time for appointments, or call your health care provider if you cannot keep your appointment. If financial needs arise, you are expected to be honest with us so we may connect you to the appropriate resources.

Figure 11-1, cont'd

There is a duty to share the information if the patient wishes this information, and withholding it can be viewed as a type of injury to the patient's trust. If information is withheld, it must be on the basis of other moral considerations deemed more compelling than the patient's right and your corresponding duty to disclose in a given situation.

⊚ SUMMARY

It is the ethical duty of the health professional to balance hope and disclosure, while respecting the dignity and rights of each individual patient.

 Reflection
Give an example of when you think it is benevolent to share difficult information with a friend. What principles or dispositions guide your thinking?

_____

_____

_____

_____

Let us return to the story of Beth Tottle and Mrs. Uwilla. Now that Beth has gathered the facts and identified the type of ethical problem, she must continue in her ethical decision-making process.

Step 3: Use Ethics Theories or Approaches to Analyze the Problem

This step is designed to encourage you to reflect consciously on your basic ethical approach to complex problems, such as moral distress, illustrated by the story of Beth Tottle and Mrs. Uwilla and her family.

That we are drawn to an ethics of care approach for analyzing this issue is not surprising. As the relationship between Beth Tottle and the Uwilla family further develops, we come to understand how this relationship, the context surrounding the Uwilla's complex situation, and the overriding cultural significance drive the decision making. Communication is relational. The ethics of care is a need-centered and individualized relational approach. It involves analyzing the Uwilla's situation with care, empathy, involvement, and the maintenance of harmonious relationships.[14] Beth reflects on how the team's communications have impacted the relationship with Rene Uwilla and sees the ethical significance of a more patient-centered approach. The moral distress is embedded in the relationship with the Uwilla family.

You probably have also recognized that a heavy reliance on the duties and rights that come into conflict in this story places the analysis within the deontologic framework or approach to this issue. Much of the traditional health care approach to ethical problems relies on an understanding of our various duties, commitments, rights, or loyalties. Do you also find yourself thinking as a deontologist about this problem?

If you depend solely on neither duties nor rights, your approach may look more to the consequences that will be brought about by this unsuccessful communication. In this case, you are reasoning as a utilitarian.

Reflection

> Which consequences are relevant for your consideration in the story of Beth Tottle and Mrs. Uwilla? Which ones would weigh the most heavily? Why?

_____

_____

_____

_____

Once you have identified relevant duties, rights, and consequences and have determined the approach you will use, you are in a position to determine an ideal course of action for Beth and the team to take. This ideal course also should be guided by character traits of compassion and integrity. Compassion requires striking a balance in health care communications between providing guidance and allowing autonomy to achieve shared consensus in complex situations.[15]

Because we live in a less than perfect world, however, Beth must now begin the arduous task of identifying the several practical alternatives.

Step 4: Explore the Practical Alternatives

Seemingly good rapport exists between the members of the health care team; however, this rapport has not yet been developed with Mr. Uwilla. Building a trusting relationship and truly sharing decisions is a process that happens over time.[16] Still, the son has now directly asked the team what their intentions are in treating Mrs. Uwilla. Beth Tottle and the team now need to come up with some alternatives. We offer some possible alternatives.

Alternative A. The team could consider the information exchange complete with the clinical information as shared. This alternative is one based on diagnostic reasoning alone, and as you know from your reading in previous chapters, rarely is one mode of clinical reasoning used in isolation. This leads us to alternative B.

Alternative B. The team could offer support to Mr. Uwilla. Mr. Uwilla's anger and anxiety illustrate well that fears of abandonment can reflect a lack of respect toward the patient and family. At such times, the therapeutic encounters in which the health professionals are involved must become the vehicle for such comfort. Active gestures of caring, and just simply being there, can assure the patient that the health professional, and by implication, all the powers of the healing professions, will not abandon her or him. Beth may also decide to engage Mr. Uwilla at a deeper level in ongoing communications. The door is still open for Beth and other members of the team to clarify their intentions. Little was done before this meeting to legitimize the reality and complexity of Mrs. Uwilla's care. This led to a focus on the scientific and economic issues, but not the moral or emotional ones, leading to an obstacle in their relationship with the son. Mr. Uwilla shows resistance to the team because of these poor initial communications and trust must be reestablished. Thus, the fourth step in Beth Tottle's process of moral judgment and action may well be to offer support to Mr. Uwilla right away and tell him that these decisions do not need to be made today, rather they are ones that her colleagues would like him to begin to think about. She may take a lead in the meeting and redirect the conversation to Mr. Uwilla. She will need to use her interdisciplinary teamwork and communication skills to balance duty to the client and duty to her teammates.

Alternative C. Beth and the team can address the emotional, in addition to the cognitive, communication needs of the Uwilla family. Beth knows from her health professional training in effective communication that there are two types of patient needs that must be addressed: the cognitive and the affective. "Affective" refers to the deep emotional need. The health care team has attempted to meet Mr. Uwilla's cognitive need by giving him diagnostic information and asking questions. They have not met his affective need. Beth may choose to alter the direction of the meeting to one that ensures he feels understood by reflecting his feelings, showing respect through validation, concern, and compassion. She may use a reflective response, such as "When you say 'I can't be expected to immediately manage this, I am only one person,' what is the hardest thing about your mom's illness for you and your family?" By using her interpersonal skills, Beth will show Mr. Uwilla that she values his thoughts; this may start to close the information gap between him and the team. Beth is fulfilling her professional loyalty to the team in a way that is likely to benefit the patient as well.

Alternative D. Beth can more fully explore the cultural aspects of the case. The team has missed an opportunity to ask him the meaning of the illness for Mr. Uwilla and his family. Beth may choose to try to get to know the Uwilla family's cultural background and how that contributes to the case. What are the Uwilla's cultural expectations? What is the meaning of illness in the Haitian culture? What is the role of the healer? The caretaker? Beth will need to use her narrative and contextual reasoning to think about who Mrs. Uwilla was, who she is now, and who she may become. She must work with the team to reason about the patient's prospective story and how her son fits into that story. Narrative can give meaningful structure to life throughout time, and tapping into Mrs. Uwilla's narrative will give her son and the care team a better way to make decisions with her best interests as a guide.[17]

Reflection

Now that you have read some ideas about the practical options open to Beth, add some more of your own if you have them.

_____

_____

_____

_____

Step 5: Complete the Action

Whatever Beth decides to do, she now needs the courage to do what she reasons is a caring response in this situation. The most difficult part of her action will be if she decides to redirect the communication with the family and that results in her breaking faith with the team. Beth will need moral courage to identify the good and change the context of care for the Uwilla family. Addressing this moral distress allows for the health professionals to move forward with integrity.

Step 6: Evaluate the Process and Outcome

When Beth has completed the action, has she carried out her professional responsibility? If on reviewing her action, she realizes it followed the most thorough and careful ethical analysis that she was able to exercise in this situation, she can rest assured that she has given everyone involved her best effort. Reviewing your thinking with colleagues can further help you make an accurate assessment.

Beth may also ask an institutional resource to come and meet with the caregivers on the unit to help them learn methods to improve their communication and empathy skills. Communication is often learned during professional training, but it is a skill that must be practiced. This story highlights, as many do, that how we communicate has an impact on the quality of the relationship with an individual patient, family, and other team members. It follows that health care professionals have an ethical duty to develop their skills in communication. Many professional organizations rank communication high amongst the needed practice skills and continuing competencies. Knowledge of how to best communicate can give the provider a strong footing when interacting for a caring response. This reinforces that on a professional level, the "good outcome" is upheld when providers possess technical *and* interpersonal abilities to supplement their professional reasoning.

Communication Standards, Technologies, and Tools

National Standards

Communication is so vital to health care delivery that many national accreditation standards are in place to ensure that communication is both safe and effective. The Joint Commission, a not-for-profit independent organization that accredits health care facilities in the United States, includes communication among its top elements necessary for providing safe, quality care. Standards are currently in place that support effective communication in a variety of areas, including, but not limited to, the environment of care, provision of care, treatment and services, human resources, record of care, national patient safety goals, medication management, information management, and leadership. Two examples of such standards relate to patient education and caregiver-to-caregiver communication in patient hand offs.

Patient Education

Standards are currently in place to ensure that patients receive information about their care that they can understand, both verbally and in writing. Health professionals are morally responsible for evaluating a patient's readiness to learn and preferred learning styles. As you recall, responsibility as a moral agent includes both accountability and responsiveness. These basic distinctions support effective communications. Patient education must also take into consideration health literacy as it relates to education material. *Health literacy* is defined in Health People 2010 as "the degree to which individuals have the capacity to obtain, process and understand basic health information and services needed to make appropriate health decisions."[18] Health literacy is not just the ability to read. It is a complex set of reading, listening, analytic, and decision-making skills *and* the ability to apply these skills to health situations. Health literacy is a function of an individual's skills and social demands. It varies by context and setting and greatly impacts health professional and patient communications. According to the American Medical Association (AMA), poor health literacy is a stronger predictor of a person's health than age, income, employment status, education level, and race.[19] Many communications are limited in that the patient or family does not understand the advice being presented. Health providers must attend to and accommodate for health literacy in their professional communications.

Hand Offs

No one can care for a patient 24 hours a day. *Hand offs* by definition involve the transfer of rights, duties, and responsibilities from one provider or team to another.[20] As of 2006, The Joint Commission has required hospitals to establish standards for hand off communications. As you recall from your reading of Chapter 9, patients have multiple care providers. The authors can recall situations during which a patient was handed off to them for care. They can recall times when this was done with great care, and times when it was haphazard. Members of health care teams use various methods to ensure good communication during hand offs. Most organizations and agencies use both verbal and written hand off procedures. The hand off process is vitally important because it is the main way to communicate the patient's plan of care to help ensure coordination of efforts.

Team Communication

As you learned in Chapter 9, care is almost always provided by teams of clinicians. Good communication between members is critical to safe and effective delivery of care. Communication failures between providers often cause system failures and human errors that lead to preventable harm to patients.[20] Communication barriers are complex within health care teams. Some communication difficulties are transmission based; however, more often, there are hierarchical gradients, conflicts related to roles and plans of care, and human factors that influence successful communication. Lack of time, use of jargon, multitasking, and the team culture are all barriers to optimal team communication. Effective teams have leadership, mutual respect, cohesion, and high levels of collaboration with reliable communication amongst the team.[21] The story of Mrs. Uwilla highlights how a team of people share responsibility for good patient care throughout the process of the relationship and help to ensure a result that meets the criterion of a caring response.

New Technologies

Earlier in this chapter, we talked about modes of communication. Evolving communication technologies such as blogs and social networking sites are alternative points of connection. These connections create new communication demands and cultures. E-mail, for example, has challenged long-standing norms by crafting a culture in which some individuals are expected to be available 24/7. Social networking sites allow individuals to build and maintain relationships, communicate with users of similar interests, and feel more connected.[22] Facebook and other social networking sites present even more questions regarding boundaries and the mixing of personal and professional lives.[23] They have an impact on communication from a privacy, safety, and professional reputation standpoint. Given the popularity of these sites, as indicated by the large number of visits (at the time of this book's writing, Facebook was the number 2 visited site on the web, second only to Google[24]), use of these connections will continue to evolve.

 Reflection

Vanessa is a 25-year-old social worker practicing in a mental health clinic. Recently, the clinic supervisor proposed that all providers who use social networking sites must cease to do so while working on the unit. Vanessa has been using a site for 4 years now and has many questions related to this proposal. What do you think of this proposal? Use your ethics knowledge to help Vanessa support or reject the proposal.

_____

_____

_____

_____

Tools for Communication

Research studies have found that effective patient-professional communication is associated with better health outcomes and greater patient satisfaction and compliance. It can also prevent ethical dilemmas.[25] In an ideal world, all communications would go well, but we know that in reality that does not happen. We all lose our cool. We all encounter conflicts and differences of opinion. Conflict creeps in and, when not addressed, interferes with a caring response. Several tools can assist the health professional in achieving more effective communication. We have shared several throughout the chapter but add this list to help fill up your toolbox.

- Value and appreciate what the patient or family member communicates.
- Acknowledge the patient's emotions by using reflective summary statements.
- Talk less and listen more. Listen for content, meaning, and emotion.
- Watch nonverbal messages.
- Seek to understand the other person's position.
- Understand the patient's story. Understanding the patient as a person can help you reason narratively and give you insight into the patient's illness experience.
- Encourage other members of the health care team to give communications the time they deserve.

Summary

Effective health care communication is vital to a caring response. You have learned about various components of communication throughout this chapter. It is a complex topic that is often at the root of many ethical issues in health care. Our hope is that as you learn more about essential elements of communication, you will be better prepared to actualize your role as a moral agent. Communicating as a health professional is about being and doing. Skilled communication will help you uphold your ethical duty to treat patients in a dignified, courteous, and respectful manner.

Questions for Thought and Discussion

1. Anjali works as a nurse in the pediatric oncology unit. She has just finished working a 12-hour shift. She is tired because it has been a busy and stressful day. Two of the children she was caring for needed intense interventions, and she had a family meeting for a client with a recent diagnosis of terminal cancer. On top of it all, Anjali is worried that she will be late to relieve her mother-in-law, who is caring for her daughter while she is at work. She must now communicate with Dacy, the incoming

nurse, to hand off her patients at change of shift. The unit is noisy, and the secretary has just overhead paged Anjali. Dacy is ready for report but is socializing with the unit secretary.

What are the potential interferences with Anjali's ability to communicate?

If hand off of her patients is ineffective, what are some of the potential results?

Are there any strategies that Anjali or Dacy can use to help improve the quality of the hand off process?

2. Pooja is an occupational therapist working in an outpatient hand clinic. She has just met her new client Darren, who has arrived at the clinic for evaluation and treatment of a radial nerve injury after an open reduction and internal fixation of an elbow fracture. Darren is concerned by his lack of hand motion and sensation as a result of the nerve injury. He talks with Pooja about his injury and operative course. He had full hand use before the surgery. He reports having minimal conversations with his surgeon to date. He was sedated after the procedure, and his follow-up visit was quite brief. He asks Pooja what her opinion is, saying, "I get the feeling something went wrong during my surgery. I asked why my hand is like this now, and they gave me some technical jargon. Do you think the surgeon made a mistake?"

If you were Pooja, how would you handle this communication? What would be your first step? Why?

Role play your response with a student colleague or out loud. How did you do? Was it easy or hard to respond to?

3. Is there a right not to know the truth? Under what conditions might such a right be argued?

References

1. Taylor, R., 2008. *The intentional relationship: Occupational therapy and the use of self.* F.A. Davis, Philadelphia, PA.
2. Levetown, M., American Academy of Pediatrics Committee on Bioethics, 2008. Communicating with children and families: From everyday interactions to skill in conveying distressing information. *Pediatrics* 121 (5), 1441–1460.
3. Kuehn, B.M., 2009. States explore shared decision making. *JAMA* 301 (24), 2539–2541.
4. Drake, R.E., Wilkniss, S.M., Frounfelker, R.L., et al., 2009. The Thresholds-Dartmouth partnership and research on shared decision making. *Psychiatric Services* 60 (2), 142–144.
5. Karnieli-Miller, O., Eisikovits, Z., 2009. Physician as partner or salesman? Shared decision making in real time encounters. *Social Sci Med* 69, 1–8.
6. Purtilo, R.B., Robinson, E.M., Doherty, R.F., et al., 2008. *Maintaining compassionate care: A companion guide for families experiencing the uncertainty of a serious and prolonged illness.* MGH Institute of Health Professions and Kenneth B. Schwartz Center, Boston, MA.

7. Haddock, J., 1996. Towards further clarification of the concept 'dignity.' *J Adv Nurs* 24, 924–931.
8. Gallagher, A., 2004. Dignity and respect for dignity—Two key health professional values: Implications for nursing practice. *Nurs Ethics* 11 (6), 587–599.
9. DePalo, R., 2009. The role of hope and spirituality on the road to recovery. *Exceptional Parent* 39 (2), 74–77.
10. Eliott, J.A., Olver, I.N., 2009. Hope, life and death: A qualitative analysis of dying cancer patients' talk about hope. *Death Studies* 33, 609–638.
11. HarrisInteractive, 2008. *Number of "cyberchondriacs": Adults going on-line for health information has plateaued or declined.* Available from: <http://www.harrisinteractive.com/harrispoll> (accessed 8.10.09).
12. Kübler-Ross, E., 1969. *On death and dying.* Macmillan, New York.
13. US Department of Health and Human Services, 1999. *The patients' bill of rights in Medicare and Medicaid: fact sheet: April 12, 1999.* Available from: <http://www.hhs.gov/news/press/1999pres/990412.html> (accessed 23.10.09).
14. O'Sullivan, E., 2009. Withholding truth from patients. *Nurs Standard* 23 (48), 35–40.
15. Sanghavi, D.M., 2006. What makes for a compassionate patient-caregiver relationship. *J Quality Patient Safety* 32 (5), 283–292.
16. Karnieli-Miller, O., Eisikovits, Z., 2009. Physician as partner or salesman? Shared decision making in real time encounters. *Social Sci Med* 69, 1–8. 17.
17. Mattingly, C., Fleming, M.H., 1994. *Clinical reasoning: Forms of inquiry in a therapeutic practice.* F.A. Davis, Philadelphia, PA.
18. Glassman, P., 2009. *Health literacy: National Network of Libraries of Medicine.* Available from: <http://nnlm.gov/outreach/consumer/hlthlit.html> (accessed 19.10.09)
19. Ad Hoc Committee on Health Literacy for the Council on Scientific Affairs, American Medical Association, 1999. Health literacy: Report of the Council on Scientific Affairs. *JAMA* 281, 552–557.
20. Denham, C.R., Digman, J., Foley, M.E., et al., 2008. Are you listening. . . .are you really listening. *J Patient Safety* 4 (3), 148–161.
21. Mickan, S.M., Rodger, S.A., 2005. Effective health care teams: A model of six characteristics developed from shared perceptions. *J Interprofessional Care* 19 (4), 358–370.
22. Cain, J., 2008. Online social networking issues within academia and pharmacy education. *Am J Pharmaceutical Educ* 72 (1), 10, 1–7.
23. Schwartz, H.L., 2008. Facebook: The new classroom commons. *Chronicle Review,* B12–B13.
24. Alexa Internet, 2009. *Top sites: Top 500 sites on the web.* Available from: <http://www.alexa.com/topsites> (accessed 9.10.09).
25. Mueller, P.S., Hook, C.C., Fleming, K.C., 2004. Ethical issues in geriatrics: A guide for clinicians. *Mayo Clinic Proc* 79, 554–562.

12

Informed Consent in Treatment and Clinical Research

Objectives

The reader should be able to:

- Describe three basic legal concepts that led to the doctrine of informed consent.
- Describe three approaches to determining the disclosure standard for judging that a patient or client has been informed.
- Discuss three major aspects of the process of obtaining informed consent.
- Differentiate between the never competent and the once-competent patient and the challenges posed by each in regard to informed consent.
- Compare informed consent as it is used in health care practice and in human studies research.
- Define the terms placebo and placebo effect, and explain why placebo use is a challenge to the general idea of informed consent.
- Discuss the possible benefits and harms of placebo use and the ethical principles that are important in analyzing placebo use.
- Identify three general guidelines for information disclosure of genetic information and the challenges to informed consent that genetic testing raises.
- Describe some considerations one must always take into account to be sure one is being culturally competent and honoring cultural difference when informed consent is the standard.

New terms and ideas you will encounter in this chapter

informed consent	voluntariness	once competent
battery	mental competence or	surrogate/proxy
disclosure	mental capacitation	consent
fiduciary relationship	limited English	legal guardian
contract	proficiency (LEP)	best interests standard
disclosure standards	capacity	substituted judgment
general consent	competence	standard
special consent	never competent	advance directives

assent

vulnerable
  populations

therapeutic research

institutional review
  board (IRB)

placebo

placebo effect

genetic information

right not to know

genomics

Topics in this chapter introduced in earlier chapters

Topic	Introduced in chapter
A caring response	2
Trust	2
Character traits	4
Virtue	4
Principles approach	4
Autonomy	4
Beneficence	4
Nonmaleficence	4
Shared decision making	11
Health literacy	11
Rights and responsibilities	11

Introduction

One important avenue to your success as a professional who has learned how to arrive at a caring response is to perfect the communication, listening, and interpretive skills necessary to honor *informed consent*. Informed consent is one of the cornerstones of the current U.S. and Canadian health care systems. Although the doctrine is the most formalized in these countries, it is an important concept in most Western health care systems. Whether with patients or research subjects, basic principles of respect for the person undergird informed consent. By going step by step through the ethical decision-making process, the importance of several aspects of informed consent in achieving your goals as a moral agent should become apparent. To inform your thinking, consider the story of Jack Burns and Cecelia Langer.

🐚 The Story of Jack Burns and Cecelia Langer

Jack Burns, a 74-year-old retired cross-country truck driver, came to the emergency department of his hometown hospital because of "kidney problems" and dehydration. The health care team quickly decided that he should be admitted for further tests. He balked, saying he was "allergic" to hospitals, but after talking to the doctor in the emergency department, agreed to "stay overnight—that's all." Cecelia Langer, a nurse practitioner from the renal unit, came down to the emergency department and accompanied him to the admissions area because he seemed weak and a little disoriented. When the intake clerk presented him with the general hospital admissions informed consent form he retorted, "You got a noose around my neck. I know I gotta sign this thing to get treated." Cecelia encouraged him to read it and went over the main points with him.

Jack was admitted to the general medical unit because no beds were available in the renal unit. The next day, he was presented with another consent form by the medical unit nurse, this one for the tests themselves, and he became belligerent. He asked for "that nurse that helped me last night." Cecelia was called from the renal unit and came into his room. He said he could not understand what they were trying to get him to do. She patiently explained the procedure he would undergo, referring to the informed consent form each step of the way. Although she herself thought it seemed quite well written, it took almost 20 minutes of talking with him before he decided to sign it. But when the imaging team took him to prepare him with contrast dye for the test, he again became agitated, claiming he had never been told that they were going to "inject poison" into him. The imaging team leader took out the form and showed him the place where it had been discussed. He still seemed disgruntled but just shrugged his shoulders and said, "Okay. But I hope that woman who explained it to me knows she did a terrible job because I would have never signed it."

The imaging team gave some consideration to postponing his test, but when they asked him if this is what he wanted, he grunted, "Go ahead! Do the test!" The team also thought about whether to tell Cecelia about his comment and decided to do so. At first she was annoyed, but later she found herself thinking about what to do to avoid this kind of thing happening to a patient again. Maybe he really did not understand!

 Reflection

Before you continue, take a minute to jot down your own response to this situation in regard to Cecelia's and the other health professionals' role in explaining the procedure. Can you think of anything else they could have done to help Jack?

_____

_____

_____

_____

You will have an opportunity to revisit their situation as you study this chapter. You can begin to assess it by comparing it with any experience you may have had in which you were asked to give your informed consent for a treatment or diagnostic intervention or for participation as a research subject.

 Reflection

If you have ever been asked to sign an informed consent form, could you understand it easily? Did you have to sign your name? Was someone on hand to answer questions you may have had at the time, or was there a telephone number where you could reach someone later? Did reading and signing the form make you feel more reassured about what you were about to experience? Why or why not?

_____

_____

_____

_____

Now that you have a story to refer to and have considered your own experience, if any, you are ready to read on about informed consent.

The Goal: A Caring Response

Informed consent is founded on basic legal-ethical principles. It entails a process of decision making and is both a process and a procedure. The idea is that you can perform your professional tasks better and in a morally praiseworthy way by bringing the person's informed preferences into your plans. In summary, it is another tool to assist you in your skillful search for what a caring response entails.

An example of a procedure consent document is provided for you in Figure 12-1. You can see from this example that an informed consent document spells out how the health professionals intend to use specific diagnostic or treatment interventions for the purpose of improving a patient's condition. If designed appropriately, the document enables the person to become well informed before entering into the decision-making process. Informed consent, then, becomes a vehicle for protecting a patient's dignity in the health care environment, the fundamental belief being that such consent should foster and engender trust between the health professional and the person receiving the services.

Tingsboro Hospital Procedure Consent Form	Patient Label Name Medical Record # DOB

Procedure: _____

I,_____, consent to the above treatment procedure as deemed medically necessary by my medical provider. My care provider,_____, has explained to me the nature of my condition, the procedure, the risks and the expected benefits of the above procedure compared with alternative approaches.

My provider has also explained to me the likelihood, and some possible complications of this procedure including, but not limited to, bleeding, infection, loss of limb or organ function, drug reactions or possibly death. I also understand that I may need a blood transfusion during or after this procedure.

I understand that Tingsboro Hospital is a teaching hospital and that students and other trainees may participate in this procedure as permitted by law and hospital policy. I also understand that tissues, blood, body parts or fluid may be removed from the body during the procedure. These materials may be used for diagnostic, therapeutic or research reasons.

Any additional comments:

_____

_____

_____

_____

_____   _____
Signature of Patient   Printed Name

_____   _____
Signature of Provider   Printed Name

Date:_____

Figure 12-1. Informed consent document.

1 *Reflection*

What strengths and difficulties do you see in using the informed consent document in Figure 12-1 to foster the ideal of engendering trust?

1. Strengths

_____

_____

2. Difficulties

_____

_____

To help better understand how informed consent became so central to the health professional–patient relationship, we invite you to engage in the six-step process of ethical decision making, with your focus on informed consent.

The Six-Step Process in Informed Consent Situations

The most important thing to bear in mind as you analyze the specific informed consent–related challenges facing Jack Burns and Cecelia Langer is that the informed consent document, process, and procedures can support important ethical dimensions of the relationship. Its importance can be better understood by examining some aspects of the development of the idea.

Step 1: Gather Relevant Information

As you may recall, when the six-step process was introduced in Chapter 5, we provided a long list of types of information that you would need to help you arrive at a caring response. We also warned you that other types of information could help as well, information not related to the patient's specific situation. Information about the legal principles underlying informed consent is one example; elements of the process related to disclosure in informed consent are another. Let us examine each before identifying the type of ethical problem facing Cecelia Langer.

Relevant Legal Concepts That Support Informed Consent

Among the most important legal concepts that have given rise to our thinking about informed consent are battery, disclosure, and the fiduciary relationship. The common law legal right of self-determination and constitutional right to privacy also are instrumental in legal thinking. You will consider self-determination for its ethical implications in another section of this chapter.

Battery, based on common law in the United States and other Western countries, is the act of offensive touching done without the consent of the person being touched, however benign the motive or effects of the touching.[1]

Disclosure guarantees the legal right of a person to be informed of what will happen to him or her. Several landmark legal cases have set precedents for current thinking on the importance of disclosure. Some practical challenges encountered regarding the appropriate standard of disclosure to use are discussed in the next section.

One of the earliest legal cases in the United States related to disclosure is Schloendorff v. Society of New York Hospital, which emphasized the relationship of disclosure to autonomy. This 1914 ruling stated that every human of adult years and sound mind has a right to determine what shall be done with his or her body. For example, a surgeon who performs an operation without the patient's consent is liable on the basis of the harm of nondisclosure.[2] In the 1918 Hunter v. Burroughs case, the courts ruled that a physician has a duty to warn a patient of dangers associated with prescribed remedies so the patient is at liberty to decide whether or not the risk is worth it. Both rulings were early attempts by the courts to bring the patient's preferences into decisions regarding what would happen to his or her own body.[3]

A third related legal concept is the idea of a *fiduciary relationship*. You were introduced to this idea in Chapter 2. In such a relationship, a person in whom another person has placed a special trust or confidence is required to watch out for the best interests of the other party. Most health professional–patient relationships are considered to be this type. The physician-patient relationship in the United States was ruled a fiduciary relationship in a 1974 case, Miller v. Kennedy, on the basis of the "ignorance and helplessness of the patient regarding his own physical condition."[4] This is, of course, an outdated understanding of the patient as "ignorant and helpless," but that does not negate the basic idea of the need for faithfulness on the part of all health professionals.

The legal case that gave to posterity the term informed consent is Salgo v. Leland Stanford Board of Trustees (1957). This case stated that the physician violates his or her legal duty by withholding information necessary for a patient to make a rational decision regarding care. In addition, the physician must disclose "all the facts which materially affect the patient's rights and interests and the risks, hazard and danger, if any."[5] With this ruling, the U.S. courts firmly wedded the notion of a patient's autonomy with that of a health professional's duty to warn of known danger or harm. In other words, the courts recognized that a caring response could not be achieved without those aspects of the interaction.

Relevant Facts Regarding the Process of Obtaining Consent

Let us go on to some practical matters. Currently, the law supports that a patient should gain information about a proposed procedure and should have a voice in the decision. This constitutes a legal contract between patient and health professional. A *contract,* as you may know, is a legal agreement on which both parties claim to understand the situation they are agreeing to, including their respective responsibilities and rights.

However, the law also recognizes that there may be several challenges in attempting to implement the consent process in a meaningful manner. Some challenges are related to the standard and amount of disclosure, whereas others are related to the person's ability to grasp the situation (Figure 12-2).

Disclosure Standards. *Disclosure standards* are a key consideration. You have seen that a major legal concern is that a patient be informed. What disclosure standard can be used to judge that the level of information was sufficiently clear to be understood? One common suggestion is that "customary medical language" be the standard of disclosure. A second approach, which emphasizes the likelihood that patients will misunderstand technical terms used by the health professional, suggests that the standard be determined by what a "reasonable" person would need to make an informed

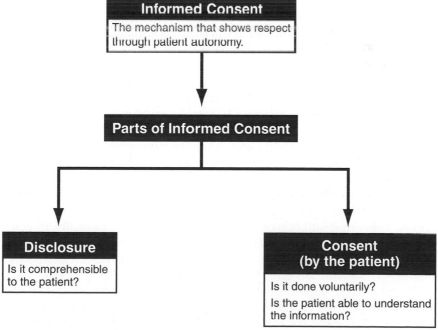

Figure 12-2. The two dimensions of informed consent.

decision. Finding one standard appropriate for everyone continues to perplex many. In fact, the courts have not settled on one standard, either. So, a third common approach is to conclude that the only alternative is to adopt an individualized standard for each patient.

Reflection

What are some practical barriers to institutionalizing any of the three suggested standards for an individual patient?

_____

_____

Do you have any ideas about what an adequate approach to the issue of a disclosure standard fitting for all would be?

_____

_____

A related aspect of ensuring adequate disclosure focuses on the appropriate amount of information that must be provided. In many health care settings, patients are directed to sign a standardized *general consent form* when they are admitted. You will recall that this happened to Jack and was the trigger for his first outburst of concern. The wording that appears on a typical general consent document states that a patient is consenting to routine services and treatment for his or her condition, the goal being the best care possible. In a teaching hospital, the person also is told that on entering the hospital she or he consents to become a participant in the hospital's educational programs. Then, when certain invasive procedures are being considered, the consent is valid only when the person signs a *special consent form*. Recall that Jack also was asked to sign a special consent form for the imaging diagnostic test he would undergo; that became the source of his second outburst of frustration. The amount and type of information deemed adequate and appropriate in the special consent form may vary tremendously from one institution or procedure to another. Traditionally, medical and other relevant clinical information is presented in both verbal and written formats. Informed consent forms constitute the written document, but the verbal give and take gives the words life.

The goal is to take the patient's background into consideration and determine the relative advantages and disadvantages of each decision choice for that patient's future well-being. How each patient achieves understanding in the consent process is unique because we all learn and process information differently. Studies show that simple verbal and written consent procedures do not always yield adequate patient under-standing.[6] Many researchers are studying the effectiveness of alternative consent strategies, such as modified written forms to combat poor health literacy, and the inclusion of teaching aides and multimedia formats (e.g., video, interactive computer animation programs).

Anxiety and fear created by the unknown or general distrust of the health care system leave many patients with the sense that unfair advantage is being taken of them. When presenting informed consent documents, you should be found on the side of "taking too much time" with each patient, all the while being attentive to the patient's cues regarding his or her level of comprehension. The best consent processes always uses shared decision making with the patient as the measure of success.

 SUMMARY

The standard used and amount of information disclosed combined with psychological factors that influence the patient's experience must all be taken into account in assessing whether disclosure is consistent with a caring response.

Voluntariness Must Be Assured. Informed consent assumes that a person voluntarily agrees to the procedure or process he or she is about to undergo. Within informed consent discussions, this is referred to as *voluntariness.* People speak or act voluntarily when no coercion compels them to do so against their own best interests and wishes. For this reason, individuals judged to be in vul-nerable situations in which their ability to say "no" or "this is what I want" is compromised should be treated with special regard. As you may recall, Jack told Cecelia, the nurse practitioner, that he felt pressured to sign the consent form. A good informed consent process (in contrast to just an informed consent form) allows him either to increase his comfort level to the point of being willing to sign the form or to go away being clear why he chose to refuse treatment.

 Reflection

What steps did Cecelia Langer and others take each step of the way to try to meet the criterion of voluntariness? Do you feel confident that they succeeded? Why or why not?

_____

_____

_____

_____

One instance that tests the limits of voluntariness as a standard of respect for a person is the psychiatric practice of involuntary commitment for mental illness. This practice long has been condoned by the medical profession, and often by society as well. The increasing awareness of the importance of voluntariness, however, has created an environment in which such patients are able to maintain control over large parts of their treatment regimen, sometimes including whether to accept or reject medications.

 SUMMARY

A conviction that the patient's consent voluntarily is given must be added to the condition of adequate disclosure for the ethical goals of informed consent to be realized.

Competence as a Consideration. Health professionals have a moral obligation to ascertain the level of a patient's ability to grasp the situation. The ability to grasp it is called *mental competence* or *mental capacitation,* two important terms we describe more fully on page 262 of this chapter. For the purposes of our discussion now, please note that the idea of competence and capacity in the informed consent context allows us to address the assumption that individuals possess certain crucial knowledge without which they are unable to engage meaningfully in an act. Take, for example, the act of making a will. The person who does not know the general value of his estate or who does not have the mental capacity to recognize the existence of a rightful heir is not in a position to sign a valid will no matter what he or she may know about himself or herself or the world in general. These two pieces of information are so essential to the making of a will that unless one is in possession of them, one cannot properly dispose of one's estate. In the same fashion, a person must be knowledgeable about certain crucial aspects of his or her health and the condition creating the problem to offer true informed consent. This formulation of competency is too narrow, however, when taken alone. It depends almost solely on the professional's clinical evaluation, how much a person is told, and how much he or she can repeat back to you. This surely is not all you wish to know concerning a patient's decision to give consent. A fundamental concern is whether the patient truly understands the nature of the illness and the basis for consenting or refusing intervention. For example, Jack may be having difficulty comprehending because of cognitive changes often associated with uremic poisoning. This is something to which Cecelia must pay close attention in the process of gathering relevant information about this patient. She will also need to obtain his medical record to determine whether any other conditions in his medical history, such as dementia or mental health disorders, may compromise his mentation.

Appelbaum and Grisso[7] propose the following four relevant criteria for ascertaining the level of decision-making capacity that patients may be exhibiting:

1. The first level is the *ability to communicate choices*. Beyond that is the ability to maintain and communicate these choices consistently over time.
2. The second, a qualitatively different level, is the *ability to understand relevant information* on which the choice is based.
3. The third level is the *ability to appreciate the situation and its consequences according to one's own values.*
4. The fourth level is the *ability to reason about treatment options*, which includes weighing the various values and relevant information to arrive at a decision.[7,8]

Ideally, a person should be able to function at all four levels. For instance, nothing we know about Jack suggests that previously he was incompetent or incapacitated. At the same time, Cecelia has knowledge about the delirium effects of uremic poisoning that may give her pause about his mental acuity at this moment in time. Key to assessing Jack's decision is the process by which his decision is reached, not just the outcome or choice itself. This is an important feature to remember when working in health care. Many patients make decisions that we as health providers would not necessarily make for ourselves. It is the patient's right to make an informed refusal of a treatment that you think they should accept; patients have the right to make unreasonable choices in health decisions, just as they do in financial and other decisions in their lives. In short, as a part of caring for Jack, Cecelia must take every precaution to ensure he is competent, a topic that is pursued in more depth later in this chapter.

Step 2: Identify the Type of Ethical Problem

Cecelia and the other health professionals seem to have little doubt about the importance of ensuring that Jack be comfortable in giving his consent for general and special intervention purposes. They recognize themselves as moral agents (A) responsible for a caring response to his concerns. They believe the appropriate outcome (O) is for him to be fully informed and willingly able to give (or refuse) consent. The challenge seems to be *how* to get to that outcome. They are experiencing barriers in the course of action (C) designed by the institution to reach the result of informed consent.

 Reflection

As a reminder, jot down the kind of ethical problem that focuses on barriers to an ethically optimal outcome.

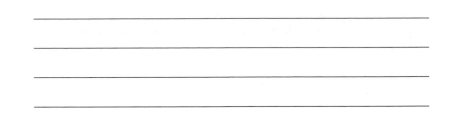

If you responded "moral distress," you have remembered well what you learned previously. In this case, Cecelia Langer (who has become the person Jack seems to trust the most) has to overcome the barriers to achieving her intended ethical goal. Because she can speculate what the range of barriers are, her distress falls into moral distress type A. Schematically, her problem looks like this:

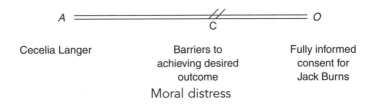

What possible barriers are there?

First, the wording of the informed consent form may be a problem itself. You have already been introduced in this chapter to the challenges that the basic idea of informed consent raises regarding standards and amount of disclosure needed for different patients The readability of informed consent forms has been shown to exceed the average reading levels of most adults in the United States. [9] Or maybe the form is so badly worded that no one is really benefited by this mechanism, and Jack is just one of the people to bring it to the attention of the health professionals.

Second, the barrier Cecelia might be facing is that Jack may have had life experiences that make him extremely anxious about giving away his autonomy. Has he been a prisoner of war or had other traumatic experiences? Did he see loved ones treated without respect for what he thought were their reasonable requests? We do not know. We certainly can observe that anxiety played a part in his reactions to the requests for him to sign the documents.

Third, he might be afraid of what he, or the health professionals, will find out if they go ahead with the tests. In other words, his reluctance may not be centered on the consent itself but rather on what it represents. His reaction at the time he is about to have the dye injected and the diagnostic test performed may be indicative of his fear of what the tests will reveal.

Fourth, although Cecelia is trying hard and believes she is doing a good job, the barrier may come from this patient not being able to comprehend what is really happening, even though he pretends to. He may be mentally incompetent, lack cognitive insight, have a reading or learning disability, or in some other way be deeply confused about this whole thing.

1 *Reflection*
Can you think of other possibilities? If so, jot them down.

_____

_____

_____

_____

Once the type of ethical problem is identified, Cecelia can use the tools of ethics to analyze it (and hopefully move toward resolution).

Step 3: Use Ethical Theories or Approaches to Analyze the Problem

Cecelia, the unit nurse, and the medical imaging team are working well together to address this problem. Cecelia, in particular, has a challenge: obviously, she has other things to do besides be concerned about Mr. Burns, who is not one of "her" patients in the strict sense of the word.

The resolution of her moral distress requires her to call on both virtues and the help of ethical principles to guide her.

Virtues Associated with Caring

In Chapter 4, you were introduced to the idea of virtue, the expression of which is in the form of character traits or dispositions. Character traits help a health professional stand firmly in her or his commitment to find a "caring response" in a great variety of situations. When we reflect on the challenge facing Cecelia Langer, the common health care virtues like honesty, compassion, or courage do not seem entirely fitting for her situation. What dispositions can help her remove the barriers that are keeping her from her desired outcome—that is, confidence that she has supported Jack's right to give (or refuse) informed consent? Character traits that come to mind in observing her at work toward the achievement of this goal include kindness, thoroughness, patience, and sympathy. We also can assume she knows that if she sloughs off on this task, the self respect needed for maintaining her own integrity as a professional will receive a blow. Hers is an apt example of how different character traits are needed for different types of ethically challenging situations.

She also will want to move toward further action, and for that she can find some guidance in the principles approach, applying the principles of autonomy, beneficence, and nonmaleficence.

Principles Approach

Patient Autonomy. Beauchamp and Faden[10] note that, "As the idea of informed consent evolved, discussion of appropriate (ethical) guidelines moved increasingly from a narrow focus on the physician's or researcher's obligation to disclose information to the quality of a patient's or subject's understanding of information and right to authorize or refuse biomedical intervention."[10] The governing ethical principle in informed consent is the right to self-determination or autonomy. It also is reflected in the legal right today.

The health professional can think of informed consent as a claim to engage in a communication process designed to free the patient to make an informed choice. One could go further and say it is a claim to honor all the conditions, including the communications process, that allow the person to make that choice. Anytime you begin communication around informed consent issues with a patient, you are inherently acknowledging an initial imbalance of information between the two of you. Because of this imbalance, the patient's self-determination is compromised; therefore, your goal as a moral agent is to set the conditions for his or her freedom of choice. Only then can both parties enter into dialogue and agreement as equals.

Because Jack Burns still seems upset after he has signed the second form, we can conclude that communication may have broken down somewhere.

 Reflection

Do you think Cecelia Langer met the conditions that would foster good communication between herself and Jack? From what you know, what, if anything, could she have done differently at the outset during their initial exchange to avoid his negative response?

_____

_____

_____

_____

Whatever your suggestion, the key is that the communication should be useful to the person in making a decision that is fitting for his or her life situation and within the context of personal values. Therefore, you are responsible for informing the person of the conditions under which a real understanding will be achieved. Only then can both parties enter into dialogue and agreement as equals.

Beneficence and Nonmaleficence. Two additional principles, beneficence and nonmaleficence, also are basic foundations on which to build your communication with the patient. As you know, these two, taken together, morally require you to do everything possible to refrain from harming patients and also meet your positive obligation of beneficence to help them do what is most beneficial. You as a moral agent can act according to these principles through trying to ensure that patients become equipped with knowledge of what they really want and what it means within the bigger context of their life. Failure to take seriously the process of informed consent constitutes a type of harm. Unfortunately, today, the informed consent form sometimes is treated as a procedural necessity and is handled carelessly, maybe even handed off to a receptionist or aide who is not trained to—and should not be expected to—fulfill this essential component of a caring response. Whatever the process in the institution where you are employed, failure to take informed consent seriously is tantamount to trashing the principle of nonmaleficence ("do no harm").

 SUMMARY

Both character traits and ethical principles can help informed consent be realized as an integral aspect of a caring response. The patient's autonomy and the health professional's duties of nonmaleficence and beneficence are important markers toward achieving that goal.

Step 4: Explore the Practical Alternatives

We are catching Cecelia "downstream" in her moral distress because we know from the story that Jack signed the form and had the diagnostic procedure. We also know that he seemed unhappy at the end and that she, too, is now concerned. However, whether we look at her predicament at the time she was first discussing the informed consent form with him, or the second time, or even now, after the fact, her concern is that there was or is a barrier to her arriving at the outcome of a caring response.

 Reflection

What do you think she should do once she learns that this patient—who was not her patient in the first place—seems to be struggling with the issue of informed consent?

_____

_____

_____

_____

Let us pick up her story at the current time, with her pondering what to do because no matter what she did in the past he seemed "dissatisfied."

She can talk with him again herself. Let him know what she heard from the imaging team and ask him what happened that led him to be so unsatisfied with the outcome of their exchange. Perhaps through that action she will be able to understand better where she let him down (if she did) or if his lingering reluctance had nothing to do with her exchanges with him.

She could go directly to the medical unit where he is a patient and discuss the whole situation with the team so that they can have insight into their own future care of him. Perhaps follow-up psychiatric or cognitive evaluations should be pursued should his mentation not clear once his uremia is treated medically.

She can also take the informed consent forms to the appropriate committees within her institution, probably the committees that designed the forms, and ask them to review the documents for clarity, accuracy, and completeness.

Finally, she can let the matter drop. It is over and done.

Steps 5 and 6: Complete the Action and Evaluate the Process and Outcome

Given Cecelia's continued concern and Jack's apparent continued unease, the first through third options combined with further reflection on her experience are warranted. Each may provide insight not only into the possible failures of the informed consent process but also into what the health professionals can do in the future to help ensure a more positive outcome.

One area for reflection will be taken care of by the institution's committees. Cecelia's experience provides them with an opportunity to review the documents, processes, and procedures of informed consent.

Another area for reflection is that Cecelia and her colleagues should try to better understand the various sources of anxiety and fear that the form, the discussion about the procedures, or other aspects of the informed consent procedure might generate in patients. Are there opportunities for them to learn how to communicate better surrounding these discussions?

A third is that the challenge of arriving at a caring response through the use of informed consent requires diligence regarding how to show respect, taking into account differences among individuals and groups of patients. For instance, the story of Jack and Cecelia probably evokes for you the picture of two Northern European white people. In fact, Jack grew up in a small village in Northern Thailand with a mother of Thai descent and a father who is half Thai and half German. He immigrated to the United States 20 years ago. Language is not much of a barrier for him in his adopted land; however, he was never formally educated in the English language. Cecelia is a fifth generation "Yankee" who married her high school sweetheart. Both she and her husband grew up in Stoningham, Connecticut. These two individuals come from different cultural backgrounds and may have different values that guide their communication and decision-making processes. The well-intentioned but autonomy-dominated principles of informed consent are not universally beneficial to all patients. There are many ways in which language and related cultural barriers can diminish positive effects.[11] Although Jack did not have a perceived language barrier, there may be cultural ones that make obtaining informed consent more complex. U.S. federal antidiscrimination laws require that health care facilities receiving federal funds provide professional interpretation services for patients with *limited English proficiency (LEP)*. LEP refers to individuals whose primary language is not English and who have limited ability to read, write, speak, and understand English. In their 2007 study examining whether the basic criteria for informed consent were evident in prenatal genetic counseling practices in Texas, Hunt and deVoogd found that patients who needed translation were consistently disadvantaged in the quality and content of their consultations.[12] Many providers feel the burden of additional time and effort to obtain consent when a language barrier is present; however, given how central informed consent is to the practice of safe, legal, and patient-centered care, providers have an ethical obligation to ensure successful information exchange during the consent process. Each case warrants the professional's most vigilant attention if a caring response is to be achieved.

Reflection

If you can, list some cultural or ethnic groups who would not find the idea of informed consent for each individual member of their group consistent with their moral norms. If you know of none, you have an important task to do in acquainting yourself with the rich diversity of patients and clients you are bound to see.

_____

_____

_____

_____

    Much of informed consent presupposes that a patient desires to be independent and in control of his or her own individual destiny. Your professional goal and privilege of arriving at a caring response goes beyond assuming this. The differences can cause such profound mistakes that a later section of this chapter is devoted entirely to the topic.

SUMMARY

The health professional providing the patient with pertinent information for informed consent inevitably must personalize the amount and the type of information provided, despite the difficulty in doing so. Even then, the process of arriving at a caring response has but begun.

When Cecelia engages in Step 6 of the ethical decision-making process (i.e., evaluating the process and outcome), she may conclude that she "missed the mark" somewhere. If not, she will have at least been diligent in her commitment to finding a caring response in this dimension of her professional role. We ask you to turn now to additional important considerations relevant to your skillful use of informed consent as an ethical tool.

The Special Challenge of Incapacity or Incompetence

Incapacity and incompetence are two terms used to describe the condition of patients for whom the process of truly informed decision making and consent to such decisions are not possible. Capacity and competence mean different things, although they are often used interchangeably. Capacity more commonly refers to clinical judgments, and competence to legal ones.[8] *Capacity* is a medical concept that implies that a patient has the ability to understand and weigh medical information to make health decisions.[13] Capacity can fluctuate when patients experience certain medical conditions; for example, fever can temporarily compromise a patient's decision-making capacity. In contrast, certain medical conditions, such as Alzheimer's disease, can progressively worsen a patient's decision-making capacity. *Competence* is a legal term. All persons are presumed competent until legally judged otherwise. Most writing and reflection on the subject urge extreme caution and diligence in discerning how far to proceed with evaluation and treatment if a patient is incapable of making a competent decision. Many patients have decision making and functional abilities that are task and context dependent. The patient's actual performance along a continuum is key in the determination of capacity. It is not what patients say they will do but rather what they actually do when completing the task. The authors recount many clinical cases where the patient could verbalize how to do a task, such as using a stove, but when taken to the actual kitchen and asked to prepare a hot beverage could not safely perform the task. This is why it is so essential that health care delivery be a well-coordinated team effort. Whether referred to as capacity or competence, the patient's decision-making abilities are of greatest importance. Wettstein[14] summarizes this distinction well as "a person is considered incapacitated when the person is no longer able to perform that specific function and incompetent when a court has ruled so."[14]

The two types of incompetent patients are those who were *never competent* and those who were *once competent*. Some examples of patients who were never competent include newborns, small children, and individuals who have been severely mentally impaired from birth. In such instances, *surrogate* or *proxy consent* usually is sought, meaning that someone is appointed to consent on their behalf. When never competent persons become patients, a *legal guardian* is appointed. These patients usually have a guardian for other purposes, and in most instances, the same person is appointed. The next of kin is usually but not always considered the most qualified to be the guardian. The goal here is to determine who can speak for the best interests of this person who has never been in a position to voice her or his informed wishes. (This is called the *best interests standard*.) In contrast, for individuals who were once competent (e.g., those who have organic brain damage that developed in later life, or adult psychoses), a guardian also may be appointed. The guardian must then attempt to make a decision on the basis of what a person would have wanted when competent. (This is called a *substituted judgment standard*.) Sometimes a next of kin or other person makes statements that reflect what the guardian believes the patient said when he or she was competent. Often, this is helpful evidence of what a now incompetent person would want. Other signs are letters, past conversations, comments in the past about other people who became incompetent, or the person's general lifestyle.

In recent years, proxy consent for once-competent persons has been further formalized by the advent of *advance directives*. The general idea is to allow each person while still competent to make his or her wishes known regarding decisions that will be made at a time when he or she becomes legally incompetent, especially in illnesses that will end in death. Some types of advance directives include living wills, durable power of attorney documents, medical directive documents, and values histories. They are discussed further in Chapter 14. Because these documents vary in focus, you are encouraged to check with your place of employment and also with any state laws that may guide the legal use of such documents where you live.

In most regards, the bottom line remains the same regardless of whether a patient is competent: they have a right to assent to health care decisions through informed participation. *Assent* is a term that arose to cover situations where a person is not in a position for his or her consent to be legally honored but puts the onus on the caregivers to try to discern what that person wants in regards to decisions profoundly affecting his or her life. Assent in children and adults with impaired decision-making capacity honors respect for persons and ensures autonomy (or remaining autonomy in the case of adults). It asserts that the patient is part of the decision-making process by being informed of and included in discussions regarding their care. This ensures that they can, in their own way, communicate a choice and have a say in what happens. Alderson, Sutcliffe, and Curtis highlight this nicely:

"The person who is in the body, and is the body, can have unique insights that may be essential for informed decision-making."[15]

Different countries have established different ages at which children can provide independent consent. In the United States, the legal age of consent is currently 18 years; however, children assent to medical decision making with their families and care providers at much earlier ages. Children often express their deep preferences through their body language, words, and actions. Children need intellectual capacity for true informed and voluntary consent; however, the process is complex because it calls on moral maturity, autonomy, reason, and emotions.[15] Many parents and providers struggle with the balance of asking children to take responsibility for weighty medical decisions given the burden that is often associated with them, knowing that things may not go as expected. That being said, many health professionals, including the authors, feel strongly that, especially in instances of chronic conditions, children should be invited to be active participants in the care planning process; it is through this participation that they learn the life skills necessary for successful management of their chronic condition. These experiences essentially help teach self-determination and illness management.

There is reason for serious concern over what happens when adult input capacity is diminished or missing because informed consent is not always taken as seriously as it should be. Patients often are asked to sign such forms with little more than a perfunctory explanation: "You have to sign this so we can do the operation." In all cases, a professional should be present who is able to explain the procedure and its risks to the patient (or, if incompetent, the surrogate) and to answer any questions. Many people have the misconception that if a patient or surrogate signs the form, consent is legally binding no matter what. The form alone is only evidence that they have signed a piece of paper. But in a busy health care setting, where patients' lack of willingness to move quickly may be getting in the way of the efficient operation of the institution, there is a great risk that the consent form becomes an empty substitute for truly informed consent.

---

⑥ SUMMARY

Incompetence and incapacity point to the medical and legal situations in which patients are judged unable to make informed decisions on their own. Due respect for their autonomy and well-being is attempted through the use of surrogate decision makers, best interests and substituted judgment legal procedures, advance directives, and the idea of assent when fully informed consent is not possible.

Informed Consent in Research

Clinical research is essential to scientific discovery. Clinical trials provide health professionals with new knowledge in how to best prevent and treat illness. As a health professional, you may find that you are a principal investigator or a member of a research team. Obtaining informed consent is a fundamental ethical and legal requirement for conducting human subjects research.[16] To help focus your attention on this important aspect of informed consent, consider an informed consent form used for research, as shown in Figure 12-3.

Reflection
Would you sign this form? Yes_____ No __
What is clearly stated?

_____   _____

_____

What, if anything, should be written differently?

_____

_____

Almost every experimental procedure within the health care setting necessitates some infringement on a person's physical or psychological independence. If the dignity of a person being subjected to an experimental procedure is to be preserved and his or her personal autonomy recognized, he or she must be allowed to grant consent to the procedure. In summary, individuals must not be involuntarily submitted to experimental procedures. Rather, they must freely and willingly give their consent to the procedure, even though little personal risk may be involved. By granting consent, the patient agrees to the means used to bring about the investigator's desired end and expresses willingness to participate in bringing about that end.

Following are the basic ethical and legal stipulations involved:

- An investigator cannot perform a research procedure, even of no or minimal risk, without the subject's consent.
- Consent is meaningful only if it is based on relevant information and is not coerced.
- Consent may be a necessary, but not sufficient, condition for the investigator to proceed. (An extreme but true example, homicide is not justified despite a subject's consent.)[17]

RESPONSIBLE INVESTIGATOR:

TITLE OF PROTOCOL:

TITLE OF CONSENT FORM *(if different from protocol):*

I have been asked to participate in a research study that is investigating *(describe purpose of study)*. In participating in this study I agree to *(describe briefly and in lay terms procedures to which subject is consenting).*

I understand that

a) The possible risks of this procedure include *(list known risks or side effects; if none, so state)*. Alternative treatments include *(list alternative treatments and briefly describe advantages and disadvantages of each; if none, so state).*

b) The possible benefits of this study to me are *(enumerate; if none, so state).*

c) Any questions I have concerning my participation in this study will be answered by *(list names and degrees of people who will be available to answer questions).*

d) I may withdraw from the study at any time without prejudice.

e) The results of this study may be published, but my name or identity will not be revealed and my records will remain confidential unless disclosure of my identity is required by law.

f) My consent is given voluntarily without being coerced or forced.

g) In the event of physical injury resulting from the study, medical care and treatment will be available at this institution.

   For eligible veterans, compensation (damages) may be payable under 38USC 351 or, in some circumstances, under the Federal Tort claims Act.

   For non-eligible veterans and non-veterans, compensation would be limited to situations where negligence occurred and would be controlled by the provisions of the Federal Tort Claims Act.

   For clarification of these laws, contact the District Counsel (213) 824-7379.

_____   _____
DATE   PATIENT OR RESPONSIBLE PARTY

                       _____
                       PATIENT'S MEDICAL RECORD NUMBER

                       _____
                       AUDITOR/WITNESS

                       _____
                       INVESTIGATOR/PHYSICIAN REPRESENTATIVE

Figure 12-3. Human studies consent form.

Protocol C.A.V.: A pilot study to evaluate short-course irradiation to small cell bronchogenic carcinoma with combination chemotherapy including the drugs Cytoxan, Adriamycin, and vincristine, and prophylactic brain irradiation. The drugs are to be started on Day 1 with the irradiation and repeated on Day 29 and thereafter every 21 days for 6 cycles.

You have been found to have a tumor of the lung which is best treated by drugs because of the extent of disease, metastases, involvement of the lymph glands, or _____ .

Antitumor drugs (chemotherapy) have been found to be effective in slowing tumor growth but are not curative as of now. New drugs and various combinations of new and current antitumor drugs are being tried in the hope of finding better drugs and more effective combinations. The aim of the treatment is to slow or to halt the spread of disease and permit you a longer period of relative well-being.

Radiation therapy is also a proven effective method of killing tumor cells. In this treatment plan for lung cancer, the affected lung will be irradiated for three weeks to maximize the potential reduction of your tumor. Your brain will also be treated with a modest dose of irradiation in order to ward off the spread of disease to this area. A temporary loss of hair may be expected within the field of irradiation.

You will also be given chemotherapy drugs (Cytoxan, Adriamycin, and vincristine) in combination with the irradiation. These drugs will be given to you intravenously on Day 1 and 29 of treatment and thereafter every 21 days for 6 cycles.

Antitumor drugs, such as the ones used in this plan, and radiation therapy may produce some damage to normal cells in the body, even though the treatments are designed to attack primarily the tumor cells. Care will be used to try to minimize the effect of the damage to your normal cells. The particular forms of damage include: nausea, vomiting, diarrhea, lowered white blood cell count, mouth ulcers, and loss of hair. The drug Adriamycin might make worse any cardiac problems you have. During the treatment you will be monitored carefully with blood tests, urine examination, x-ray examination, ECG, chemical tests, and other studies. Should any of these untoward effects occur, your treatment plan will be reevaluated and, if necessary, modified.

If you have any questions, these will be answered prior to starting the treatment program. You are under no obligation to join this study. You will continue to be treated if you refuse. You are free to withdraw your consent to participate in the study at any time without any prejudice to your continued medical care. The confidential nature of your case will be maintained.

I have read the information contained on this page and all my questions have been answered to my satisfaction. I consent to participate in this medical study.

_____
Patient's Signature   Date

_____
Witness (Investigator)   Date

_____
Witness   Date

Figure 12-3. Cont'd.

The procedure by which consent is brought about is to inform the patient of the range of benefits and risks related to the procedures. The consent form must be signed by the patient, rendering him or her also a research subject. It is also essential that patients understand the difference between being a patient and being a research participant because of a difference in goals. The goal of treatment is to improve or manage the patient's condition. The goal of research is to answer a question through use of study participants. A patient must be provided with effective treatment, whereas a research participant may receive no treatment or one whose likely benefit is unknown.

What about people who for some reason cannot give consent for experimentation? Can consent be given on their behalf by someone who is judged to have the person's interests in mind? Because of the possibilities for abuse of such persons, considerable attention has been devoted in recent years to trying to set up reasonable guidelines for ensuring their protection. Much disagreement still exists about the morally acceptable way to proceed. Most discussion has taken place within the context of research on children and individuals with cognitive disabilities or developmental delays, and on prisoners, students, or others who are in a compromised position or in no position to refuse. Sometimes they are referred to collectively as *vulnerable populations*. At one extreme is the position that people in vulnerable populations should not be subjected to research unless it is related to their own illness (i.e., it must be *therapeutic research*). This implies that a parent or other guardian cannot second guess what the person would do if given the opportunity to consent to a research project that did not also offer possible direct therapeutic benefit to the person, such as a medication or procedure for a fatal condition when no other interventions are available.

Others argue that this position is too conservative regarding experimentation in children and persons with reduced mental function. For instance, it excludes the possibility of obtaining values for various bodily fluids in healthy newborns. Without this information, newborns with life-threatening conditions may die because there are insufficient data to judge the degree of their effect on newborn survival or thriving. This may be an instance in which the minimal risks involved (taking bodily fluids from healthy newborns without their consent) are overridden by the great benefits gained by the research. The previous discussion points to the difficulty of arriving at a policy position to meet at least the basic requirements of morality for a wide range of investigators.

 SUMMARY

As in most areas of ethical reflection in the health professions, dilemmas around clinical research on patients require that professionals engage in continual weighing and decision making in their attempt to honor the subject's values. Informed consent has correctly been seen as one essential mechanism to ensure that respect is shown in this situation.

One institutional mechanism that has become a regular means of monitoring the quality of informed consent in research is *the institutional review board (IRB)*. The IRB was implemented in the 1980s to help ensure not only that persons consenting to research understood what they were getting into but also that the research project itself was ethical in its design and inception. In addition to informed consent considerations, the IRB of an institution must assess the necessity of the project, the type of findings that will result, and the way that the subjects will be treated during the study. It also assesses whether the study involves any inhumane treatment of individuals or groups. If you are asked to do a human subjects study as a part of your professional preparation, you probably will have to fill out the forms required by your local IRB.

Like the informed consent form itself, completing the necessary forms for the IRB does not assure that humane practices in human subject research will be followed. It does, however, at least submit the investigator to the rigors of review by a panel of concerned professionals and laypeople.

Placebos: A Special Case of Information Disclosure

Informed consent hits a brick wall when placebos are involved because to seek the patient's consent destroys the effect of a placebo. *Placebo* comes from a Latin word meaning "I shall please." It consists of any therapeutic procedure (or component of one) that is given for a condition on which it has no known physiologic effect. A pure pharmacologic placebo is a preparation of an inert substance that is not known to have any pharmacologic effect. An impure placebo is an active drug given for its psychological effect even though it has no known direct effect on the disorder in question, such as prescribing an antibiotic for a common cold or other viral infection. Administration of the latter type of placebo carries the risk for real side effects, as well as the interpersonal and professional risks we will discuss in regard to pure placebos.

The issue of placebo use has received some attention from psychiatrists and ethicists, but most of the literature on this topic has been directed toward physicians. Little research has been done concerning the role of other health professionals and the use of placebo medications and procedures, and yet nurses and pharmacists, in particular, play a direct and essential part in this particular form of deception in health care practice. To think clearly about the ethical problems that may arise in such a situation, it is important to understand the reasons for prescribing a placebo and some of the history and psychology of the placebo response.

Why would any professional give this type of medication? It seems to defy the best of clinical discernment and belie the possibility of obtaining consent. One important reason is what is called *the placebo effect*. Virtually all treatments (and also some diagnostic studies) have positive effects for some patients over and above the specific effects of their pharmacologic mechanisms. In other words, contrary to the immediate response of rejecting the practice, in some cases, the practitioner may judge it to be clinically beneficial for the patient. Beecher[18] in 1955 published the classic study that showed that placebos are effective in treating pain in 35% of patients, regardless of the source of pain or clinical condition of the patient. Over all these years, additional studies have done little to alter these percentages. Modern neuropharmacology research has discovered that the brain produces its own chemicals, which can act as analgesics and relaxants. These chemicals, called endorphins, seem to work better for some people than for others, which may explain scientifically why some people respond positively to placebos and others do not. A common error made by health professionals has been the assumption that a symptom (e.g., pain) successfully treated by a placebo is therefore not real or is "only psychological."

 SUMMARY

Although the administration of a placebo involves withholding informed consent and therefore often is held in question from a professional ethics viewpoint, the discovery of endorphins gives us a scientific way of understanding some of the powerful physiologic effects of placebos.

The placebo effect may be partly responsible for the success of ancient remedies given by shamans or medicine men. Some of these remedies contained pharmacologically active agents, but others did not, and much of the healer's work consisted of rituals and symbols. That the medicine men often were successful is a tribute to the power of the therapeutic partnership.

Modern examples of the placebo effect are the effects of suggestion in decreasing stomach acid in patients with ulcers, alleviating bronchospasm in asthma, and decreasing blood pressure. The phenomenon of the placebo effect is widespread and powerful enough so that no research trials of new medications or even surgical procedures are considered truly rigorous unless the element of suggestion has been effectively eliminated, as in randomized, double-blind, clinical trials.

Some ethicists and others oppose the use of placebos in health care because they see it not only as an end run around informed consent but as an example of deception or outright lying.

 Reflection

Do you think there are times when placebo use would justify the deception? If no, why? If yes, what are they?

_____

_____

_____

_____

A utilitarian approach to the use of placebos supports that their ethical acceptability can be determined by weighing the positive effects against the possible negative ones that could result from placebo therapy. We have said that in some specific instances relief of pain has resulted, by anyone's standard, in a positive effect.

 Reflection
Thinking as a utilitarian, what do you think are some of the potential harmful consequences?

_____

_____

_____

Now that you have listed some consequences, the following are two that often are cited.

Loss of trust in the therapeutic relationship is viewed as one harmful consequence. Deception preempts the patient's opportunity to share freely in the responsibility for his or her health. Allowing deception in our professional and private relationships tends to diminish the overall basis of trust that is so key to the quality of those relationships.

Inadequate diagnosis is another dangerous consequence.[19] If a physician is too quick to use a placebo for treatment of a patient's aches and pains, and it seems to having a positive effect, a potentially serious and treatable medical disorder may be overlooked. Thus, a thorough medical and psychological evaluation is important before the use of placebo therapy.

Much of the harm attributed to placebo use comes when it is given without respect for the patient as a person. Physicians may prescribe placebos to prove patients wrong when they feel too angry to give the patient real medication, to punish "problem" patients, or to release staff frustrations.[20] Health professionals may find it difficult to respect patients who respond to placebos because of our emphasis on mechanistic physiologic explanations. Many health professionals believe that a patient's positive response to a placebo indicates that the symptom is not real, even though this has been disproved by many studies, such as Beecher's, and by the recent discovery of endorphins. A positive response to placebos does not indicate that the patient is a hypochondriac. Patients in perfect mental health with real pain and illness may respond to placebos.[21] In fact, cooperative patients who have stable relationships with their caregivers are more likely to respond well to placebos than are the more difficult or less cooperative patients. Thus, significant risks ought to be kept in mind, but it seems unwise to rule out the possibility of placebo use completely. We are beginning to learn more about the therapeutic powers (psychological and chemical) of the mind, but we must also remember that we live in a society that has become dependent on pills and potions—symbolically and actually. Compassion allows us to use placebos in situations where a patient may be respectfully benefited and where that patient is likely to be unable to produce the desired effect without the symbol of the medication or other medical procedure.

Disclosure of Genetic Information

Informed consent also arises with interesting challenges in genetic conditions and prediagnostic genetic testing. Because disclosure of *genetic information* almost always is sensitive, it makes sense that each person who comes for testing provide consent for participating in a diagnostic procedure that identifies one's genetic profile and risk of genetic disease. What to do in regards to others who are affected raises complex questions of disclosure.

🐌 The Story of Meg Perkins and Helen Williams

Two years ago, Meg Perkins was diagnosed with ovarian cancer. Recently, she was diagnosed with breast cancer. While scanning the Internet to learn more about her condition, she learns about ovarian-breast cancer syndrome, a genetically linked condition that manifests itself in ovarian and breast cancer. This is sobering news to her because she has two daughters of child-bearing age and wants to share any information she can with them about her condition if she has this syndrome and also what it may mean for them. She learns that some women who have this syndrome undergo prophylactic mastectomy or removal of their ovaries, although this is still controversial. She tells her daughters about what she has learned from her research and that she plans to be tested. One daughter is anxious to learn everything she can; the other says that she "wants nothing to do with this nonsense" and that she does not want to know the outcome of her mother's genetic testing.

Helen Williams is the genetic counselor that Meg visits after her test. Helen is faced with the difficult task of telling Meg that because her tests reveal the genetic conditions that put her at an 85% risk for having this syndrome, she is correct in thinking about how this involves the whole family. She also tells her that at least one of her two daughters is at a very high risk for development of cancer. The genetic counselor offers to provide Meg's husband and daughters with accurate information elicited from Meg's test findings and to do so in language they can understand so that they will be able to make informed decisions; she will need Meg's and the other members' informed consent to do so. She explains to Meg that this is the job of the genetic counselor and that Meg is not different from many patients who, because of the expansion of genetic information, have found the need to seek professional counsel on this issue.[22]

Meg reveals that she sees a bumpy road ahead and asks Helen what she thinks is best for the family. Helen tells her that this is entirely up to the family and then engages Meg in a discussion about how and what kind of information would be shared if the family members do consent.

In brief, genetic counselors can be expected to be guided by the following points.

How the information is conveyed matters. If Helen had said, "You have an 85% risk for a serious defect," it would convey a different story than, "You do have an 85% chance of a condition that has the following characteristics, generally speaking, but you also have a 15% chance that you do not have it." This illustrates that the profession of genetic counseling has as one of its ethical tenets to try to convey information in as neutral and encouraging language as possible. The goal is to optimize the autonomy and respect of all family members in their decisions and is a posture that all health professionals guided by the goal of a caring response must exercise.

The extent of information shared also is important. Today, unexpected findings often accompany a genetic screening or laboratory test; therefore, health professionals are faced with the challenge of deciding how much of the unexpected information should be included. In fact, Helen says this happened in Meg's case. The desire to determine the appropriate limits of sharing this additional information is not restricted to genetic information. Due regard for the patient and the significance of the additional information for the patient's health are always a consideration. Meg seems to want to know as much as possible, and Helen has been guided by this knowledge.

Genetic information sometimes creates a particularly unique situation because the disclosure of this information has ethical, legal, and social implications. A longstanding concern of genetic testing is discrimination. Many patients find that once they are identified as having (or at increased risk to have) a medical condition, they are faced with denial of health insurance or employment. The federal Genetic Information Nondiscrimination Act (GINA) was passed in 2008 to prohibit such discrimination.[23] Knowledge can also raise concern regarding the future of one's health and, as scientists gain a better understanding of genetic-environmental interactions, the need to prepare patients for probable life changes.[24] In the case of Meg Perkins, genetic information has a multigenerational dimension with deep relational implications for her offspring.[25] Some individuals with genetic conditions may not want other family members to feel guilty, may have fear about their possible contribution to the syndrome, or may fear that the news will cause psychological harm if the condition will lead to more challenges or suffering for loved ones. Because of the potent nature of genetic information, it also raises the question of whether a patient and his or her family members have a right not to know.

With these weighty considerations in mind, Meg tells Helen that she is going to encourage her family to come in to talk with her.

The Right Not to Know

Genetic information has enhanced the questions about the possibilities that individuals have a *right not to know* about information that could be harmful, shameful, or embarrassing about themselves and that they would choose not to know.

Suppose that Meg's daughters are identical twins. If one consents to testing and is found to have the gene composition that gives her a high probability for the development of breast and ovarian cancer, and she decides to take the drastic measure of a prophylactic radical mastectomy before the appearance of cancer, her sister (who has the identical genetic makeup as her twin) who did not want to know her genetic profile inevitably will know that she has the gene. What she will not know is the aspects of the illness such as time of onset, severity, duration, or treatability.[26]

Let us assume that the two sisters consent to meet with Helen and discuss their conflict. Twin A says she will consider it abandonment if she is not tested and allowed to make this choice. Twin B says that she will be betrayed if, having been offered the opportunity and refused, Twin A is given the opportunity for testing then takes the steps that will in fact reveal the status to Twin B. Is there any moral claim on the genetic team not to proceed with the genetic testing of Twin A? Most ethicists and clinicians would argue "no"; their duty is to provide services to those who are in need of it, but they will do their best to help minimize the amount of hurtful information that trickles to Twin B and also to offer their services to her if she wishes to seek it at another time. Unfortunately, the psychological well-being of one twin (A) appears in direct conflict with the other (B), but the resolution between them probably cannot be solved satisfactorily by the health professionals refusing to offer testing, counseling, and treatment to

Twin A. More generally, the possibility of a patient's right not to know certainly supports the idea that a patient's informed consent to a procedure does not give the professional the prerogative to force the findings on a patient, compromising her or his psychological defenses and well-being.

 SUMMARY

> Genetic information is especially powerful because of its ability to involve whole kinships. Informed consent for such testing must involve the professional's sensitivity to how deeply the resulting information can impact not only the patient but the whole kinship. Not only can genetic information disclose essential secrets about individuals, it can challenge familial roles, stigmatize, and lead to social injustices. This has raised the relatively new idea in health care ethics that there is a right not to know.

The clinical field that is emerging based on genetic information is called *genomics*. Genomics will raise new clinical and ethical debates regarding the questions of informed consent and information sharing regarding genetic tests, gene therapy, and genetic enhancements. Health providers must collaborate as a team to balance the client's needs and requests with conflicting demands.[24] Using the six-step process of ethical decision making helps coordinate your ethical reasons with your clinical reasoning in such situations.

Summary

Informed consent in health care and human subject research has become a standard part of Western health care practice and policy. Addressing the shortcomings and adopting varying approaches in different situations are challenges that must be met. Schematically, the idea of informed consent in both health care and human subject research has two dimensions: the information disclosed and the decision-making capacity and voluntariness of the respondent. The advent of advance directives and surrogate decision making is an apt reminder of your responsibility for understanding and abiding by the patient's considered wishes.

Informed consent in health care should be yet another means of facilitating communication between patient and health professional. Consent-related documents are supposed to be tangible evidence that informed consent was, in fact, given. But health care professionals generally place too much emphasis on the form and too little on the informed consent process. Even when the process is emphasized appropriately, the ethical principle of individual autonomy that sometimes dominates must be placed within the larger context of respect for all individuals. At times, respect requires that the partici- pation of the patient be conducted with respect for cultural or other norms that do not place individual autonomy in the prime position. The special challenges of informed consent and information disclo- sure related to placebo use and in genetic testing and interventions will continue to be the topics of lively debate as you enter into pro- fessional practice and will provide an opportunity for you to help shape ethical principles and guidelines consistent with a caring response.

Questions for Thought and Discussion

1. Scott is a 32-year-old man admitted to an acute psychiatric hospital for suicidal ideation in the setting of noncompliance with his psychotropic medications. Scott voluntarily presented to the hospital that he knew from many years of coping with his chronic schizophrenia as he was becoming increasingly psychotic. Scott is refusing to take the recom- mended psychotropic medications that the weekend staff prescribed. He has begun yelling and throwing medication cups back to the nurses stating, "You guys know you can't make me take this junk! This is what is made me crazy in the first place. Get the hell out of here before I call my lawyer." Scott's mental status has been fluctuating greatly, and you arrive to care for him. The medical team asks you to try to convince him to "be compliant" and take some medications to help get his condi- tion back under control. What do you think about Scott's case? How can the team ensure informed consent in this patient? Can you ethically justify medicating Scott against his will? If so, explain.
2. Suppose you are asked to serve on a national commission to develop guidelines for informed consent for adolescents. What age do you think an adolescent should be viewed as capable of providing full and inde- pendent informed consent for treatment? What reasons do you have for your position on the matter? Why are these reasons important from the standpoint of the professional's liability? Of the adolescent patient's well-being?
3. It has been maintained that patients have a right to complete informa- tion about their conditions. But what happens when the diagnosis reveals a genetic disorder that can have known harmful effects on the children? Should the spouse automatically be told? The children? Other relatives? Who is "the patient" in such situations? What guidelines do you think should guide such information disclosure?

Topics in this chapter introduced in earlier chapters

Topic	Introduced in chapter
Ethics committee and ethics consultation	1
A caring response	2
Locus of authority problem	2
Moral distress	3
Quality of life	3
Utilitarianism	3
Principles approach	3
Nonmaleficence	3
Beneficence	3
The health care team	9
Communication	9
Shared decision making	11
Informed consent	12
Assent	12

Introduction

With more than 100 million people in the United States who have at least one chronic condition, chronic care is demanding the attention of health professionals, families, and the health care system more than ever before.[1] Many factors contribute to the increase in the number of chronic conditions and symptoms when compared with even a few years ago. Among these are advances in neonatal intensive care, the increasing incidence rate of long-term survival after traumatic brain injury occurring anywhere across the life span, and an increase in adult longevity. These are just some sources of this growing population of patients nationally and globally.

The term *chronic condition* (from *kronos*, which means "time" in Latin) focuses attention on long-term management of a condition in contrast to one that is either quickly addressed or is at the end of life. It does not denote that the person eventually will die of the condition, although some do. Examples of the latter include cystic fibrosis, amyotrophic lateral sclerosis, muscular dystrophy, multiple sclerosis, Parkinson's disease, Huntington's disease, and severe chronic obstructive pulmonary disease. The common denominator in chronic conditions is that the symptoms persist over time, some for months, years, or a lifetime. You may know someone (or be a person) with one of the previous conditions or someone who lives with symptoms of arthritis, diabetes, clinical depression, schizophrenia, dyslexia, or one of the dementias. The presence of all these forms lends support to the idea that in your generation of the health professionals, most of you will be deeply involved in the treatment of chronic symptoms and the functional impairment that often accompanies them. Currently, the clinical management of patients with chronic conditions often lacks coordination among specialties, providing plenty of room for you to become advocates for improving the quality of care for such persons.[2] This chapter focuses directly on the ethical challenges this population presents and relevant details for achieving a caring response to this condition. A caring response is not unique in comparison with other types of conditions, but at times, the challenges present in slightly different forms. It is noteworthy that in almost all chronic conditions the patient interacts with a whole team of people, sometimes with a *chronic care team* specifically, but other times with teams devoted to a particular disease or injury. This in itself creates an environment of multiple relationships that affect the patient and, very often, include the family or others who provide care besides health professionals.

 Reflection

Do you have a friend, family member, or colleague who has a chronic condition that necessitates ongoing clinical interventions? Perhaps you have one yourself. What are the major challenges that you think, or know, face this person? Are there disruptions in everyday activity that they experience? How are their daily routines different from others'? Jot down a few notes so that as you go through the chapter you can relate that person's situation back to the opportunities health professionals have to provide patient-centered care.

_____

_____

_____

_____

   As you have experienced in previous chapters, to further help set your thinking, you have an opportunity to examine a narrative, this one of a family who is interacting with the health care system because one family member is in a situation that requires ongoing care.

 The Story of the McDonalds and the Cystic Fibrosis Team

The pregnancy had been without complication, and the delivery was much easier than Megan had imagined it would be. She and Gerald beheld the screaming newborn with the wonder that only new parents can feel. Mary

Elizabeth McDonald had entered this world with all the gusto her parents presumed she would need as a second-generation immigrant in their adopted land.

And so it came as a shock to parents and clinical staff alike when shortly after her birth Mary Elizabeth had serious respiratory distress develop. She was placed in the pediatric intensive care unit, and after several series of tests, the clinicians told her parents that Mary Elizabeth had cystic fibrosis. The parents asked many questions about this condition, and nothing they heard sounded encouraging. Gerald went online to find out all he could from the Internet, which plunged them into despair. The health care team in the intensive care unit, including a genetic counselor, social workers, and others, tried to console and encourage them, highlighting the great strides in treatment and longevity that individuals with this incurable chronic condition have enjoyed in the past several years. But Megan and Gerald feared that they had brought this long-awaited and beloved child into the world to endure a life of suffering if, indeed, Mary Elizabeth lived beyond infancy.

That was 12 years ago. Today, Mary Elizabeth is a bright, beautiful child, small and thin for her age, but with a happy spirit. Her inner vitality is a joy to all that meet her, although her life includes long periods of hospitalization and home schooling (and treatment) because of the seriousness of her symptoms. She begins and ends each day with bouts of severe coughing, sometimes for an hour at a time, and several times she has had bacterial infections and pneumonia so serious that the family's parish priest has administered the sacrament of Last Rites, provided only for persons who are believed to be imminently dying. Her school schedule is arranged so that only a few of her classmates surmise where she goes when she leaves daily for the school clinic for the vigorous chest percussion needed to loosen the thick brown mucus that continuously gathers in her lungs. The entire family agrees that it was worth the expense to move to a larger city where they have access to the ongoing availability of an excellent cystic fibrosis team. Given their repeated encounters with the health care system, they find it a wise choice. Among the most helpful is team member Betty Mortimer, a respiratory therapist whose own family has a history of cystic fibrosis and who has been on the team treating Mary Elizabeth for years.

Mary Elizabeth excels in school and is seen as a leader among her peers. Over the years, all three McDonalds have learned to live a day at a time to see what it holds for them as a family. Some days, Megan's activities are completely given over to tending to Mary Elizabeth; other times, she almost forgets that there is any difference between her daughter and other children. Gerald has taken a second job to help defray expenses. Currently, both parents are concerned that Mary Elizabeth is entering puberty and fear that the teen years will present her with new challenges exacerbated by her chronic symptoms. They have long belonged to a parent support group and know that some young people with cystic fibrosis have less difficulty than others making the transition into the teen and adult years, succeeding in their social life and studies, having satisfying careers, and finding a life partner. They also have learned more about the genetic component of cystic fibrosis and know that soon they will have to discuss with her the probabilities of her own children having the condition or being carriers of it. Given their strong religious position on abortion, Megan was shocked to overhear Mary Elizabeth say to a friend recently, "If I got pregnant, I'd have to have an abortion so my child wouldn't have to go through what I'm goin' through." Megan wept all day.

Unbeknown to the McDonalds, the cystic fibrosis team is having a crisis of its own. The head pulmonary specialist on the team, Dr. Abraham Levy, who has managed Mary Elizabeth's care for 8 years, is a world-renowned expert in the field. He announces to the team that he plans to persuade the family to put Mary Elizabeth on an *experimental treatment* in the form of an intravenous medication that the team has used in two other cases rather than having her undergo a lung transplant. The experimental treatment has passed the test of safety and effectiveness standards set by the federal government and has been tested on animals. Now it is being attempted on select patients as part of a phase II clinical trial. A visible pall falls over the room. Three members of the eight-member team assent to his decision, but the second most experienced physician on the team begins to argue with Dr. Levy about this decision. What all of them know is that although this experimental intervention has been heralded in reputable journals and medical circles as a "miracle drug," decreasing the rate of breakdown of the respiratory system in some patients, the first time it was attempted at this institution the patient died shortly after the treatment was administered. Since then, two additional serious deleterious responses to the drug have been reported in the literature. Dr. Levy says that Mary Elizabeth so perfectly fits the criteria for inclusion in the clinical trial that he feels confident of its success and on that basis, the patient's informed consent will be easy to obtain. Some of the team conclude that he will emphasize the benefits of the drug choice only and overemphasize the (to be sure) serious risks of a lung transplant option for the patient.

The next day, Dr. Levy announces to the team that he raised the issue with the McDonalds and obtained their informed consent. Mary Elizabeth was there, assented, and was very excited. "Maybe I can play soccer like my friends!" he reported her as saying. Although the McDonalds were more cautious, he relayed, they decided to go ahead, hoping that she might be among the first to benefit from this new intervention. Mary Elizabeth mentioned also maybe being able to help other girls like herself who will suffer from the effects of cystic fibrosis in the future. Looking around the room and seeing their questioning eyes, Dr. Levy says, "Come on, you doubters. We all have the same goals in mind, and we have to pull together!"

After the team meeting that day, the five members who question Dr. Levy's decision lag behind in the lounge. To put it lightly, they are very upset and unsure of what to do. They pride themselves in being a well-working team and have great respect for Dr. Levy and each other. They have traditionally made such decisions as a full care team. Betty in particular is concerned as she recalls Mary Elizabeth saying that she saw a television program where some doctors were experimenting on patients behind the patients' backs and that of all the things she could not handle, it would be that. They tried to assure her that situation seldom happens and is completely unethical. It would not happen to her here. She could count on that. They are aware that Dr. Levy has little time for what he calls the "armchair philosophers" on the ethics committee, and he prides the team in being able to work out their differences in a reasonable and respectful manner. So he will be upset with them if his decision goes to the ethics committee, an alternative one of them suggests. Another member thinks in this case it is appropriate for each of them to do more research on their own, both about the effects of the experimental medication and also about what the McDonalds were told. Because the treatment is not scheduled to begin until the next week, they agree to all go home and sleep on it and then reconvene after work the next day.

This care team, the patient, and the family are in a relationship that is not unusual for patients with chronic conditions. Some characteristics of this type of team relationship are:

- the shared concern for and loyalty to the patient;
- the long experience of working with each other;
- knowledge that the family caregivers are very much affected by the patient's condition; and
- the care being provided is by the multidisciplinary team, which is designed to provide coordinated care but also can lead to fragmentation at times.

In addition, the complexity and uncertainty facing all of them about what to do next is not unusual. Chronic, long-term conditions always continue to evolve over time, unlike more acute conditions. We turn now to the challenges they face together.

The Goal: A Caring Response

The means by which the goal of a caring response in this situation can be realized is, in many regards, similar to those in any other type of situation. For instance, the care must be personalized to the needs of the patient's specific situation. However, as we already noted, a key consideration that distinguishes a chronic care situation from many others is that collectively the interventions extend over a long period, sometimes from the patient's birth to her or his adulthood and old age. Figure 13-1 outlines several dimensions of the range and possible lifelong duration of chronic conditions.

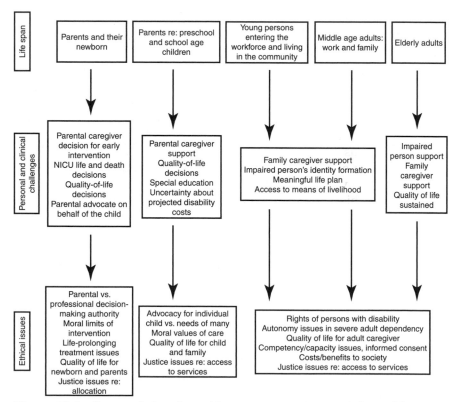

Figure 13-1. Scope of chronic and long-term care issues. *Adapted from a schema developed by Ellen Robinson and Ruth Purtilo to illustrate disability issues across the life span.*

We can predict that in Mary Elizabeth's case, she (and until she reaches adulthood, her parents) will be in relationships with health professionals on a regular basis. For her, there is a high probability this will continue throughout her entire life.[3]

There also are several generic considerations that apply to all patients with chronic conditions.

First, for most patients, their expectations of the health professional or team is not to effect a cure, although if a cure would become known, the focus obviously should shift in that direction.

Second, the point of accepting clinical interventions is to protect or improve the quality of life, whether it be through prevention of secondary symptoms, freedom from pain or other discomfort, or rehabilitation designed to help build or sustain important functions, relationships, and roles. The health fostering and health maintenance interventions for the patient with one ongoing condition (complete with its evolving symptoms over months or years) casts the challenge in a somewhat different light than those directed to acute symptoms. It is a balance of periods of illness and wellness. Persons with a chronic condition have been found to experience challenges to life meaning, needing to balance freedom to do as they want and feel they need to do with loss of control.[4]

Third, and related to the second, the patient counts on the professionals to design treatment programs with the idea that the family (or other significant personal caregiver) is an essential consideration. More than in most other types of treatment planning, the health professional team must take the family caregivers' well-being into account (see later for further discussion of this point) In Mary Elizabeth's or other children's situations, a parent or other adult guardian is the legal spokesperson. The same is true for adults with limited capacity, as discussed in Chapter 12. There are not only ethical but also economic and other practical reasons for making decisions that are appropriate for the family caregivers' needs, and the patient's.[5]

Fourth, clinically and socially, the patient needs the professionals to be acutely aware that "the chronically ill" may have difficulty harnessing appropriate long-term care services. A caring response on the part of the professional must include concerted advocacy efforts designed to counteract and denounce such discrimination and dehumanizing experiences. This extended role of the health professions is discussed in Section V of this book.

 Reflection

Can you think of other considerations that should inform health professionals who are working with chronic conditions but might not be as important in acute care settings? List them here.

_____

_____

_____

_____

 SUMMARY

In chronic condition situations, a factor that affects treatment decisions is that cure often is not the goal, whereas quality of life is.

Again, the six-step process of ethical decision making can be called on for assessing and discerning an ethical course of action in chronic care situations.

The Six-Step Process in Chronic Care Situations

Let us return to the McDonalds and the cystic fibrosis team; we pick up the story at the juncture where the team has become divided about the decision made by the team leader. The first step is to gather relevant information.

Step 1: Gather Relevant Information

The team is paying attention to information that has caused them concern. They know that the drug has been approved for human use in selected situations, such as Mary Elizabeth's case, and that the alternatives for Mary Elizabeth are few. They know all too well that a lung transplant is a high-risk surgery and that for some patients the symptoms of cystic fibrosis grow more serious during the changes of puberty and adulthood.

Evolving Clinical Status over Time

Unlike most health professionals who work in acute care situations, the chronic care team (in this case, the specialized cystic fibrosis team) is in a position to assess a patient's status over a period of time. The members have been working with the McDonalds for several years; therefore, they have a reasonable understanding of Mary Elizabeth's current clinical condition compared with previously. Her condition can be characterized as stable, with the only big unknown being the patient's prepubesence; however, they can compare her condition with conditions of other similarly situated patients because their clinical expertise is in cystic fibrosis and respiratory disease.

Like many teams, they are now faced with a situation in which their certainty is faltering. They know that so far the team has been able to help the

McDonalds manage Mary Elizabeth's symptoms. Unfortunately, at this pivotal moment in the team's relationship, they themselves are divided because of the uncertainty of what is best for Mary Elizabeth, a challenge that so often creates distress for teams working with chronic conditions. Their firsthand experience with the proposed course of action for Mary Elizabeth is limited to the serious negative outcome it had for their one other patient on the unit, an 8-year-old child. They will have to do their homework regarding this ongoing clinical trial and also regarding the surgical option of lung transplant. Is the experimental approach appropriate for a young patient just entering puberty? There is no evidence of long-term effects because the intervention is so new. How does this weigh in the decision?

Team Effects

Fortunately, overall the professionals believe they are privileged to work with a group of outstanding colleagues in this field of medicine, at one of the world's top academic medical centers specializing in respiratory and pulmonary disease. The team is a "dream team" (most of the time!), hitting the rough spots with their common goals to guide them and with deep respect for each other's competence.

It is relevant information that similar to most chronic care situations, the family caregivers have developed a deep trust in the team as a unit. The family must feel free to raise questions, express their emotions, and in other ways show their concern within the current situation. When this trust breaks down, the negative effects on the family may haunt them for years.[6] For the McDonalds' well-being, all activity should be pursued in a manner that allows that trust to be sustained, no matter the actual treatment approach, experimental or transplant. This, of course, means the team be totally trustworthy (Figure 13-2).

The whole team must reckon with the knowledge that this patient's immediate family is an excellent support system. Mary Elizabeth can count on both parents to be there for her. Knowing that, the team should use every means to discern the decision that will best keep this tightly knit family unit strong and optimally functional. Theirs is a long and arduous road ahead, and the opportunity for the patient to take the experimental medication is but a moment in their lifelong relationship. Not only is respect for the parents' wishes warranted, they also must be protected against any outside influences that will create needless guilt, unnecessary resignation, burnout, or other debilitating events in their life.

Quality of Life Focus Is Paramount

Chronic care team members who believe a patient's quality of life is being compromised by activity within the health care environment have good reason for consternation. In the story of the McDonalds, some members of their team are feeling stressed about the planned course of intervention. In

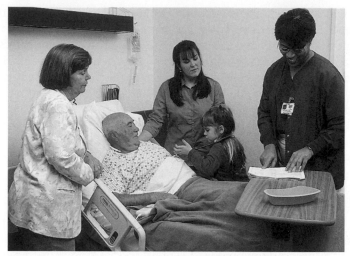

Figure 13-2. The trust between the team and family is essential.

part, this is an informed consent worry that the preteen and her family are not keenly enough aware of the risks associated with the experimental treatment protocol, or of all the alternatives. The whole family's quality of life may be compromised by their not being fully informed agents in the type of important decision they are used to making as shared decision makers.

The team needs to get a better idea, if they can, about the full basis of the McDonald family's enthusiasm regarding the proposed experimental drug. Even if Mary Elizabeth fails to benefit appreciably in terms of her own physical symptoms, the whole family may feel better in the long run if each believes they also are contributing to ongoing research for a means by which the debilitating effects of the disease will be decreased.[7]

In taking quality of life considerations into account, each of the doubters must look beyond the specific symptoms of cystic fibrosis to consider the positive aspects of Mary Elizabeth's current social situation. Examined in this more general context, they have consistently believed that Mary Elizabeth's quality of life is quite good; she appears to be successful academically, seems well accepted at school, and has the benefit of a devoted and capable health care team with back-up clinical support in her school system. However, she also is approaching an age at which her paroxysms of coughing, the exhaustion it can cause, and other signs of pulmonary compromise may make it difficult for her to participate in the rigorous everyday activities that teens enjoy. She may start to feel the negative effects of one who is viewed as "disabled" in some regards. In other words, as she becomes a teenager, she may experience greater teen pressure in her peer group because of her physical difference and may be discriminated against, openly or subtly, in the social activities appropriate for her age group. She is at risk of being labeled as "disabled." She may begin to experience discrimination in the workplace if she looks for an after-school job. None of these negative effects would be surprising because there is a tendency for society overall to show such disrespect to persons with physical or mental impairments, no matter their age.[8] Although the two treatment protocols may seem similar medically, does the family believe one would emphasize Mary Elizabeth's difference from other girls her age more than the other? Is there any way that this information, too, can help the team to make the right decision?

External Factors

Chronic care teams need to have knowledge of the various financial supports available to patients and their families. Especially in the United States, but also in some other countries, insurance or other coverage can run out, either because the patient reaches a certain age, or school level, or the source of coverage caps out at a certain financial figure. Moreover, a confusing variable in insurance coverage for different chronic conditions is that a diagnosis may slip from one coverage category to another. For example, elsewhere we have raised a worry that chronic conditions with a genetic component that necessitates long-term or even intergenerational interventions may become "lost" between two categories of coverage.[9] Cystic fibrosis often falls into that group. What is the McDonalds' situation regarding insurance coverage? Were any of these considerations taken into account, influencing both the physician's and parents' decision? The team must have this information, too.

1 *Reflection*

Can you think of other information that the team members have—or if not, should have—in their reflection on Dr. Levy's decision? If so, jot them down here.

_____

_____

_____

_____

Step 2: Identify the Type of Ethical Problem

This story presents you with an interesting question about the moral agent. Obviously, there are several agents, namely, Dr. Levy, the other team members, and of course, the patient's parents. Therefore, on the one hand, this issue could be viewed as a locus of authority ethical problem. Who should have the say about what? Medically and legally speaking, it is clearly the physician in cooperation with the family of this preteen who are responsible for the outcome. But the rub is that the proposed course of action appears to some other team members to be running slipshod over extremely important social and contextual considerations that they feel professionally qualified to follow up on further to be sure each is taken into account. We encounter these key players at a point where each justifiably feels responsible as a moral agent whose specific expertise is informing their disturbing responses to Dr. Levy's course of action.

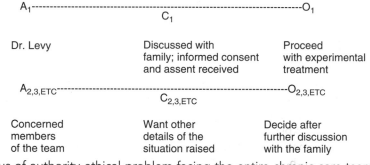

A_1--O_1

C_1

| Dr. Levy | Discussed with family; informed consent and assent received | Proceed with experimental treatment |

$A_{2,3,ETC}$--$O_{2,3,ETC}$

$C_{2,3,ETC}$

| Concerned members of the team | Want other details of the situation raised | Decide after further discussion with the family |

Locus of authority ethical problem facing the entire chronic care team.

It should be clear by now that the team also is facing moral distress. It is a good time to go back and review the two types of moral distress. In type A, the moral agent or agents knows the right thing to do, but there are external (or internal) barriers to moving ahead to the ethically appropriate outcome. As you learned in the previous two chapters, an essential ethical feature of the health professional and patient relationship is shared decision making; this, in turn, depends on informed consent because this process ensures that the patient's autonomy has been honored. When the decision involves families, the challenge increases.[10] Type A moral distress in this situation is being generated by some of the team's doubt about whether Dr. Levy gave the McDonalds adequate information to make a fully informed decision. Without suggesting that he has been negligent or uncaring, it is not unreasonable for the doubting members of the team to raise this worry. With so many decisions about a patient over months or years, and often into old age, the process of informed consent in chronic care and rehabilitation can get overlooked. Some have criticized that, in this area of health care, informed consent is more often minimized than in any other.[11] The patient and family may agree on goals at the outset, but sometimes the health professionals then proceed without taking due vigilance as the process moves forward.

Each member of the team has information they believe should be included so that the McDonalds' decision will incorporate all the areas of their life that may be affected.

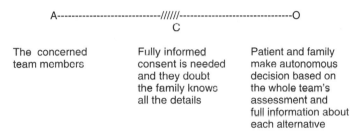

```
A----------------------------//////--------------------------------O
                             C
```

| The concerned team members | Fully informed consent is needed and they doubt the family knows all the details | Patient and family make autonomous decision based on the whole team's assessment and full information about each alternative |

Type A moral distress facing the "doubting" chronic care team members.

Type B moral distress is expressed through emotional discomfort and anxiety when a professional or team is working from a place of high uncertainty about the clinically correct way to proceed. Interestingly, the team members as individuals are experiencing deep disquiet in part because none of them are fully confident that the duress occasioned by a lung transplant will serve Mary Elizabeth well either. They are aware that Dr. Levy has had to make a wager based on his clinical reasoning about the likely best clinical course for this young patient even though there is a relative lack of data about the success of the experimental treatment and a known high risk of survival and thriving with a lung transplant. Because of all this uncertainty as it relates to the well-being of their young patient, the emotional upheaval and doubting carries the moral weight of their duty to affect the most positive outcome possible.

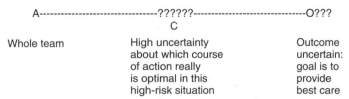

```
A------------------------------??????--------------------------------O???
                               C
```

| Whole team | High uncertainty about which course of action really is optimal in this high-risk situation | Outcome uncertain: goal is to provide best care |

Type B moral distress facing the entire chronic care team about the best course to take.

Step 3: Use Ethics Theories or Approaches to Analyze the Problem

All the members of the team have learned that they need not remain in a state of moral distress. They can each reflect on the situation from the point of view of the ethics theories or approaches available to them.

Utilitarian Reasoning

The team members who are experiencing moral distress could appeal to their knowledge about the consequences they believe will be brought about by various courses of action and try to conclude which will bring about the most good overall. In so doing, they would be acting as utilitarians, trying to optimize the balance of benefits for everyone involved over the burdens brought about.

> ### Reflection
> Reasoning as a utilitarian, which outcomes do you think should take precedence as the doubting team members decide how to proceed?

_____

_____

_____

_____

You may have listed such things as keeping the trust of the family on the heath professionals' judgment high, keeping the team working well together, and giving the McDonalds every reason to believe they have all of the necessary information to make the decision. The overall desired outcome, of course, is to provide the ethically best treatment approach based on the most clinically advisable and fully informed course of action.

Whatever your response, as almost always with a simple weighing of overall benefits and burdens, the team is faced with several unknowns about the consequences of their possible action. Reliance on this weighing alone seems insufficient to bring about the most morally supportable outcome. At the very least, the team members have the additional tool of ethical principles to help them in their ethical reasoning

Principles Approaches

As you know by now, ethical principles can help you to determine the kind of action that your moral duties and attitudes require, not solely the outcome brought about.

⌐ Reflection
Name at least two principles you think the team can rely on in their deliberation about a course of action.

_____

_____

_____

_____

We propose that the principles of nonmaleficence and beneficence provide additional guidance for them. Informing the professionals is their understanding of this patient's autonomy. As dependency increases and social roles change, patients with chronic conditions must adjust their spheres of autonomy.[12] Chronic care balances debility or illness with wellness, taking into account that these change as time goes on. Obviously, the ways in which nonmaleficence and beneficence must be expressed also will change.

The Principle of Nonmaleficence. As you may recall, the principle of nonmaleficence means that health professionals must "do no harm." In the discussion at hand, the obligation to do no harm requires the team members to look closely at the means they are using, not just the consequences. It includes not causing harm directly, removing it when it is present, and preventing it from happening. Each of these aspects of nonmaleficence is briefly examined.

Causing harm could result if the doubting members of the team engage in actions that cause the family, who needs the team over a long haul, to experience the direct harm of distrust. The McDonalds will be lost if they cannot trust the motivation and judgment of the team leader and members. Therefore, nonmaleficence includes deciding how the family should be approached again, if at all, regarding the decision they have already consented to about the experimental treatment regimen.

Removing harm also is necessary. The doubters are worried that harm already has been done by virtue of the McDonalds acting on information that some team members believe is incomplete. If Mary Elizabeth and her parents have made their decision without all the available relevant knowledge, everyone on the team should be supportive in helping to rectify the shortcoming. Viewed from this perspective, nonmaleficence also requires that Dr. Levy and the team members who supported his decision be willing to listen to the genuine concerns of the other team members and, if necessary, revisit his handling of the situation with the McDonalds. Each member has an opportunity and moral duty to act from a disposition of the compassion this family deserves.

In addition, harm must be prevented. In most chronic care situations, the health of the whole family is so intricately connected to the patient's well-being that the caregivers (in Mary Elizabeth's case, her parents) must never be put in a position to believe they have done anything but the best for the patient. This dimension of nonmaleficence supports the idea that the team collectively must ensure the parents have all the pertinent facts for true informed consent and give the McDonald family the support they need in their decision. At this juncture, the parents' autonomy as decision makers becomes a key to preventing harm.

The Principle of Beneficence. The principle of beneficence requires the professional not only to do no harm but also to seek the very best outcome possible for the patient. That is the job of the entire team. Again, the patient–family caregiver unit comes into central focus. The best possible outcome for the patient also must take seriously into account what constitutes the well-being of the family caregivers. This is true not only for instances such as the McDonalds, where the patient is a minor, but for all situations of serious chronic and long-term care situations. Obviously, some people with chronic conditions can live independently, but many need assistance with some aspects of their daily functioning. To complicate matters, many today are living at home with serious impairments that necessitate complex technology. Doherty[13] highlights that the health professional's advocacy designed to ensure that patients and family caregivers have the information they need for the operation of these "machines" is an important part of beneficence. Care giving in the home traditionally has fallen to women, and in the most recent estimate (a decade ago), seven of 10 caregivers were women. However, currently an increasing number of men also are becoming family caregivers for chronic conditions associated with impairment, especially as the population ages and the dementias and other chronic conditions take their toll on both men and women.[14] In a recent project, the authors helped organize a handbook directed to family caregivers. A part of it addresses the range of common stresses on them. We share a portion of it here in Box 13-1; we believe it will give you insight into how to provide a caring response when family or other volunteer caregivers exhibit behaviors associated with stress.

In short, the "best decision" for the patient cannot be made in isolation from what will sustain and nourish the relationship of the caregiver as an individual and in relationship with the patient, whether the caregiver be a family member, friend, or other layperson.[15]

Box 13-1   FAMILY CAREGIVER HANDBOOK
   A Helpful Outline for Addressing Family Stresses

Coping with the Stresses of a Prolonged Trajectory for Your Loved One

Prolonged illness situations, particularly where the outcome is uncertain, are very stressful for family caregivers. An illness may present a variety of stressors. Different individuals may experience stress differently because of their personalities, their relationship with the ill person, their role in the family, or their financial or employment situation. Sometimes family members do not realize how stressed they are or why—they may feel generally anxious or "just not right."

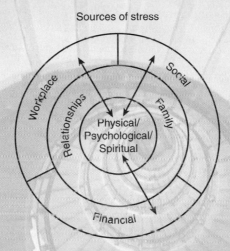

The diagram shows different kinds of stressors. Psychological, spiritual, and physical stressors are shown at the center because of their role in our general well-being. The arrows show the interaction between the layers of stress. The list below details different types of stressors. Take a look at the list and try to identify the stressors you currently feel.

Types of Stress

Physical

- Extra demand on time and energy
- Lack of sleep/altered sleep patterns; can lead to chronic overtiredness or exhaustion
- Changes in appetite: undereating or overeating
- Lack of ability to fight colds and illness
- Headaches, upset stomach, back and other body aches

(Continued)

Box 13-1   Family Caregiver Handbook—*cont'd*

Psychological

- Anxiety
- Guilt
- Fear
- Anger
- Sadness, depression
- Helplessness
- Loss of control

Spiritual

- Anger at God, leading to feelings of guilt
- Feelings of being abandoned by God
- Life losing meaning
- Loss of faith

Family/Relationship

- Marital stress
- Children may act out in reaction to loss of time with parent
- Intrafamily fighting due to family members seeing loved one's illness differently and feeling they would make different decisions

Social

- Decreased interaction with family/friends due to lack of time or decreased physical and emotional energy
- Feelings of isolation
- Unwelcome increase in interaction with family/friends
- Less time/interest in usual recreational pursuits

Financial

- Loss of wages due to absence from work
- Expenses related to hospitalization: travel, parking, meals out, childcare
- Anticipated cost of health care for loved one: hospital bills, potential home care

Workplace

- Missed work time
- Decreased ability to concentrate when at work
- Decreased job performance leading to decreased self-esteem
- Threatened loss of job

(From 2006. Coping with the stresses of a prolonged trajectory for your loved one. In Compassionate care handbook: a guide for families experiencing the uncertainty of a serious illness. Boston: The MGH Institute of Health Professions. Used with permission from MGH Institute of Health Professions, with special thanks to Dr. Ellen Robinson, managing editor; Marion Phipps, RN; and Mary Zimmer, MSW, who contributed the major substance of this section.)

Summary

In chronic condition situations, every ethical consideration must attend to the long-term course of decisions and how it will affect the family or other support network.

Weighing benefits and burdens in a purely utilitarian fashion is insufficient as the situation must meet the test of taking into account specific harms and benefits this patient, this family, and this team face. The principles of nonmaleficence and beneficence provide a path to discerning the most morally supportable course of action and helping to ensure the patient's and family's autonomy.

Step 4: Explore the Practical Alternatives

By now you know that one difficulty professionals face in moral distress is deep emotional upheaval. Under such conditions, the range of alternatives often seems small. However, in your study of ethics, you have an opportunity to think broadly about the alternatives; hopefully they will prepare you for the real life situations you are bound to encounter.

We suggest several alternatives for the concerned members of the team.

1. Support Dr. Levy's decision unequivocally by letting the matter drop. What is done is done, and he is the one who will shoulder the ultimate burden of responsibility about the decision with this family.

2. Take the issue up with Dr. Levy again before the drug is implemented so that the concerned team members can bring their concerns to the table and ask him for further details about the procedure, how his decision was made, and what he actually discussed in detail with the three McDonalds. As discussed in Chapter 9, showing team loyalty to Dr. Levy solely to keep the team running smoothly may not be sufficient reason to let his decision rest without further discussion.

3. If Dr. Levy will not meet with the whole team or they still feel unsettled after the meeting, tell Dr. Levy that they plan to request an ethics consultation so that some objective third parties can help the whole team reexamine the doubters' causes for concern. Their goal is to help discern, from an ethics point of view, which course most fully supports the principles of nonmaleficence and beneficence toward the patient. This consult also could provide insights into how they might coalesce around a mutually arrived at next step with the least fallout among the team members. The team can then follow up immediately with the results of the ethics consult as further guidance.

4. Each concerned team member goes directly to the McDonalds to express their specific concerns about the procedure and what they know about it and to give the McDonalds an opportunity to raise questions. This helps ensure that the McDonalds have an opportunity to directly

provide feedback about the information they have and the conditions under which they gave consent or assent for the procedure. Then the team will be in a better position to decide whether to call an ethics consult before the experimental procedure is begun.

 Reflection

List any other alternatives you think the team members can take to help ensure that the McDonalds receive the most appropriate caring response.

1. _____

2. _____

3. _____

Of all of the alternatives, including ours and yours, which do you conclude is the most morally supportable course of action for the doubters to take?

_____

_____

_____

_____

Step 5: Complete the Action

The team has several alternatives from which to choose. Once the principles of nonmaleficence and beneficence are included in the mix of considerations, they will see that their course of action must fall on the side of the patient's (and her family's) best interests over the course of action that will be the least stressful for the team. When push comes to shove, the team's comfort cannot be honored over the patient's well-being.

We do not believe that the first alternative of letting the matter drop is advisable. There is too much agitation in this situation, and to let it carry over into the treatment procedure cannot serve either the patient or team well. This matter has to be addressed.

On that basis alone, we conclude that the second, and if necessary, addition of the third alternative, is the most morally supportable. At the same time, the team is divided, and the more it becomes so, the more likely some other negative side effects of that division will spill over to the McDonalds. The doubters have a responsibility to approach Dr. Levy in a way that does not unnecessarily put him in conflict with the rest of the team. How they approach him, who approaches him, and when are relevant considerations to making the team meeting work to everyone's benefit.

What do you think about the fourth alternative, having each member of the team go directly to the family? We see it as a morally risky approach because the information that might be transmitted to the McDonalds may sound contradictory to them or become fragmented. The intent of the team is positive, but this action may backfire. Moreover, Dr. Levy has a right to know that the information being provided to and evoked from the family is not unnecessarily raising doubts in the McDonalds' mind about the good intent that the whole team actually shares.

Our support for the second and, if necessary, third alternative, then, comes from some things we know about this situation. The team is a long-standing and well-working team. They have their history of trust and mutual respect going for them, so the team members who have doubts now must muster enough courage to bring that trust into this difficult moment. They must be confident in their abilities to handle this difficult conversation using the communication skills introduced in Chapter 11. In addition, we have no reason to believe that Dr. Levy (or any member of the team) had ulterior motives in mind when recommending the experimental drug regimen. At the same time, the doubters have a right to be heard completely, too. We know how Dr. Levy feels about the ethics consultation, so he should certainly first be given an opportunity to meet with the team and then be informed that the doubting members of the team are exercising their right to take their concern to the ethics consultation service in the hospital if necessary.

Step 6: Evaluate the Process and Outcome

As in every difficult ethical situation, the team members should take time to reflect back on whatever does happen next and how their own dispositions, emotions, reasoning, and conduct played in the final decision. Because they will again have been reminded that in the end the chronic care team's role is first and foremost to get behind the patient's best interests, they will have an opportunity to glean from their experience how those interests were honored and why, at times, they seemed not to be. It will serve them well to reflect on the special challenges of working in a setting where the patient, family or other caregivers, and health care team will be together for a long time. A caring response to each other is as fundamental to the patient's positive experience as that response is to the patient directly.

SUMMARY

In the management of chronic conditions, team approaches dominate; therefore, an effective team is essential to a caring response. An effective team is one that always holds the patient's well-being as the gold standard against which all their activity is measured.

Summary

The increase in scope and number of patients who present to the health care system with chronic symptoms and illnesses, together with the increasing range of interventions available to them, creates an opportunity for you to meet the goal of a caring response for this population. Actual interventions include prevention of new symptoms or decrease in their severity when they do appear, rehabilitation and health maintenance within the constraints of the disease or injury, and vigilance not to assume every new symptom is part of the constellation of symptoms associated with the original chronic condition. Some key factors to take into consideration while arriving at a caring response are the persistence of the patient's symptoms and the generally predictable evolution of a specific chronic condition. The importance of nurturing the family or other caregiver relationships cannot be underscored enough. Promoting patient and family autonomy is a big factor. In Chapter 14, you will have an opportunity to carry some of these considerations over into the area of end-of-life care, demonstrating the similarities and differences when working with this population.

Questions for Thought and Discussion

1. Saul is 47 years old and has recently been diagnosed with Parkinson's disease. As a movie producer in Hollywood, he knows he has all the benefits of modern medicine at his disposal. Still, he slowly is acknowledging that nothing he has read or learned from his sources of information promise him anything but increasing loss of physical and cognitive faculties over time.

   You are a therapist working in a sports center where a number of movie stars, producers, and other notables of the film industry work out. Saul has grown quite fond of you and often stays after his workout to chat. But today he is sad and depressed. He tells you of his diagnosis, about which you had not known, and asks you "as a member of the medical world" if you think there is any hope for him or whether he should just give up now. How will you respond to this man who is reaching out to you in your role as a health professional but who is not your patient per se? How will you help him balance hope and a realistic approach to what you know he may be facing? What, if anything will you say to other people with whom you work that may help him through this initial phase of reckoning with his diagnosis?

2. A leading cause of pain and functional impairment in the United States is arthritis, which affects one of every six people. You are asked to serve on a national commission because of the role your profession plays in the clinical management of arthritis. The charge to each commissioner is to identify how your profession can contribute to a greater quality of life for individuals with the pain and dysfunction of arthritis. Each profession will be advocating for policies that allow them to be reimbursed for beneficial services rendered by its members. You believe you have a moral obligation to advocate for patients as the representative of your profession. Examine how your profession factors into the overall picture of symptom management in arthritis. What arguments will you bring to the commission on behalf of your profession?

3. Chronic conditions and disability often are treated as one and the same. Still, many individuals with disabilities do not have illnesses or symptoms that necessitate health care interventions. One downside of this conflation of the two ideas is that persons with disability often are treated as if they are "sick." Discuss the problem from the flip side of the coin: namely, the ethical issues that arise when a person with a chronic condition is treated as if he or she has a disability, not an illness or clinical symptom. Name some chronic conditions in which there is likely also to be disability.

References

1. Elmore, R., 2009. *Chronic care: Wagner's chronic care model*. Healthcare technology news. Available from: <http://news.avancehealth.com/2009/03/chronic-care-wagners-chronic-care-model.html> (accessed 14.01.10).

2. Bodenheimer, T., 2009. Coordinating care: A perilous journey through the health care system. *N Engl J Med* 358 (10), 1064–1071.

3. Rothenberg, L., 2003. *Breathing for a living: A memoir*. Hyperion, New York.

4. Delmar, C., Boje, T., Dylmer, D., et al., 2008. Achieving harmony with oneself: Life with a chronic illness. *Scand J Caring Sci* 19, 204–212.

5. Blustein, J., 2007. Integrating medicine and the family: Toward a coherent ethic of care. In: Levine, C., Murray, T.H. (Eds.), *The cultures of caregiving: Conflict and common ground among families, health professionals and policy makers*. Johns Hopkins University Press, Baltimore, MD, pp. 127–146.

6. Pinch, W.E., 2002. Four candles on the birthday cake. In: Pinch, W.E. (Ed.), *When the bough breaks*. University Press of America, Lanham, NY, pp. 141–176.

7. Coleman, L., 2007. The legal ethics of pediatric research. Duke Law School Legal Studies Paper No. 186. *Duke Law J* 57 (3), 517–624.
8. President's Council on Bioethics, 2005. *Taking care: Ethical caregiving in our aging society*. US Government Printing Office, Washington, DC, pp. 53–91, 95–150 (Chapters 2 and 3).
9. Purtilo, R., 2004. Genetic labels and long-term care policies: A winning or losing proposition for patients? In: Magill, G. (Ed.), *Genetics and ethics: An interdisciplinary study*. St. Louis University Press, St. Louis, MO, pp. 153–163.
10. Hyun, I., 2003. Conceptions of family-centered medical decision-making and their difficulties. *Cambridge Q Healthcare Ethics* 12, 196–200.
11. Zehr, M.D., 2002. Informed consent in the long term care setting. *Clin Gerontologist* 25 (3–4), 239–260.
12. Mars, G., Kempen, G., Widdershoven, G., et al., 2008. Conceptualizing autonomy in the context of chronic physical illness: Relating philosophical theories to social sciences perspectives. *Health Interdisciplinary J Soc Study Health Illness Med* 12 (3), 333–348.
13. Doherty, R., 2005. The impact of advances in medical technology on rehabilitative care. In: Purtilo, R.B., Jensen, G.M., Royeen, C.B. (Eds.), *Educating for moral action*. F.A. Davis, Philadelphia, PA, pp. 99–106.
14. US Department of Labor Womens' Resource Division, 2000. *Report on the working group on long term care: Nov. 14, 2000*. Employee Benefits Security Administration, Washington, DC.
15. Levine, C., 2005. Acceptance, avoidance and ambiguity: Conflicting social values about childhood disability. *Kennedy Institute Ethics J* 115 (4), 371–383.

14

Ethical Issues in End-of-Life Care

Objectives

The reader should be able to:

- List six ways that a caring response can be achieved in end-of-life care.
- Define palliative care and give at least three examples of how it is expressed.
- Identify some practical means by which a dying patient's trust can be fostered and reasonable expectations can be met by health professionals.
- Discuss how abandonment affects people with life-threatening conditions.
- Describe four guidelines that can help you continue to "abide with" a patient who is dying.
- Identify some basic ethical concepts that have special importance in the treatment of patients at end of life.
- Identify three "faces" of the virtue of compassion.
- Discuss the professional's duty of nonmaleficence for its relevance in end-of-life care.
- Distinguish ordinary and extraordinary or heroic interventions and list two criteria for deciding that an intervention is extraordinary.
- Describe the idea of medical futility and its role in the ethical debate about appropriate end-of-life interventions.
- Describe the ethical principle of double effect.
- List three mechanisms to assist patients and professionals in discerning the proper moral limits of intervention.
- List and discuss the merits and limitations of advance directives.
- Summarize the ethical debate about clinically assisted suicide and medical euthanasia.

New terms and ideas you will encounter in this chapter

end-of-life care	hospice	psychological
palliation	hospice care	abandonment
palliative care		abide

compassion
supererogation
life-prolonging
 interventions
withholding and
 withdrawing
 treatment
ordinary versus
 extraordinary
 means

usual and customary
 treatment
benefit-burden ratio
 test
medical futility
killing
principle of double
 effect
time limited trial
advance care planning

living will
durable power of
 attorney for
 healthcare
U.S. Patient Self-
 Determination Act
 (PSDA)
clinically assisted
 suicide
medical euthanasia

Topics in this chapter introduced in earlier chapters

Topic	Introduced in chapter
Ethics committees	1
Ethics consultation	1
Care and a caring response	2
Patient-centered care	2
Quality of life	2
Ethics of care approach	4
Virtue	4
Benevolence	4
Fidelity	4
Nonmaleficence	4
Autonomy or self-determination	4
Six-step process of ethical decision making	5
Health care teams	9
Hope	11
Do not resuscitate (DNR)	11
Shared decision making	11
Informed consent	12
Surrogate decision maker	12
Substituted judgment standard	12
Best interests standard	12

Introduction

Working with patients and their loved ones when the patient has a condition that carries a medical prognosis of being incurable poses special ethical challenges. How should you, the health professional, treat such persons with the dignity they deserve? The terminology often encountered in the health care literature (e.g., terminal, fatal, irreversible, incurable) adds anxiety when health professionals use it in conversation with patients and their families. At the same time, your work with these patients can be the perfect opportunity to be a positive influence in their lives. For this and other reasons, we will address ethical issues that come sharply into focus when a person is going to die because of his or her medical condition. The current term in the literature and in practice that you will encounter is *end-of-life care.*

Throughout this textbook, you have been reminded of the importance of care in the ethics of the health professional–patient relationship. In no situation does this apply more than in the treatment of persons who are coming to the end of their life. Most health professionals want to convey to patients who have incurable illnesses, "I care," and the examples in this chapter illustrate ways in which that message can be meaningfully conveyed. It requires a clear understanding of special ethical considerations that emerge in this type of situation, rigorous application of your technical competence, and personal adaptability to each patient. To help focus your thinking, consider the following story.

The Story of Almena Lykes, Jarda Roubal, and Roy Moser

Mrs. Almena Lykes is 42 years old and was diagnosed with amyotrophic lateral sclerosis (ALS) about 18 months ago. When she was admitted to the hospital with severe pneumonia and shortness of breath, she had some movement in her arms and could get around in the wheelchair. Despite physical, occupational, and respiratory therapy and good nursing care, she has become weaker since being hospitalized. Test results indicate that her pneumonia probably developed because of weakness of the swallowing muscles (which allowed aspiration of mouth contents into the lungs). She is discouraged, knowing that her condition is going to get progressively worse and that she will eventually die. She also believes that her husband is not willing to care for her at home any longer, a fact that the staff cannot confirm because he has not called or appeared since she was admitted.

After a 2-week course, Almena's condition takes a decisive turn for the worse. Dr. Jarda Roubal, her physician, believes that she is not going to be able to bounce back from this pneumonia even with vigorous treatment with antibiotics and respiratory therapy because of rapid deterioration of her swallowing and breathing muscles. Dr. Roubal discusses the seriousness of her prognosis and the options open to her for interventions regarding her pneumonia (e.g., medications, respiratory therapy) and predicts that she is near to the time when she will have to make a decision whether or not she wishes to be placed on a ventilator permanently. He answers all questions directly about the seriousness of her prognosis. He asks her nurse, Roy Moser, to place a respirator in her room for quick initiation of ventilator support should it be needed.

Yesterday evening, Mrs. Lykes asked Roy to sit down with her by her bed. Tearfully, she told him that she really was ready to die. She requested that her treatments in physical, occupational, and respiratory therapy be discontinued and that she not be placed on a respirator unless it would mean she would suffer less while she was dying. She said she had seen a movie in which a woman was given morphine to speed up the dying process and make it painless and explained that was what she wanted. She also requested a Do Not Resuscitate (DNR) status. "Dr. Roubal means well, but he will make a vegetable out of me," she says, breaking down. Roy said he would be sure to talk to Dr. Roubal about her wishes but that the final decision would be made by her and the team caring for her. Then Roy documented the conversation in her clinical record.

That evening when Dr. Roubal came through to check on the patients, Roy Moser took him aside and conveyed the whole conversation as best he could recall it. Dr. Roubal listened intently and said, "What do *you* think?"

"I think we should do what she suggests. She isn't going to get better."

After a moment, Dr. Roubal said, "Well, you are right about her not getting better, but I think she is depressed and once she gets on a respirator and over the pneumonia she will see it differently. She still has a lot of life in her." Dr. Roubal then went to visit Almena. He said to her, "The nurse has told me about your concerns. I would like you to think it over. There's still a lot we can do for you."

Later that evening, Roy went back to Almena Lykes's room. Almena looked extremely sad and alone, her eyes puffy from crying. Now she was dry eyed and made an attempt to lift her limp hand. "I don't know what to do," she said.

Before continuing, take a minute to think about Dr. Jarda Roubal's and Roy Moser's response to Almena Lykes.

 Reflection

What is each doing to show a caring response to her problems?

Do you think one or the other is more correct in their judgment about whether to continue treatment? On what do you base your opinion?

_____

_____

_____

_____

In this story, you can quickly discern by now that several important ethical dimensions of professional practice come into full view. As in previous chapters, we will guide you through the six-step process to highlight some of them, knowing that you may identify others.

The Goal: A Caring Response

Suppose that you are Dr. Jarda Roubal or Roy Moser. It goes without saying that Mrs. Lykes deserves all the respectful consideration from you that you would give to any patient. She needs to feel confident that you are competent because her life literally may be in your hands. In a word, she expects you to give her your best attention consistent with a caring response.

As discussed in previous chapters, caring is a balancing act. The very purpose of your professional role is to be technically competent and show the appropriate personalized nurturing also necessary for true care. This becomes even more important in end-of-life care. The health professional who is committed to patient-centered care at end of life will do at least the following:

1. Maintain vigilant attention to clinical interventions appropriate for the person's condition, whether preventive, rehabilitative, or comfort enhancing. The diagnosis of an incurable condition does not mean that the whole range of interventions may be prematurely dropped from the clinician's resources for optimal treatment.
2. Take enough time to communicate with the patient (and loved ones) to get a "feel" for the person's values, strongly held beliefs, habits, cultural and ethnic characteristics, and personality. This also helps facilitate discussion amongst patients, their support systems, and the care teams regarding how they would like to receive clinical information and handle decision-making tasks.
3. Listen carefully to what the person has to say. A focus on the patient's quality of life governs you in your attempt to create a warm, personal environment. Only the patient's (or if the patient is incapable of indicating preferences, the surrogate's) interpretation of what makes life worthwhile counts, not yours or anyone else's. Sometimes concerns that are important to the patient seem insignificant to a health professional.
4. Recognize that a patient's perception of quality of life is fluid near the end of life. Many research studies (and clinical cases) verify the fact that perception of quality of life often undergoes revision as an individual's condition evolves.[1] Patients should be given information, choices, and control whenever possible.
5. Understand that the final phase of a condition brings with it a myriad of emotions. Patients facing end of life may experience shock, anger, fear, grief, denial, pain, and depression; others may express readiness

or relief. In the words of Hank Dunn, "Facing the reality of death is like encountering a wide river that must be crossed . . . None of us can force one another across."[2] And not all patients believe there is another side. These emotions take time to process and work through. Patients need your comfort, patience, and assistance to effectively do so.

Reflection

What might you expect would weigh heavily on Mrs. Lykes's mind right now?

_____

_____

_____

_____

How can you respond in a warm and supportive manner to her concerns?

_____

_____

_____

_____

SUMMARY

A caring response in end-of-life situations requires apt attention to quality-of-life issues for the patient and family.

Palliative Care

As we come to realize that health care includes the provision of comfort measures to people who are dying, and attempts at curative and restorative treatments until they are shown to be futile, the notion of palliative care becomes integral to a caring response. *Palliation* means to reduce the severity of or relieve symptoms without curing the underlying disease.[3] *Palliative care* is patient-centered and family-centered care that optimizes quality of life by anticipating, preventing, and treating suffering.[4] Palliative care is not limited to individuals with incurable conditions that lead to death, although that is the focus of our discussion.

Some objectives of palliative care include the following general guidelines:

- People with advanced, potentially fatal conditions and those close to them should expect and receive skillful and supportive care not focused on curing the patient.
- Health professionals must commit themselves to using their professional knowledge effectively to prevent and relieve pain and other disturbing symptoms.
- Health professionals should regain awareness and humility about what modern medicine can and cannot do so that patients can deal with their own death realistically, not as the enemy but as a part of life.
- Health professionals must recognize that the patient's continuing downward course may be a time of anxiety for the health professional, too, which poses a challenge to the whole team.[5]
- Providing the best care possible means that as much imagination, competence, and energy must be directed to palliative interventions as would be devoted to care of a patient without an incurable condition.

Throughout the patient's illness, the goal of providing the best palliative care possible includes giving emotional support to people closest to the patient. This helps encourage the patient, although you might find yourself frustrated with the patient's relatives and close friends because they are angry and confused or feeling intense sorrow and may transfer their feelings to you. Their demands, worries, questions, and interference with treatment can be disconcerting, especially when their actions call into question your own best judgment or exacerbate your own anxieties about the patient's plight. (This may be a good moment to review Figure 13-2, which lists the sources of stress families experience when faced with caring for a loved one with a chronic condition. The sources are similar when end-of-life care goes on over a period of time). Remember that any time the patient's most intimate sources of support are alienated or harmed, the patient also inevitably suffers deleterious consequences. At best, family and close friends are a great assistance to your efforts; at worst, they should not be unnecessarily excluded from your support and deprived of relevant information. Although their behaviors differ according to culture and other family practices, they have a right to be included.[6]

In palliative care, stopping intense efforts to effect a cure must be coordinated with an even more intense effort to engage in a regimen of clinical intervention aimed at reduction of discomfort. The words of a talented physician some years ago still have great relevance today:

> *"Even when we decide that our advanced technologies are no longer indicated, we can still agree that certain extreme measures are indicated—extreme responsibility, extraordinary sensitivity, heroic compassion."*[7]

These words are especially valuable because often at the moment that you admit the person is indeed beyond medical intervention aimed at cure, you may momentarily feel at a loss as to how to continue to express your caring. We can imagine that Roy Moser had this feeling when he walked into Almena Lykes's room and noticed she had been crying or when she confessed she did not "know what to do." Your own imagination may be thwarted by the knowledge that the patient's time is limited. This could deter you from setting attainable goals that may be of importance to the patient. Tonight is the future. Tomorrow is the future. Mrs. Lykes can be encouraged toward the goal of using the bathroom unassisted tonight or sitting up to write some letters tomorrow. Sometimes, too, patients are hesitant to offer information about their desires because they fear the goal will seem irrelevant or even silly to someone else. For example, one young woman confided to the chaplain that she longed to go to the chapel for religious services but was afraid it was too much work for the nurses to get her there. Another woman who needed large doses of pain-reducing medication told the medical technologist she was concerned that the "fuzziness" created by the medication would impair her judgment when her lawyer came to discuss her estate. The technologist relayed the information to the woman's physician, and the physician arranged to have the medication withheld during the lawyer's visit, with the grateful consent of the patient. Another aspect of palliative care is to adjust your approach according to the probable time left before the patient's death. One has to be an artist of "good timing." The person who senses that the end is near often will ask to be left alone with only a few select people or, in some cases, with no one at all. To be cheerfully intrusive at such times denies a person the need to determine the use of last moments. In contrast, to treat a person who may live for months or years with a slowly progressing illness as if he or she is about to die at any moment robs that person of the sense of belonging among the living. A balance is needed to plan and attend to life tasks amidst what may be an uncertain disease trajectory. A 42-year-old woman dying of a slowly progressing leukemia went into her local hospital for her monthly blood tests. A laboratory technician who had not seen her for several months greeted her by saying, "You still around?" The woman told her husband later, "She was just teasing, but it made me feel funny—like maybe I was supposed to have died already or something."

Anyone who has experienced the ordeal of a loved one's prolonged dying knows that some of the tensest moments are those related to not knowing how long the person will be alive, to being afraid that one will prematurely die, and to not knowing how to make appropriate plans for the future. The art of palliative care includes being as sensitive as possible to the time frame the patient and family are living with and adjusting your own approach accordingly.

Hospice Care

One highly successful alternative for patients with conditions beyond medical cure is *hospice,* which originated in England and has spread to many countries in the world.[8] *Hospice care* focuses the entire staff and institutional structure toward maintaining the patient in as comfortable, pain-free, alert, and humane an environment as possible.[9] Hospice teams are interdisciplinary. They recognize the dying process as a part of the normal living process and provide support and care for the patient during this phase. Hospice programs provide a unique set of benefits for patients and their families. Evidence shows improved pain assessment and management, improved bereavement outcomes, better overall satisfaction, and lower mortality rates among family members of patients who received hospice care.[10] Patients are generally eligible for hospice when they forgo curative treatment and have a life expectancy of 6 months or less, although as the concept continues to evolve, these regulations may change.

 SUMMARY

Palliative care has many dimensions, among them your concerted effort to maximize quality of life through decreasing physical, psychological, and emotional pain and attending to the patient's own timing and life situation.

Now that we have laid the general groundwork for what a caring response entails in this type of situation, we invite you to turn to the by now familiar process of ethical decision making to consider Almena Lykes's story in more detail.

The Six-Step Process in End-of-Life Situations

The art of caring requires that health professionals be keenly aware of when the moral aspects of the relationship hit a snag and an ethical problem appears.

Reflection

Do you think Dr. Jarda Roubal and Roy Moser are faced with an ethical problem? If so, jot down why or why not and how their respective roles as physician and nurse are similar and different.

_____

_____

_____

_____

We believe they do have an ethical problem, given the seriousness of Almena Lykes's clinical condition. The life or death decision about life-prolonging measures must be negotiated to her satisfaction, and her present anxiety must be taken seriously into account. We begin here by reviewing the salient facts of her story to help highlight some details of the problems in her particular situation.

Step 1: Gather Relevant Information

The most important fact we have is that Mrs. Lykes has a progressive, incurable condition, the pathology of which will continue to cause her muscles to grow weaker. She will experience greater functional impairment and ultimately failure of her heart and respiratory muscles. She will lose control of her throat muscles, resulting in an inability to swallow. Eventually, she will die of her condition.

Dr. Jarda Roubal is monitoring this clinical course and trying to maintain her respiratory functions. Roy Moser is a central, coordinating figure of the team of therapists, technologists, and others who gauge how various interventions are helping to maintain the health she has remaining. They also are trying to stay in touch with her feelings and keep her optimally functioning and comfortable. We know that all three of the key players in this story are at a crossroads. Should Mrs. Lykes's expressed wish to give up now be honored, or should the health professionals listen to her confusion in the lonely evening hours and again encourage her to hang on? Dr. Roubal will be the one to make the final call, medically speaking, about how to proceed with technologic and medical interventions. However, from an ethical viewpoint, that call must be made with as much certainty—and in as much accord with Mrs. Lykes's real wishes—as possible.

One key to her suffering is that she may be abandoned by her husband and may be (or already is) left alone by someone she deeply counted on. The fear and reality of such abandonment is common enough that it warrants your further consideration here. Almena, like many patients who face death and dying, may fear isolation, pain, dependence, and the family's response to her deteriorating condition. Not only do patients experience betrayal from their own body, they often experience physical and emotional betrayal from those closest to them. Some patients like Almena with progressive neurologic conditions may feel they are living with dying. This awareness of death can prompt one to reflect on life's meaning and to seek closure in personal, practical, and spiritual matters.[10]

Abandonment: A Patient's Reasonable Fear

Almena Lykes knows that things are not going to get better, clinically speaking. We have just mentioned how sometimes spouses, other loved ones, and friends fall away during the patient's process of dying. Some challenges that face family and other loved ones in regard to their role during a long-term course were mentioned in Chapter 13. Mrs. Lykes has a chronic, disabling, and incurable condition. For whatever reason, Mr. Lykes has disappeared; it is not possible to ascertain whether his absence is because of fear, weariness, disgust, or anger at her situation, or his own pathology.

In addition to abandonment by loved ones, patients also sometimes detect that health professionals are distancing themselves, which exacerbates the patients' anxiety and suffering. Health professionals seldom physically abandon patients who have an incurable medical condition. Sometimes, however, they are caught in policies that prevent them from giving a patient as much of or the type of treatment the professionals believe that person needs. For instance, in the United States, some health plans have been accused of shortchanging patients by not paying for needed treatment for some groups.[5] Because health plans vary widely in their practices, you should check out the conditions of your employment site before signing a contract so as not to be forced into what seems to be abandonment by policy dictate.

Psychological abandonment is the greater danger that sometimes leads a health professional to physical neglect of the patient. Why? For one thing, their concepts of what health care interventions should accomplish may lead professionals to distance themselves because the patient continues to "get worse." Others are repulsed by the appearance, smells, or other disturbing manifestations of a patient's condition.[11] Psychological preparation for the pain of loss when a patient dies is advisable, and sometimes health professionals distance themselves to protect against the pain of that loss and feeling of failure. But psychological abandonment is distancing that far exceeds the use of necessary defense mechanisms. It follows that no matter what Mrs. Lykes's husband chooses to do, the responsibility for not abandoning her also falls on Dr. Roubal, Roy Moser, and the other health professionals working with her. Together they can support each other to overcome their tendency to abandon her physically or psychologically.

Reflection

Suppose you are Roy Moser that evening in Almena Lykes's room. What aspects of this situation might make you feel like fleeing? What steps can you take to help ensure this type of harm does not befall her? What additional information from Mrs. Lykes might be helpful or necessary to provide appropriate care for her, thereby remaining faithful to your role?

_____

_____

_____

_____

Abiding: A Patient's Reasonable Hope

The idea of abiding with a patient may help you to think about what the opposite of abandonment looks like. To *abide* means "to endure without yielding," "to bear patiently," and "to remain stable."[12] Sometimes, good care simply requires digging your heels in and standing firm.

The following are some general guidelines that can help you to maintain an attentive position toward Mrs. Lykes that she will experience as your abiding with her. You will recognize them as having themes similar to the ones you were introduced to as a part of personalized care and good palliative care in these situations. The guidelines include:

- Recognize your own feelings of fear, disgust, and repulsion. They are embarrassing, and the inclination is to pretend that they do not exist. Denial does not make them disappear.
- Encourage sessions in your workplace where everyone can share their feelings in a safe, constructive environment.
- Make efforts to talk to patients so that you will know them better and can focus on who they are personally. In many instances, the troubling feelings become less important.

You deserve assurance that you have appropriate policies in place to help you show respect for Mrs. Lykes the way you are expected to do for all patients. You deserve assurance that the type and number of interventions you are offering do honor her considered wishes and her body's capacity for responding positively to them.

 SUMMARY

Physical or psychological abandonment of a person who is dying can be countered by professionals who choose to abide with the patient. Professionals need support themselves in this situation.

Having touched on some salient features of the patient's situation, please turn to the ethical decision-making process again.

Step 2: Identify the Type of Ethical Problem

Both the physician, Jarda Roubal, and the nurse, Roy Moser, are faced with ethical problems that come from a high degree of uncertainty about the best course of action to take for Mrs. Lykes.

Locus of Authority Problem

This juncture of their quandary is an apt place for you to consider a locus of authority problem.

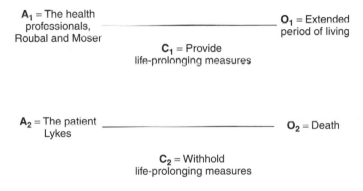

A_1 = The health professionals, Roubal and Moser

C_1 = Provide life-prolonging measures

O_1 = Extended period of living

A_2 = The patient Lykes

C_2 = Withhold life-prolonging measures

O_2 = Death

A = Moral agent
C = Course of action
O = Outcome

Locus of authority ethical problem.

You recall that the locus of authority prototype of ethical problem requires two or more moral agents in the situation to decide which of them should be the final appropriate moral voice in the decision. To the extent that Almena Lykes is competent to make her own decisions, and the diagnosis of an incurable condition is confirmed, the ultimate answer is easy: she is. The physician has requested something that is potentially lifesaving, so we want to be sure she is not making a decision to refuse it on partial knowledge or because she is depressed. She must not make a decision that she will not only regret but that is irreversible.

Talking to her further is an obvious next step both the physician and nurse want to pursue. In Chapter 12, you were introduced to informed consent. The goal is to be sure that she is competent to make, and is making, an informed decision. Dr. Roubal believes she might be refusing the ventilator because she is depressed and that she will change her mind, suggesting that she will want to be put on the respirator when her depression lifts. Although many patients with chronic conditions suffer from depression at some point during their illness, this is not a judgment he should make lightly. A visit by the liaison psychiatrist can help ascertain whether she is clinically depressed to the point of being unable to make this important decision. The position he apparently is holding, that of a paternalistic authority who will try to talk her into accepting the respirator, should not be maintained without the additional information about her mental status.

Moral Distress

At the point we enter their picture, Jarda Roubal has made a clinical judgment that he believes is in Almena's best interest, but he certainly is shaken by Roy's report. Roy, too, must be in a situation where he cannot be sure what is going on. Both have additional work to do as moral agents; therefore, the health professionals also face moral distress. They, like she, are emotionally unsettled, apparently because of their own uncertainty about how to proceed. They know she is approaching the end of her life and has a right to request the discontinuation of therapies. However, Dr. Roubal and others also want to be sure she is not making an impulsive decision because the stakes of the outcome are literally life and death. Almena has stated that one of her concerns regarding this phase of her condition is that if Dr. Roubal puts her on the ventilator it will "make a vegetable out of her." Roy has worked with many patients with ALS who have chosen ventilation as a pulmonary support and who have done quite well. Some only need ventilation at night. It is possible that once Almena's pneumonia clears that she would be in this category. Would she be okay with this as an option? Roy Moser also wonders if Almena has ever seen other patients with ALS who use assistive devices such as computerized communication systems or environmental control units. Her knowledge of these technologies as possible options to help her live better in the end stages of ALS would ensure that she is has all the needed information to make a truly informed decision.

 Reflection

Recall that there are two types of moral distress. From the description we have given, is the team faced with type A or type B?

_____

_____

The uncertainty about the obvious best clinical way to proceed is so tied to the life and death consequences of their decision that they are experiencing type B moral distress. This often happens around end-of-life care, although one of the values of the ethical study you are engaged in is to decrease the margin of uncertainty with salient facts and the other steps of ethical decision making.

Step 3: Use Ethics Theories or Approaches to Analyze the Problem

What resources does each of these professionals need to arrive at a caring response in this type of situation? The ethics of care approach places virtues in a central place and provides a useful means of assessing the ethical issues here. Much has been written about the virtue of compassion in health care, and nowhere is it more important than when the patient has an incurable condition. The term *compassion* often is used in everyday language to indicate a warm or positive feeling toward the patient, which helps to convey sympathetic involvement with the patient's plight. Although that usage is not incorrect, further attention is warranted when applied in the context of health care. From an ethics perspective, we invite you to examine it as a virtue, as a duty, and as going beyond duty.

Compassion: Three Moral Faces of an Idea

The three powerful components of compassion are[13]:

- the character trait or virtue of sympathetic understanding recognized as a virtue;
- the willingness to carry out your professional responsibilities toward the patient, recognized as moral duty; and
- the readiness to go beyond the call of duty.

We can observe these dispositions in others but may not readily recognize them as compassion.

Compassion as a Virtue. The virtues of kindness and benevolence are recognizable as promoting a desire to treat people with gentleness and to "do good" when it is in your power to do so. Being able to do good depends first on the ability to imagine vividly how another feels, so that you become aware of the needs and wants of the other person. The word compassion comes from the Latin, *passio* ("suffering") and *con* ("with"). It entails the desire to treat others with empathetic understanding. It is from this root meaning that compassion usually is understood solely as a disposition toward others, a virtue.

Reflection

Knowing as little as you do about Mrs. Lykes's situation, what do you believe are some of her needs that warrant your empathetic understanding? To aid in your reflection, write them down.

_____

_____

_____

_____

The desire to be empathetic is a resource in itself. You might find it expressed in something as simple as a reassuring arm across her shoulder, knowing she is discouraged, or a telephone call to assist Mrs. Lykes in making contact with a close friend or a person in religious life who has been a source of guidance or comfort to her in the past. To do so with understanding increases the likelihood that you will get it right in terms of the way you choose to express your empathy. Compassion is a virtue that closely is associated with what it means to care. If you recall from Chapter 2, care is an opportunity but also is a burden. In other words, it goes beyond any superficial understanding of kindness or benevolence. The additional two components of compassion help to highlight this interpretation.

Compassion as Willingly Doing Your Duty. A form of compassion sometimes overlooked is willingness to carry out your duties on behalf of the patient's best interests as you have discerned those interests through your empathetic posture. As compassion compels you to do what is right, you can see how two aspects of ethical thought (character traits and the deontologic approach of duties) are brought together in an actual situation. Compassion, as a character trait in the type of person you want to be, aids you in the desire actually to do what you discern to be right. This helps you to keep to task, to pay attention to doing your work competently, and to not be careless about the well-being of the patient when you would rather be meeting a friend or golfing or even going about some other aspect of your daily work. In a word, it helps you to abide with the patient.

Compassion as Going Beyond Duty. Finally, the motivating force of compassion positions you as a moral agent to exercise kindnesses that go beyond duty. In philosophic terms, acts that altruistically go beyond duty are called acts of *supererogation.* An example recalled by one of the authors was of the recent death of a pediatric patient. The infant was in the neonatal intensive care unit for more than 7 weeks, during which time the ups and downs of his critical condition roller coastered both the care team and the family through much uncertainty. The infant was withdrawn from life-sustaining treatment and died. The infant's funeral was attended by several of his care providers. This supererogative act brought tears to the parents' eyes. In this fast-paced health care delivery environment, such deep compassion was rarely actualized.

The Principle of Nonmaleficence

Your general duty of fidelity or faithfulness to patients includes the stringent principle not to harm them. Do you remember the more philosophic term for this duty? If you said "nonmaleficence," you are right. The deliberate and diligent efforts of many before you to put in place procedures to assist you in providing compassionate care is one indicator that your moral obligation not to harm has been taken seriously by health professionals and society.

 SUMMARY

Virtues and character traits guide the moral agent to act within an ethics of care approach. At the same time, the principle of nonmaleficence shows that the deontologic approach also helps inform what is right in this type of situation.

To learn more specifically the forms that right actions might take in end-of-life care situations, we proceed to the next step of decision making.

Step 4: Explore the Practical Alternatives

You have already noted that if you were in the shoes of Jarda Roubal or Roy Moser an ethics of care and principle-based approach will have led you to explore what Mrs. Lykes really knows about the decision to be made, if she is too depressed to make an informed decision and, finally, what her considered choice is.

So, one alternative is to discuss your (and her) quandary with other members of the health care team who have been involved in her treatment. This activity will help decrease the amount of moral distress the team is experiencing. These discussions (along with the information gathering completed in Step One) will provide clarity to the locus of authority problem and place the team in a better position to creatively problem solve alternatives. This step is a place where the *who* and *how* is broached with Almena once the decision is made about *what* is the morally correct course of action.

Once you have reached a point of greater certainty, you will have to assume a function appropriate to your professional role on the team involved in Almena Lykes's care in regard to life-prolonging interventions or, as they are often called, life-sustaining treatments. *Life-prolonging interventions* is that term applied to many technologies that assist in basic life functions such as breathing, eating, and maintenance of vital organs that otherwise will shut down. Life-sustaining treatments range from CPR to mechanical ventilation to nutrition and hydration to antibiotics, to name a few. Most of the difficult clinical and ethical issues arise around how far to go in *withholding* the start up of life-prolonging interventions or, if they have been started, in *withdrawing* them at some later time. The issues of withholding or withdrawing are so important that you will learn more about them later in this chapter.

We assume that Dr. Roubal's referral to psychiatry has deemed Mrs. Lykes to be mentally competent. As a member of the team, you are helping to determine the proper moral limits of clinical interventions designed to support an extension on the length and quality of her life. Therefore, one basic practical determination you have to make is whether interventions in this situation are "ordinary" or "extraordinary," according to what Almena Lykes believes is the balance of benefits over burdens she will receive by initiating them.

Employing Ordinary and Extraordinary Distinctions

Having introduced you earlier in this chapter to some problems that arise because health professionals stop treatment prematurely or psychologically withdraw, you now have an opportunity to consider the converse. Psychologically, withholding or stopping a treatment is sometimes difficult for a health professional. The development of DNR orders some 30 years ago marked a pivotal change in health care delivery because it was the first order to directly withhold treatment.[14] In recent years, the health professional's desire to "do all that is possible," coupled in some cases with the personal need not to "lose" a patient, has led to an overzealous approach. The ethical notion of heroic procedures or *extraordinary means* has since been developed to help protect patients from such an assault.

From an ethical point of view, even treatments that are *usual and customary* (i.e., those considered the usual treatment regimen for conditions of this type) can, under certain circumstances, be judged extraordinary or heroic. The ethical criterion for considering a treatment heroic is that it may inflict undue physical, psychological, or spiritual harm on the person even as it serves to prolong the patient's life.[15] For instance, suppose that a relatively new treatment is being used successfully for amyotrophic lateral sclerosis. It could add several months to Mrs. Lykes's life; however, it has disturbing cognitive side effects. Mrs. Lykes rejects it out of hand. You must honor a competent patient's wishes. On that basis, this new treatment becomes extraordinary.

SUMMARY

Extraordinary treatment means that when a person makes a fully informed decision to refuse further treatment, that treatment is inappropriate, even though it may prolong life or have other beneficial physiologic effects.

The "bottom line" in the ethical distinction between ordinary and extraordinary rests on the patient's decision, not the health professional's judgment. Any intervention, from the most simple and routine to the most technologically advanced, can be ordinary or extraordinary, depending on its fittingness for a particular patient. This is the most important thing you must bear in mind, not the fact of how "high tech" or, in your view, invasive or expensive or experimental the intervention is. A relatively simple, safe, routine, or inexpensive intervention also could become extraordinary.

The same test can be applied to an incompetent patient, but the surrogate decision maker bears the weight of deciding what the patient would have found an unbearable burden and what would constitute a benefit.

 Reflection

Now that you know more about the concept of ordinary and extraordinary measures, list some additional alternatives to help Mrs. Lykes and the team decide the next steps in her plan of care.

_____

_____

_____

_____

Applying the Benefit-Burden Ratio Test. Why do patients refuse certain treatments? Because they decide that treatments that may be promising from a medical point of view and that are administered routinely to others impose too great a burden on them to be worth it. Honoring the patient's assessment of benefits versus burdens in an intervention has been termed the *benefit-burden ratio test.* In the story you read, that was what Almena Lykes said at one point. Patients may refuse for many reasons. Some may detest the idea of a treatment that will cause profound memory loss, or will require amputation or other disfigurement, or has side effects that cause great discomfort, or is extremely costly to the family. At the same time, the

reasons for refusal may be the benefit of gracefully "letting go." We can easily imagine two patients who would receive similar physiologic benefits
from a medical intervention but who would assign different weight to the
personal, human benefits accruing from the treatment. Mrs. Lykes might
weigh the benefit of the experimental intervention or even permanent use
of the ventilator quite differently than we would because she believes she
has accomplished what she hoped to in life and has a sense of being at peace
with the nearness of death. She may have certain spiritual or religious convictions such as afterlife beliefs that guide her decision making.

What happens when a competent patient refuses a treatment that the
health professionals believe will be highly beneficial and effective? Health
professionals are not required or allowed to override the patient's decision,
even in this difficult situation. Competent patients can refuse any type of
treatment, even one that is life sustaining. Sometimes patients choose to
withdraw from clinical care altogether and go home, an option they have a
right to choose so long as it is an informed and competent choice.

Assessing Medically Futile Care. The notion of extraordinary care also
applies when there is no reasonable hope that the patient will benefit medically from the care even though he or she may want it. The phrase around
which discussion has evolved in recent years is *medical futility.* It addresses
the flip side of the coin of the previous discussion of how patients have a
right to refuse a treatment that health professionals think is medically appropriate. Sometimes patients (and more often families) demand interventions that health professionals judge are not designed to be of any benefit to
the patient. In recent years, the idea of medical futility has become a point
of lively social-political debate and has raised questions of what medical
and other clinical interventions actually are designed (and able) to achieve
in life and death situations.[16]

At first glance, the idea of providing medically futile care seems ridicu-
lous. Why does it even need to be discussed?

In many situations, interventions that did do some good initially are
continued because to now withdraw them appears to the family or other
interested parties to be harming, even killing, the patient. The discussion of
medical futility has created helpful guidelines for judging when health professionals justifiably may withdraw previously helpful interventions on the
basis that the patient's condition has changed.

Futility always has meant that something would not help. But today, with
so many interventions available, there is a need for a clear understanding by
everyone of what "helping" and "not helping" means. The discussion of
medical futility has led to a refined understanding of when an intervention
may be withheld even though a patient wants it. In recent years, some legal
challenges have concerned how far to accede to a patient's, or surrogate's,
demands in determining the degree or types of interventions that are
warranted. The idea of futility has been useful in clarifying that medically

useless treatments should be withheld or withdrawn, no matter how much a patient or surrogate wants them.

The ethically appropriate standard by which a procedure can be judged medically futile is the good of the whole patient, not that it can sustain a single organ or body system. The rationale for this should be clear because some medical interventions may allow an organ (e.g., the heart) to survive, but the patient's condition may otherwise be completely irreversible and devastating.

In today's exciting high-technology health care environment, the tendency to extend the arm of technical intervention can lead to a distortion of the art of clinical intervention.[17] From the earliest times, our professional predecessors warned about this type of abuse, counseling always that our practice follow not only the science but also what we know about the effect on the patient's well-being. The contemporary, technology-driven medical tendency to chase an organ or system at the cost of the whole patient's well-being can be experienced. In many instances, health professionals are responding to urgent requests of patients or families who also place their trust more in the machine than in the professional and who subsequently fail to see the crumbling patient who is victim to the health professionals' frantic attempts to "spot weld" together the failing organs and organ systems.[18]

The standard for declaring an intervention medically futile continues to be the subject of debate. Questions regarding prognosis and predictions of survival and eventual quality of life can be exceedingly difficult.[19] Many professionals assert that the values of a person's life that makes intervention worthwhile are not for others to determine in these complex situations.

At least three measuring rods have been applied to the idea that an intervention can be called "futile" and therefore give health professionals the opportunity to consider not honoring the patient's or family's wishes.

- *Physiologic standard.* This is most conservative approach based on the clinical judgment that an intervention will not, or no longer will, have any appreciable beneficial physiologic effect on the patient. One example would be the use of antibiotics for a viral infection.
- *Probability standard.* A second approach is to try to quantify the probability that an intervention will have an appreciable beneficial physiologic effect. Proponents of this position suggest that although the intervention may work at times, it so seldom does that it should be dropped as a realistic alternative for this patient.
- *Quality-of-life standard.* The goal is to develop either an individual or group standard of quality of life. In this position, the benefit is framed in terms of the quality of life a patient would realize. For example, should an intervention that would bring a patient to the point of responding to light and sound but never to the point of responding to the environment in a more purposive fashion be judged futile? The risks of determining whole categories of persons who

have qualities worth or not worth supporting with interventions should be apparent in this approach.

 SUMMARY

Any treatment is extraordinary if it is also futile (i.e., offers no appreciable hope of benefit to the patient).

You will be joining the ranks of the health professions at a time when this important topic undoubtedly will continue to be debated. Currently, all three standards of futility are applied in different settings. Any time such a standard is set, certain interventions are determined not to be of any benefit, in other words, to be "futile."

Let us return now to the larger framework in which this discussion is placed, namely the criteria of ordinary and extraordinary care. Whether the care will benefit this patient in this circumstance is the governing consideration.

Keeping the Focus on the (Whole) Patient

The ethical reasoning about the limits of intervention that are morally appropriate (including consideration of ordinary and extraordinary distinctions) requires a focus on the individual patient's well-being as a point of reference. There are several helpful mechanisms for approaching the difficult question of ascertaining when enough is enough; their goal is to provide a more humane approach to patients who are critically ill or have irreversible conditions that will lead to death.

The health professions team, lead by the physician, who is the appropriate person to make the clinical judgment about the patient's medical status, should make the decisions, guided by the patient's informed wishes. However, as we have been discussing, the key considerations that arise are not solely about medical status.

Ethics committees are one mechanism to guide health professionals, patients, and their families in end-of-life care decisions. There is one important difference between what you (as a current or future health professional) must do and what an ethics committee or ethics consultant does. You are in a position to carry out, or at least be on the team that carries out, the action. The committee or consultant stops with identifying the practical alternatives with the distinctions you have been reading about in this chapter. Often, the decision involves whether to withdraw or withhold measures that, under other circumstances, would be considered usual and customary to use, or, in other words, would be "ordinary treatment."

Withdrawing and Withholding Life Supports

We mentioned the function of withdrawing and withholding life supports earlier in this chapter as one way to approach the limits of what clinical care can and cannot do. On the positive side, when a condition is reversible, many technologies act as "bridges" between life-threatening symptoms and health, allowing the person to return to a healthy, or healthier, state. Further, when a condition is not reversible, life supports* sometimes act as life-sustaining bridges between severe episodes within the dying process but ultimately are a temporary bridge between life and death itself. Almena Lykes is faced with being put on life support in the form of a respirator. At this point, she is refusing this treatment, and Jarda Roubal and Roy Moser are concerned about the enormity of her decision. Her response tells us that she is at a point where to continue to ply her with more devices to assist in various organ functions such as breathing is moving from life sustaining to life prolonging. And that raises serious questions about what it means to "prolong life." Sometimes, such prolongation begins to look like an assault on the patient as a person, overriding his or her values, quality of life, and judgment about whether the artificially supported organs are indeed "life."

The proper moral limits of medical intervention described in the preceding discussion provide a general ethical framework for withdrawal and withholding of life supports. An intervention that the patient (or the patient's surrogate) finds much more burdensome than beneficial and from which is no escape may be withheld or removed ethically. A futile intervention that will not reverse the condition or symptom ("offers no appreciable hope of benefit") also may be withheld or withdrawn.

In such an act, you, the health professional, are not killing the patient. It is an ethically justifiable act, the end of which may be the patient's death, but it does not meet the criterion of "killing." *Killing* is a direct act of commission, meaning that you—the agent—intend to bring about a patient's death and actively intervene to do so. In other words, in withdrawing and withholding you are not engaging in the activity with the intention of ending the patient's life nor are you the direct cause of her death. For example, in the case of Mrs. Lykes, she has a disease that will cause her death. Her death will probably come sooner without artificial, medically applied interventions to assist her breathing, heartbeat, kidney function, ingestion of nutrition and hydration, and other bodily functions, but eventually the medical condition directly will kill her. She does not have a respirator to assist her in her breathing. Dr. Roubal, her physician, determines that she

---

*This chapter uses the term life supports as it commonly is used in the medical, policy, and legal literature—namely, medical technologies that sustain or prolong a patient's life.

will die shortly without this medical intervention, but she refuses it any-way. Her death will be brought about by the illness within her. At best, her death can be delayed by your intervention.[20]

A decision to withhold or withdraw a treatment should be made openly and communicated with the team and documented in the medical record so that all health professionals involved in the patient's care are aware of the decision. A physician may, in consultation with the patient or patient's fam-ily, decide that a patient will not receive a certain life support, but if there is no record of the decision, the nurses, residents, or others on duty will feel obligated to initiate it in the event of a life-threatening episode.

 SUMMARY

Withdrawing or withholding treatment is not to be confused with acts of directly ending a patient's life.

This type of decision is psychologically difficult for health professionals. The process of withdrawing the life-sustaining treatment of nutrition and hydration is especially challenging. Although professionals may know ra-tionally that they are not killing a patient, it seems to be true nevertheless when they disconnect the feeding tube. All the team support mechanisms discussed in Chapter 9 need to be brought into play to assist colleagues in these difficult moments.

Principle of Double Effect. The *principle of double effect* is an ethical reason-ing tool that can help you in situations in which you act with the intent of providing palliative care for a patient but, in so doing, have the unintended effect of hastening the patient's death. The most commonly cited example of this principle is the administration of a pain reliever (e.g., morphine) that has a side effect of compromising respiration. Because the patient becomes more and more tolerant of the medication, doses high enough to relieve the pain also suppress and at some point stop the patient's breathing.

The principle of double effect acknowledges that one act can embrace two effects: an intended effect and an unintended, secondary effect. The intended effect governs the morality of the act. In this case, the intended effect is the patient's comfort, with the professional acting on the presump-tion that the quality of life must be preserved. The inescapable but unin-tended secondary effect is that at some point in the continuum of this care the patient will succumb to the high dosage. Another aspect is that the in-crease in dosage must be the minimum necessary to achieve the patient's comfort. Finally, the unintended side effect cannot ever become the in-tended effect—that is, death cannot become the goal of the person provid-ing the medication.

In summary, the most important thing for you to learn about this tool is that the intent is key. The intent to relieve the patient's pain or other serious discomfort governs the morality of the act, not the unfortunate and unintended secondary consequences (i.e., the patient dies). The second most important thing to learn is that the proportion of increase in the comfort-enhancing intervention must be only the minimum needed to achieve the intended effect, namely, the patient's relief of suffering from pain or other symptoms. Although only the prescribing professional has authority to order such medication, nurses almost always must implement the procedures, and other team members also may be involved in ensuring the patient's comfort.

Steps 5 and 6: Complete the Action and Evaluate the Process and Outcome

Returning to the story as written, Dr. Jarda Roubal and Roy Moser have several considerations to take into account before they decide whether to withhold the respirator and other life-prolonging measures. We noted that their first action is to get Almena Lykes's wishes as crystal clear as possible through continued conversation with her and to take whatever steps are necessary to learn whether she is so depressed that she is not in a reliable state to know her true wishes. Further action regarding intervention cannot justifiably be completed without knowing her informed preferences. Once they know this important information, they will have an opportunity to work together with her and the team to continue each portion of her care motivated by the goal of a caring response. Oftentimes, in cases such as Almena's, a *time-limited trial* of life-sustaining treatment is warranted. A time-limited trial designates the use of a life sustaining treatment or other therapeutic intervention for an agreed-on trial time period. The time period generally ranges from 1 to 3 weeks, depending on the clinical scenario. The purpose of such a trial is to ascertain the true benefits and burdens of an intervention.[21] At each decision point, the team, in collaboration with the patient, is well advised to use the tools of evaluation and reflection on the portion of the action they have just completed. These conditions help ensure that she does not become abandoned and that her care remains competent and personalized.

Assessment of Mrs. Lykes's circumstances and the health professionals' considerations should provide you with a good general framework for a caring response in end-of-life care. However, before leaving the subject, you will benefit from considering two additional facets of such care: first, informed consent in situations where a patient clearly is no longer competent to make decisions; and second, a brief discussion of clinically assisted suicide and medical euthanasia.

Advance Care Planning in End-of-Life Care

What should happen when persons are, or become, incompetent? Recall from Chapter 12 that their wishes then are "heard" through the voice of an appointed surrogate. One modern societal mechanism to assist surrogates and professionals alike in important decisions under such circumstances is *advance care planning*, a process that includes discussion and documentation of advance directives.

Advance directives are processes accompanied by forms that have been developed to help reassure patients that their end-of-life wishes will be honored as much as possible. They become effective only when the patient no longer is able to make her or his wishes known regarding the types and extent of medical intervention that the patient thinks appropriate.

Reflection

Because of their emphasis on the patient's wishes, what ethical principle forms the foundation for advance directives?

_____

_____

_____

_____

If you responded "autonomy" or "self-determination," you remember well what you have learned so far. If you did not answer correctly, now is a good time to go back and review the discussion of autonomy in Chapter 4.

There are basically two major types of advance directives, although some documents bear slightly different names or combine the two:

- *Living will* documents are designed to enable a patient to specify the types of treatment he or she would want to have and, more importantly, not have.
- *Durable power of attorney for health care (DPAHC)* documents are designed to enable a patient to specify a surrogate or proxy decision maker who he or she wants to make the treatment decisions when he or she is no longer able to make them. This document may also be called a health care proxy.

Reflection

As you look at these two types of advance directives, what do you think are the major strengths and drawbacks of a living will?

_____

_____

_____

_____

By comparison, what are the major strengths of a durable power of attorney? What are its major drawbacks?

_____

_____

_____

_____

Surrogate or proxy decision makers must use substitute judgment, addressed in Chapter 12, when deciding what their loved one would want. Recall that this means they must make a decision as the patient would have based on the patient's values and preferences, not their own. This is what makes proxy decision making so complex. Many surrogates say that they do not know what the patient would want. In such cases, surrogates are often asked to recall previous medical experiences that the patient went through and related discussions that the patient may have had regarding desired values, goals, and preferences. In absence of knowing what decision the patient would have made, a surrogate can collaborate with the care team to use the best interest standard. This entails making a decision that is in the best interest of the patient. It is often used in pediatrics and in situations where the patient was never competent. The living will and durable power of attorney are legally binding in all 50 U.S. states, but their wording may differ. You should familiarize yourself with those in the area where you live and work (and, by the way, where your loved ones live).

In January 1990, a nationally mandated *United States Patient Self-Determination Act (PSDA)* made it necessary for every patient in the United States to be asked on admission to a health care institution whether he or she has an advance directive or wants to prepare one. For those who have one, it is placed in the patient's permanent health care record in that institution. If the person desires one but does not have one, the institution has forms for the person to complete. Other countries do not have similar nationally mandated mechanisms such as the PSDA, although many share the task of trying to ascertain what is best for the patient in our current era where life can be prolonged almost indefinitely in some instances.

Although these forms are helpful in making an incapacitated patient's wishes known, far more important is that the patient talk to loved ones and professionals long before the moment of decision making arrives. There is no substitute for having had a long time in which to prepare loved ones for the challenge of making a life or death decision and for making decisions that honor the patient's understanding of the quality of life. Advocates of advance care planning suggest that the best place for these discussions to take place is in the primary care or home setting. This setting provides opportunities for end-of-life discussions because its outpatient, noncrisis environment can best set the stage for defining patient values, goals, and expectations. As mentioned in Chapter 13, such discussions and decisions impact both the patient and the family care providers. Research with end-stage cancer patients has shown that more aggressive medical care was associated with worse quality of life and a higher incidence rate of major depressive disorder in bereaved caregivers.[22] Patients and families often look to health professionals to bring up these difficult conversations. As a future health professional, you should seek to develop strategies for talking with your patients and families about this topic. It is difficult at times to balance prognostic realities with hope; however, good communication at end of life is an essential skill for a caring response.

Clinically Assisted Suicide and Medical Euthanasia

No modern discussion of end-of-life care is complete without a discussion of clinically assisted suicide and medical euthanasia.

Although assisted suicide often is called "physician-assisted suicide," we choose these words purposefully in calling it *"clinically assisted suicide"* because almost all health professionals who have interactions with patients could face patients who are contemplating this course of action and ask for assistance. Some health professionals, such as nurses, social workers, and pharmacists, work directly with doctors in the chain of events that lead to a patient's suicide when it is treated as a medical option in end-of life-care.[23] Many health profession organizations have issued position statements affirming their opposition to the practice on the basis that it is incompatible with professional ethics.

In the United States, the most decisive cases against this type of action occurred over a decade ago. In 1996, the Supreme Court ruled on two cases involving physician-assisted suicide and ruled against the rationale set forth for permitting assisted suicide in these instances.[24] What many people do not understand is that although the rulings are important in setting precedents against this practice, they do not (and did not) preclude individual states from passing legislation permitting clinically assisted suicide. In fact, at the time this book is being published, legislation permitting it currently exists in the states of Oregon, Washington, and Montana.

Most ethical debate identifies intent and consequences as key factors, distinguishing withdrawing and withholding life-prolonging measures from assisted suicide and direct euthanasia.[25] In all these cases, the patient dies after the act. As you now know from earlier discussions in this chapter, the intent is a morally relevant distinction between withdrawing or withholding life supports with death ensuing and those interventions designed to end a patient's life mercifully. In the former, the intent is not to cause the patient's death but rather to honor the patient's right to have certain invasive, life-prolonging interventions withheld or stopped. In assisted suicide, the health professional is the direct agent of administering the means by which a patient can effectively end her or his own life. The most commonly discussed form of clinically assisted suicide is the health professional who provides information about and a prescription for the lethal dose of a medication. In actual cases, the health professional may or may not be physically present at the suicide. The question then is how involved the health professional must be to be judged an agent in the patient's death. More fundamentally, the ethical debate steps back to a discussion of whether assisted suicide should be permitted at all.

Proponents of clinically assisted suicide probably are in a minority among health professionals, although it is impossible to ascertain how strong the support really is. Those in favor of legislation that decriminalizes assisted suicide argue that respect for a patient is determined, first and foremost, by a respect for the patient's autonomy. They also argue that the professional promises to abide with a patient, show compassion, and be committed to providing comfort when cure is no longer possible and that these commitments extend to helping a patient gain information or access to the medical means to take her or his own life.

 Reflection

Suppose Mrs. Lykes requests that Dr. Roubal give her the information and means necessary for her effectively to end her own life. What might her reasons be?

_____

_____

_____

_____

If you said things such as, "she cannot imagine going on in this condition; for her, life is no longer worth living" or "she knows it is going to get worse and she can't take it," you would be identifying the reasons given by patients and the themes that therefore often are used in support of this procedure.

Opponents argue that lethal prescriptions should never substitute for compassionate, palliative end-of-life care.[26] They object to the idea that respect for persons is embraced fully by honoring their wishes, important as they are. Respect for persons must entail a respect for life, and the appropriate moral role of the health professional is to save life, not to assist in any way in taking it. Choosing to become an advocate of death is a distortion of the age-old ethical mandate of the health professions to save life. Neither faithfulness nor nonmaleficence can be honored once the line between being an advocate of life and being an advocate of death has been crossed. Opponents also assert that compassion never can be expressed by having a part in intentionally ending a patient's life.

Medical euthanasia, that is, ending a patient's life with medical means administered by a physician, requires the direct moral agency of the physician.

The patient is truly a "passive bystander" while the health professional's intervention is carried out with the goal of ending the patient's life.

Assisted Suicide

1. The physician provides the medical means (instead of some other means, such as a gun).
2. The physician is necessary but not sufficient for the act.
3. The patient needs to do the final act (take the lethal medication).

Medical Euthanasia

1. Physician commits the act by medical means.
2. The physician is necessary and sufficient for the act.
3. The patient's condition provides the context.

Proponents and opponents in the ethical debate about medical euthanasia draw on arguments similar to the ones described earlier regarding assisted suicide. Proponents also often draw the line between voluntary medical euthanasia (where a competent patient requests euthanasia) and involuntary medical euthanasia (where requests cannot be made because the patient is incompetent). In countries where medical euthanasia legally is permitted (e.g., the Netherlands, Belgium), proponents reject advance directives as a legitimate mechanism for continuing such a request into a period when a patient no longer can speak for himself. Opponents add to their other objections that voluntary euthanasia inevitably slips into involuntary euthanasia.

Concerns from opponents to both types of procedures are that the trust health professionals accrue from their willingness to take the patient's life seriously when others devalue the patient will be fatally compromised and that health professionals themselves may become less diligent in seeking comfort measures for a dying patient if it is permissible, instead, to assist a patient in "ending it all." There also are serious concerns that minority patients and other socially marginalized members of society will be encouraged to end their lives (or have them terminated), whereas others will be offered alternatives. Alternatives in the form of diligent end-of-life care that stops short of assisted suicide then become the mandate that guides a professional's approach.

Summary

Decisions about life and death in the health professions are among the most challenging from an ethical and a practical viewpoint. There is much we do not understand, so awesome is it to look at the death experience. You will do yourself a favor to take some time to be introspective about your feelings toward death. Just as the light and heat from the sun are useful and necessary in small doses, so it is true that health professionals must dare to look at death closely enough to gain insight into their roles as humble mediators between life and death, sickness and well-being. By so doing, we all will better learn how the ethical tools of character traits and duties based on principles of nonmaleficence, autonomy, and faithfulness can help to build and sustain the moral foundations of the health professional–patient relationship in this challenging situation. Conceptual distinctions, such as ordinary and extraordinary, withdrawing and withholding, double effect, and the role of the health professional *vis à vis* allowing or intending death, can help. The ethics of care counsels each of us to keep the lens of professional treatment focused on what constitutes a caring response.

Questions for Thought and Discussion

1. Laura Penman works in a nursing home with a specialty in dementia care. She floats from the units that provide care to patients with mild dementia to the locked floor for those with severe end stages of the

disease. Today she is assigned to care for Sandra McKendrick. Sandra is an 82-year-old woman with end-stage Alzheimer's disease. Laura remembers her from when she was admitted to the facility several years ago. Last month, Sandra's daughter Kate agreed to placement of a feeding tube to get her mom through an acute hospitalization for flu-related pneumonia. She completed her course of intravenous (IV) antibiotics, but her cognitive and self-care (particularly feeding and eating abilities) abilities have not improved. Kate is visiting tonight and says "I don't know what to do for my mom. I wish I never agreed to the tube. She is not better, but if I ask the doctors to take it out now, my sister says I will be inhumane because my mom will starve. I don't know why my mom picked me as her health care proxy. This whole situation stinks!" How would you respond to Kate's statement? Is it ethical for the family to withdraw the feeding tube? What would you say to Kate's sister during this difficult situation?

2. Is there a living will or durable power of attorney act in your state or province? What are its provisions? What are its limitations? What is the legal significance of such a document, and how does that differ from its psychological and ethical significance?

3. A patient with a rare, progressive liver disease that is invariably fatal after a long and arduous period of debility has stated several times that he wishes to end his life by his own hand "when the time comes." During his most recent visit to his physician, he asks the physician to write him a prescription for "an assuredly lethal dose" of the medication he has been taking. The physician writes the prescription, then tears it up and says, "I can't do that." Then, he tells the patient how many tablets would be needed for "an assuredly fatal dose." Did the physician do the right thing? Describe some of the legal and ethical ramifications of this conduct by the physician.

REFERENCES

1. Gruenwald, D.A., White, A.J., 2006. The illness experience of older adults near end of life: A systematic review. *Anesthesiol Clin North Am* 24, 163–180.
2. Dunn, H., 2005. *Light in the shadows: Meditations while living with a life threatening illness*, 2nd edition. A and A Publishers, Inc., Herdon, VA.
3. Stedman, T.L., 2008. *Stedman's medical dictionary for the health professions and nursing*, 6th ed. Wolters Kluwer/Lippincott, Williams, and Wilkins, New York, p. 1144.
4. National Quality Forum, 2006. *A national framework and preferred practices for palliative and hospice care quality*. Washington, DC.
5. Rushton, C.H., Reder, E., Hall, B., et al., 2006. Interdisciplinary interventions to improve pediatric palliative care and reduce health care professional suffering. *J Palliative Med* 9 (4), 922–933.

6. Crawley, L.V.M., Marshall, P., Koenig, B.A., 2001. Respecting cultural differences at the end of life. In: Snyder, L., Quill, T. (Eds.), *Physician's guide to end of life care.* American College of Physicians, Philadelphia, PA, pp. 36-45.

7. Cassem, N., 1978. Treatment decisions in irreversible illness. In: Cassem, N., Hackett, T. (Eds.), *Massachusetts General Hospital handbook of general hospital psychiatry.* Mosby, St Louis, MO, pp. 573–574.

8. National Hospice and Palliative Care Organization (NHPCO), 2009. History of hospice care. NHPCO, Alexandria, VA. Available from: <http://www.nhpco.org/i4a/pages/index.cfm?pageid=3285&openpage=3285> (accessed 25.01.09.).

9. Lynn, J., 2001. Serving patients who may die soon and their families: The role of hospice and other services. *JAMA* 285 (7), 925–932.

10. Casaret, D.J., Quill, T.E., 2007. "I'm not ready for hospice": Strategies for timely and effective hospice discussions. *Ann Intern Med* 146 (6), 443–449.

11. Toombs, K., 1997. Review essay: Taking the body seriously. *Hastings Center Report* 27 (5), 39–43.

12. Random House (Ed.), 2001. Abide. In: *Webster's unabridged dictionary.* Random House, New York, p. 4.

13. Dougherty, C., Purtilo, R., 1995. The duty of compassion in an era of health care reform. *Cambridge Q* 4, 426–433.

14. Burns, J., Edwards, J., Johnson, J., et al., 2003. Do not resuscitate order after 25 years. *Crit Care Med* 31 (5), 1543–1550.

15. Prendergast, T.J., Puntillo, K.A., 2002. Withdrawal of life support: Intensive caring at the end of life. *JAMA* 288 (21), 2732–2740.

16. Stanley, K., Zoloth-Dorfman, L., 2001. Ethical considerations. In: Ferrell, B., Coyle, N. (Eds.), *Textbook of palliative nursing.* Oxford University Press, New York, pp. 75–91.

17. Cassel, C., Purtilo, R., McFarland, E., 2003. Ethical and social issues in contemporary medicine. In: Dale, D. (Ed.), *Scientific american medicine,* vol. 1. WebMD, Inc., New York, pp. 3–7.

18. Jacobs, B.B., Taylor, C., 2005. Medical futility in the natural attitude. *Adv Nursing Sci* 28 (4), 288–305.

19. Wainwright, P., Gallagher, A., 2007. Ethical aspects of withdrawing and withholding treatment. *Nurs Stand* 21 (33), 46–50.

20. Randall, F., Downe, R., 1999. The moral distinction between killing and letting die. In: *Palliative care ethics: A companion for all specialties,* 2nd ed. Oxford University Press, New York, pp. 270–277.

21. Johanson, G.A., 2009. The defined trial period in ethical decision making. *J Pain Symptom Manage* 38 (3), 473–476.

22. Wright, A.A., Zhang, B., Ray, A., et al., 2008. Associations between end of life discussions, patient mental health, medical care near death, and caregiver bereavement adjustment. *JAMA* 300 (14), 1665–1673.

23. Altman, T.K., Collins, S.E., 2007. Oregon's death with dignity act (ORS 127.800-897): A health policy analysis. *J Nurs Law* 11 (1), 43–52.

24. *Quill v. Vacco*, 80 F3d 716 (2nd Cir., 1996) and *Compassion in Dying v. State of Washington*, 79 F.3d 790 (9th Cir. 1996) (en banc).
25. Troug, R.D., Campbell, M.L., Curtis, J.R., et al., 2008. Recommendations for end of life care in the intensive care unit: A consensus statement by the American College of Critical Care Medicine. *Crit Care Med* 36 (3), 953–963.
26. Ganzini, L., Goy, E.R., Dobscha, S.K., 2009. Oregonians' reasons for requesting physician aid in dying. *Arch Intern Med* 169 (5), 489–492.

Ethical Dimensions of the Social Context of Health Care

15

Distributive Justice: Clinical Sources of Claims for Health Care

Objectives

The reader should be able to:

- Understand how the concept and function of distributive justice affect the health care environment.
- Describe what a caring response involves in situations that require the allocation of scarce resources.
- Compare the concepts of microallocation and macroallocation.
- Distinguish the contexts in which fairness and equity considerations apply to everyday professional practice.
- Evaluate the function of procedural justice assumptions as a device for enabling further discernment about allocation of a cherished resource.
- Describe some situations in health care in which fairness considerations are required for a just allocation of resources.
- Discuss the relevance of the philosophic starting point of deliberation in distributive justice: treat similar cases similarly.
- Compare the ideas of allocation based on a right to health care, on need, and on merit.
- Discuss the concept of equity in allocation decisions.
- Define the term rationing.
- List and critique five criteria for a morally acceptable approach to rationing of health care resources.
- Critique situations in which random selection has been argued as a just approach to allocating resources.

New terms and ideas you will encounter in this chapter

allocation of health care resources	"first come, first served"	material principles of justice
distributive justice	procedural justice	social justice
microallocation	principle of equity	health disparities
macroallocation	formal principle of justice	entitlement
principle of fairness		positive right

health care as a commodity	very important persons (VIPs)	proportionality
negative right	rationing	random selection/ lottery approach
merit justice	dire scarcity	

Topics in this chapter introduced in earlier chapters

Topic	Introduced in chapter
Hippocratic oath	1
A caring response	2
Moral agent	3
Moral distress	3
Ethical dilemma	3
Principle of beneficence	4
Principle of justice	4
Deontology/duty reasoning	4
Rights	4
Utilitarian reasoning	4
Medical futility	14
Extraordinary (heroic) care	14

Introduction

As this book goes to press, the United States legislature and public have again been embroiled in a health care reform debate. Among the issues are whether health care is a right and whether we have a responsibility to care for persons who are not in our immediate circle of intimacy and relationship.

All nations face questions of limited health care resources and escalating costs. These issues worldwide create ethical challenges that involve the *allocation of health care resources*. Allocation is a term that suggests intentional decisions about how a good is distributed. In ethical deliberation, such challenges fall within the category of distributive justice, the topic of this chapter, and compensatory justice, discussed in Chapter 16.

Distributive justice purports that humans have the capacity to make nonarbitrary, reasonable bases for distributing goods and services that are in at least moderately scarce supply but desired by many. For our purposes, health care resources are those goods and services. Some justice issues are best addressed by examining your direct care giving role. For example, you may be faced with a personnel shortage in your workplace and will have to decide where to cut corners and why. You may work where there is not enough equipment or space or money to fully satisfy what your best effort requires. In operating under that extenuating circumstance, you are forced to make decisions about how to spread out the desired good or service. In society, claims for goods are taken into account according to individuals or groups of people who are judged to be similarly situated according to need, merit, or other considerations. The resulting decisions about who gets what are termed *microallocation* decisions.

Some of the most critical issues regarding allocation of resources also remove you from the arena of direct patient care to considerations of policy, where whole groups of similarly situated people are implicated. For instance, in the United States and globally, current lively policy debates surround such issues as how to distribute limited supplies of medicines for treatment of AIDS, immunizations in times of epidemics or pandemics (e.g., for new strains of flu), and organs for organ transplantation.

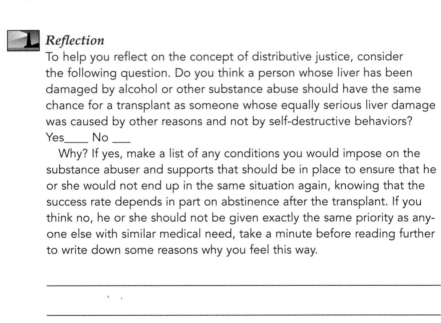

Reflection

To help you reflect on the concept of distributive justice, consider the following question. Do you think a person whose liver has been damaged by alcohol or other substance abuse should have the same chance for a transplant as someone whose equally serious liver damage was caused by other reasons and not by self-destructive behaviors? Yes____ No ___

Why? If yes, make a list of any conditions you would impose on the substance abuser and supports that should be in place to ensure that he or she would not end up in the same situation again, knowing that the success rate depends in part on abstinence after the transplant. If you think no, he or she should not be given exactly the same priority as anyone else with similar medical need, take a minute before reading further to write down some reasons why you feel this way.

_____

_____

_____

_____

Currently, in most countries where liver transplants are offered, there is a waiting period for alcoholics to demonstrate that they are successfully abstaining from alcohol, a criterion that appears to reduce the recidivism rate among those fortunate enough to be chosen for an organ. This wait is above and beyond the wait that other similarly needy potential organ recipients experience. Whatever the outcome, the decision about organ transplantation points out that in the allocation of health care resources conscious choices are made, and the choices do make a difference in the lives and well-being of whole groups of similarly situated people.[1]

⊚ SUMMARY

Distributive justice helps us find morally justifiable criteria for the distribution of desired and needed resources. Microallocation debates regarding the priority list for allocation of scarce resources revolve around considerations of need and likelihood of benefit and often include considerations of lifestyle.

Some policy decisions require that different types of societal goods be compared, recognizing that a society does not have infinite resources to cover all of them. For instance, such allocation decisions may involve trade-offs between more roads being built, or military installations provided with better facilities for troops, or existing national parks maintained. These judgments are called *macroallocation* decisions. Although these decisions are extremely important, we leave this aspect of your study to other courses.

For your discernment about distributive justice, the following story will assist you in your thinking about your role in these complex practice and policy issues.

🍃 The Story of Christopher Lacey and the Contenders for His Bed

One Monday morning, as John Krescher, a critical care nurse specialist, is going into the intensive care unit (ICU), he is stopped by Mr. Christopher Lacey's sister, a nurse. John often has seen her and her husband at her brother's bedside, although he has not had any lengthy discussions about Christopher with them. This morning, Mr. Lacey's sister says angrily that Christopher's attending physician, Dr. Sidney McCally, is planning to transfer her brother prematurely to the general medical unit. She believes it is because Dr. McCally is being urged to do so by the hospital utilization committee and the case manager for Mr. Lacey's medical coverage plan. She and her husband are threatening a lawsuit against the hospital unless her brother is allowed to remain in the ICU and receive what she believes is optimal medical care for him there. John expresses his surprise and is about to ask her some further questions, but she rushes out of the unit, apparently on the verge of tears.

John goes over to Christopher Lacey's bedside and puts his hand on the man's shoulder. He studies the patient's face for some sign of response, but there is none. John's mind is flooded with thoughts. Mr. Lacey is a 28-year-old, divorced postal employee with no children. "He is only a year older than I am," John thinks. Initially, Christopher was admitted to the hospital with severe, acute abdominal pain. After several days of tests that yielded no clues, the physicians did an exploratory laparotomy.*

At that time, an ischemic segment of bowel was resected. In the post-operative suite, Christopher experienced respiratory arrest for reasons the doctors could not explain and was transferred to the ICU under Sidney McCally's care. Since that time, 3 weeks ago, his condition has been fluctuating neurologically and he has never fully regained consciousness.

In fact, Christopher Lacey has had a stormy course characterized by multiple serious medical complications. A systemic infection developed immediately after surgery, at which time it was thought he would die. He was treated with massive doses of antibiotics and appeared to be recovered. But the antibiotics were severely toxic to his kidneys. He now shows signs of kidney failure, which may necessitate renal dialysis.

Some members of the health care team have become progressively more pessimistic about Christopher Lacey's prognosis. In the ICU rounds 2 days ago, Sidney McCally shared with the ICU nursing staff that she had had several discussions with the patient's sister and had tried to explain to her the likelihood that his condition would not improve. "But," Dr. McCally said, "she and her husband wish aggressive treatment as long as there is any hope of meaningful recovery or survival." Mr. Lacey had left no living will or durable power of attorney and had never expressed an opinion about long-term life support.

John goes back to the ICU desk where his colleague, Janet Cumming, is at the computer entering data in the patient's medical record. Janet says, "Mr. Lacey's sister is so upset because Dr. McCally has decided to discontinue intensive care therapy despite the family's objections. I guess we will be transferring him back to the regular medicine unit later today. Of course, we are 100% full, so I can see why there is a push to get him out, but I question if he is being ousted from us before he is ready." Janet then adds, "Actually, the situation is worse than you think. We have three people in this hospital on the ICU waiting list, all of them at risk of dying soon if we cannot open up any of our ICU beds for them."

The Goal: A Caring Response

Discerning a caring response in situations of distributive justice creates special psychological and ethical challenges for health professionals. Many bioethicists have suggested that the demands of justice and care are at odds

---

*An exploratory laparotomy is a procedure in which a surgeon enters the abdominal cavity to discover the source of a serious problem not detectable by other means.

with one another. In his recent assessment of the challenge, ethicist Leonard Fleck[2] places his hope on the democratic process in a society that has both justice and caring as two of its founding values and assumptions. We take that more optimistic approach in this text, based on reasons we describe in more detail, and invite your own reflection and conclusions. If Fleck and we are correct in embracing the good news that we can arrive at a caring response while taking microallocation decisions into account, the task is to apply our clinical and ethical reasoning about what is best for an individual patient from the perspective of also acknowledging the overall resources available. This does not only include reimbursement limits for services offered to the patient but also limits in your own energies, clinic schedule-imposed limitations, availability of clinical modalities or professional expertise, and space. The strength of this perspective is that it keeps us crisply cognizant of what can best be done within the reality of human limitations. It uses all aspects of a health professional's clinical reasoning discussed previously in this text, with a balance of procedural, contextual, and interactive elements of the situation. Take the story of Christopher Lacey, his family, and their health professions team. A seemingly healthy younger man becomes a victim of a series of events that leave him in a coma and dependent on extensive medical life supports for his life and sustenance. What should be done for this man whose condition shows no improvement and seems to be getting worse? On an individual patient basis, a widely recognized goal for health professionals is to do whatever is clinically and ethically best. In this story, the entire team understandably has been working to ensure that Christopher Lacey is receiving the most caring response consistent with the professional skill that each is able to provide. It is what we expect of the health professional and patient relationship.

But this chapter confronts you squarely with the reality we often are facing as moral agents: namely, that what we actually can offer him threatens to fall short of the optimum. In the story as we have it, Dr. McCally has not clearly indicated her reasons for wanting to move him out of the ICU to a general medical unit, but we do not have reason to believe that this physician has a less than pure intent. Maybe she is being pushed by the bed utilization committee of the hospital because his medical coverage no longer will support ICU level treatment, or maybe she judges deeply that a disproportionate amount of extremely expensive life support measures are being expended on him in view of his serious prognosis. She may be haunted by the knowledge that three other patients who may benefit more from ICU interventions are waiting in the wings for a bed to clear. All of these reasons fall within the purview of justice considerations that this team is facing. You can again rely on the six-step process of ethical decision making as a tool to assess ethical problems that arise when viewed through the lens of distributive justice.

The Six-Step Process in Microallocation Decisions

Of the many issues involved in this situation, consider the following issues that are related to the broad questions of allocation of health care resources directed to a single patient:

- Should care be continued in the ICU for patients whose progress is uncertain (e.g., whose conditions may worsen if they are transferred out but do not seem to be getting any better in the ICU)?
- Should patient care be continued in the ICU because the family has a right to require continued treatment of this sort?
- Mr. Lacey's regimen is based on pooled data derived from many other people in his health plan who were in circumstances similar to his. Should Mr. Lacey be transferred out because his health plan dictates that he has used up his fair share of the plan's resources?
- Should his financial situation be a factor at all in whether he is kept in the ICU?

In recent years, the direct relationship between health professional and patient has become strained by institutional constraints, some of which were addressed in Chapter 8. Traditional health care ethics, with its emphasis only on the private transaction between you and the patient, often has not addressed the larger institutional questions. For instance, nothing in the Hippocratic Oath, or even in most professional codes of ethics today, provides guidance for how to distribute health care resources fairly and equitably. The challenge is heightened when the allocation involves a scarce resource.

 SUMMARY

Traditional professional ethics codes and oaths have not addressed the question of how to distribute scarce resources ethically. The emphasis has been largely or solely on the individual patient.

Step 1: Gather Relevant Information

Patients such as Christopher Lacey bring the troubling aspects of resource allocation keenly into focus. Costs are often a major consideration; let us assume that is the case here. Although, as Chapter 14 suggests, it is possible to keep many clinically compromised people alive almost indefinitely, the reality in most Western countries is that the technology needed to keep patients on life supports is extremely expensive. Callahan[3] makes the argument that it is in fact the high cost of medical technology that makes our current health care system unsustainable. He notes: "In a rare instance of consensus, health care economists attribute about 50% of the annual increase in health care costs to new technologies or to the intensified use of old ones."[3] One complicating factor is uncertainty about whether Mr. Lacey's condition will deteriorate further if he is removed from the ICU, although it appears to his nurse, sister, and at least a couple members of the team that it may. We do not know for sure, but in most cases, we can safely assume that the treatment he needs is out of reach for his family financially. Therefore, most the benefits Mr. Lacey derives from treatment inevitably are at the expense of pooled financial resources in the form of revenue from taxes, insurance premiums, and other common funds. Of course, Mr. Lacey has worked since he was 16 years old, so he also has contributed to some of these pooled funds over the years. That too should be taken into account. Even if insurance denied this level of ICU care but the family could pay the full amount, other justice considerations are facing the professionals.

The limited number of ICU beds is one such consideration. We do not know the full clinical status of the patients in line for the ICU bed currently occupied by Christopher Lacey, but on the basis of John's concern, they are patients who are in equally clinically compromised situations. It does not appear in this instance that professional staff or medical equipment and supplies are in short supply to compound the allocation challenge.

When viewed from the standpoint of one person's situation in relation to another (i.e., Mr. Lacey's need for the ICU compared with Patient B), the allocations considerations draw on ideas of fairness. When a whole group of patients (Group A with, for example, AIDS) is compared with another group of patients (e.g., Group B has diabetes), the justice considerations draw on ideas of equity. We examine each briefly.

Fairness Considerations

An understanding of what often is called the *principle of fairness* in justice discussions requires us to explore two issues raised by Mr. Lacey's situation.

"First Come, First Served" and Procedural Justice. First, there is the idea of *"first come, first served."* As we noted, the resources Mr. Lacey needs may keep someone else from receiving this valued, life-saving therapy in the ICU. Generally speaking, once a patient is in an ICU, he or she will not be removed for another similarly situated person who comes along afterward. Fairness considerations often rely on this culturally derived "first come, first served" idea as a device of arbitration. The assumption is that there is something in the nature of the procedures we adopt that may have a moral prescription in them. Such is the case here. Our procedures for determining who gets priority attention in a queue (when everyone's need or desire is judged to be the same) is understood to lend insight into the deeper aspects of an overall just society. In the United States and most Western cultures, the

procedural justice rule is accepted whether queuing up for an ICU bed, standing in line for concert tickets, or taking a number at a deli counter. If you happened to get there first, it constitutes a moral claim on the spot, something like a "squatter's right." You can see how this rule can help to mitigate constant bickering over a resource that would equally benefit many who want or need it.

There is a caveat here. While "first in line" covers a lot of people who present for health care services, it is not always the case. As Western countries become more diverse ethnically and in other ways, the idea of who should have top priority may fall to the eldest, to males, to tribal leaders, or to others, not to whoever happened to get there first. In each case, however, the procedural justice idea that the person with top priority should be able to remain in place seems to hold.

The Identified One Versus the As-Yet-Unidentified Many. Consider a second type of fairness issue. Theoretically, resources that Mr. Lacey is using to be sustained in his bodily functions could be channeled into other kinds of programs that could save the lives of hundreds or at least improve their level of well-being (e.g., in screening or immunization programs).

 Reflection
Should the idea that transferring a patient out of the ICU to save money that could be channeled into, for example, immunizations for hundreds of children, enter the ICU personnel's decision about what to do in a particular case? Why or why not? Jot down your comments here.

_____

_____

_____

_____

In everyday circumstances, this type of reasoning that pits the identified patient against an unidentified many in a group is a morally questionable guide for action at the level that decisions are made about a particular patient by his or her health care team. You have learned that a fundamental promise of professional ethics is that the individual patient's well-being is your appropriate focus; therefore, your patient cannot be placed in a faceless pool with risk for jeopardy. For one thing, the health care team cannot ensure that funds and other resources "saved" by removing Mr. Lacey from the ICU will be channeled into saving more lives or increasing the level of health care overall because of the fragmentation that exists in the policies of health care financing. Even if we did have that assurance, the respect for this person's dignity as a human should preclude the health professional's willingness to compromise a single patient's well-being for the sake of others "out there." Later in this chapter, we consider what happens to this general ethical rule of thumb in crises of great proportion that create situations of dire scarcity. In those cases, priority must be given not to those in the most need necessarily but on the basis of how to protect the good of the whole. Although the usual thinking that governs in situations of relatively moderate scarcity is overridden in dire scarcity situations, the goal is to bring the situation back to a place where the usual norms of fairness can be applied.

Equity Considerations

You now have an opportunity to consider Christopher Lacey's story from the angle of similarly situated groups of individuals vying for a limited health care resource.

Policies should be designed to protect the rights and interests of everyone equitably. From a standpoint of justice considerations, *the principle of equity* means that policy decision makers must make every effort to set guidelines that allow that each person in a similarly situated circumstance be treated alike, with differences among groups based on criteria that are ethically acceptable. Health professionals often become involved in the development of policies that help to guide clinical practice, an issue addressed in Chapter 8. In Christopher Lacey's case, the health care ICU team should not have to take his situation from scratch and try to figure out who is and who is not eligible for what. The policy may be in the form of federal or other government guidelines, or institutional policies. It might dictate types of treatment that will or will not be covered by insurance, Medicare, or other third-party payers, or it might provide guidelines for types of patients who will not be treated because of excessive cost or unlikelihood of medical response to treatment. Understandably, much thought should go into determining ethical allocation policies to help health professionals implement good decisions. You are entering the health care environment in an era where "evidence-based" outcomes of treatment based on pooled data involving many similarly situated patients are being used as a major criterion both to guide clinical care and to ensure the distribution is equitable. Critical analysis of such themes as the difference between policies based on insurance companies' assessments of what equity requires and those based on more traditional notions of professional ethics is helping everyone understand better what an "equitable" course of action requires.[4] Your ability to think critically about unique patient cases is essential in these times to implement best practices.

SUMMARY

The justice-related principle of fairness deals with ethically support-able types of allocation among individuals, and the principle of equity, deals with allocation among groups.

Step 2: Identify the Type of Ethical Problem

The ICU team surely is experiencing emotional distress in their worry about whether Christopher Lacey will survive outside of the intensive care treat-ment environment. But although some of them who are certain he will not survive outside the ICU are experiencing moral distress, ultimately this team's basic ethical problem is not moral distress, even though they are experiencing the emotional distress that can be an important trigger for it. Their problem is more deeply rooted in the competing clinical claims that they face from other similarly situated patients who are waiting to be ad-mitted to the ICU. In other words, they have butted up against the most challenging aspect of whether care and justice are reconcilable. In Chapter 3, you were introduced to the schematic representation of the basic type of ethical problem that addresses justice-related issues.

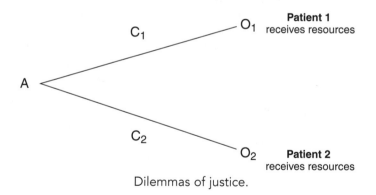

Dilemmas of justice.

This was identified as a special type of ethical dilemma.

 Reflection

To refresh your memory, describe what makes an ethical dilemma differ-ent from ethical problems of moral distress or locus of authority problems.

_____

_____

The concept of justice itself has been the subject of rich discussion from the beginning of Western ethics. Generally speaking, it can be thought of as an arbiter, useful for analyzing and resolving ethical problems regarding what is rightfully due each individual or group who presents a claim on resources and what proportion of the burden should be borne by whom. Conditions that clue you into the fact that you are in a situation requiring justice are:

- there is a good or service that more than one person or groups wants;
- there is a scarcity of the good; and
- the moral agent has an obligation not to allocate the good on an arbitrary basis.

The starting place for ethical assessment, called the *formal principle of justice*, is that similarly situated persons must be treated similarly. On the one hand, Mr. Lacey is an individual patient, but he also belongs to a group of people who are similar in their urgent need for ICU care. You will recognize this stance as the conceptual basis from which the notions of fairness and equity, discussed earlier, are derived. Obviously, the idea of simply treating similar cases similarly presents some difficulties because already in this story you have four people who deserve similar treatment. Moreover, taken alone, this formal principle of justice does not prevent you from treating whole groups of people poorly (e.g., slaves in the United States and elsewhere).

The reasoning underlying the idea of justice is that moral agents must attempt to show due respect for people by not making arbitrary or capricious distinctions and by not discriminating against some groups.

 SUMMARY

Justice requires that decisions about the distribution of goods and imposition of burdens among individuals or groups be based on consideration that can be agreed on as being morally justifiable.

Step 3: Use Ethics Theories or Approaches to Analyze the Problem

The concept of justice is so highly regarded that the principles approach has incorporated it as one of the ethical principles. So everything that follows in our analysis goes back to using this aspect of a principles approach. At least three ways of viewing the situation can help you as a moral agent to participate confidently in allocation decisions even though the professional's clinical role of doing what is beneficial for each individual patient necessarily may be compromised when resources are scarce. Once one has accepted the formal principle of justice that similarly situated persons should be treated similarly, the questions move to a more strategic level called *the material principles of justice*. We share three of the major ones here.

Health Care as a Right

One fundamental approach to justice is deontologic. As you recall, ethical principles often have the function of duties; justice is one example. Also, duties are related to rights. A right is a stringent claim on another to respond in a certain fashion. The stronger the claim, the more an agent (whether a person or society) has a duty—and must accept responsibility—for addressing the claim. Therefore, one common approach is to treat health care of all individuals as a right and, if so, to decide how much and what kind of health care each individual or group is entitled to receive. At the societal level, health care as a right often is discussed within the context of what political scientists and others call *social justice*. Within bioethics, social justice questions focus on discussions of social responsibility, such as government-sponsored policies that provide access to health care (or other basic goods and services) for impoverished members of a society.[5] Health professionals in many fields are becoming more aware of how *health disparities* are an issue of social justice that they must help to alleviate. Impoverishment is not only financial; it also includes lack of opportunities for participation in other health-supporting aspects of society. An excellent example of an initiative to engage health disparity issues through research and interventions is being undertaken by occupational therapy professionals at the national level.[6] More about health disparities and social justice is addressed in the next chapter.

Reflection

From what you know about the current policies regarding health care in your country, do you think health care is viewed as a right or privilege? Why? Explain here.

_____

_____

_____

_____

Your answer may depend in part on your understanding of the idea of rights. The concept sometimes used in discussing a rights approach is that of *entitlement*. A person deserves the good or service simply by being a member of a group. A human right broadens the bandwidth of the group to include all humans and is called a *positive right*. This approach, adopted by many countries in the world, supports policies that make everyone eligible to receive basic health care benefits. At minimum, access has to be universally available. In this way of thinking, people such as Mr. Lacey and the other patients who need ICU beds should be able to have them. The societal challenge is to find money to support an adequate supply of ICU beds so that such a basic resource is available for those who will benefit from this type of care. A rights approach does not mean that everyone can decide they want the most expensive modality or can always choose where they want treatment. Considerations of equity in the face of limited resources must guide such decisions.

Health Care as a Response to Basic Need

A second perspective that can help to further identify different treatments that are appropriate for different persons is to base allocation on need. This also has a deontologic foundation. Health care offers a universal human good: the means to healthfulness. Therefore, everyone who lacks it ought to receive a beneficial response to this need, and those in a position to provide it have a duty to do so. In this approach, health care can still be viewed as a right, but not all who hold a needs-oriented position do so. As you can imagine, one of the greatest challenges in this type of reasoning is to define the severity of need and likelihood of benefit among different groups. How does one compare the need for functional gait training with pain relief for end-stage bone cancer with eye surgery for a detached retina? Another challenge is to determine what constitutes a truly clinical need.

 Reflection
Currently, debate exists about whether cosmetic plastic surgery should be covered as a basic health care need. What reasons can be given for the position that such surgery is morally appropriate as a health care intervention? What reasons for such surgery do you find unacceptable?

_____

_____

_____

_____

In spite of difficulties, the basic premise that we as humans have varying types of need to maintain or restore a higher level of healthfulness seems to us a humane and reasonable position from which to delve more deeply into the ambiguities that are bound to arise in any position. The health professions themselves rest largely on the idea that those with more need should have greater priority unless there is evidence that the expenditure of resources on this group would not yield positive results.

Health Care as a Commodity

This perspective moves away from the previous foundational assumptions that health care is an entitlement right or that need is the governing criterion on which to base allocation. *Health care as a commodity* means that it is treated the same as any other type of product in a free market society. Health care is something to be bought, like a summer vacation package, or trash compactor, or DVD. The informed consumer decides and makes choices. The assumption is that we are free, autonomous individuals who should make choices consistent with our own values and that in doing so we are contributing to the type of society that maximizes the greatest amount of well-being for the most people overall.

Reflection
Of the basic ethics theories, which one does this perspective best reflect?

_____

_____

_____

_____

If you answered "a utilitarian theory," you are doing well to carry through the basics of ethical theory to this type of issue.

Interestingly enough, rights language sometimes is brought into the position that health care is a commodity but that it is a different type of right than a positive right of entitlement to a good or service. This is the idea of a *negative right:* that is, the right to an opportunity to purchase a good or service. Money is the key resource that governs who buys what. In this approach, it is not the responsibility of others in society to provide money (or vouchers or employee-based health insurance plans) to help people pay for health care. Everyone buys what he or she needs and wants and, in addition, can afford. People like Christopher

Lacey are free to buy more time in the ICU if they are able to pay for it.

Sometimes this way of reasoning about justice does include a component that places a claim on government and other pooled societal resources. It is recognized that even in a free market society, some interventions are well beyond the personal means of most individuals. In such instances, societal resources should be spent on individuals or groups viewed as a "good investment." In the context of justice discussions, this "investment approach" falls into the idea that *merit justice,* rather than justice according to relative medical need, is the key to allocation decisions. Western societies see merit in a person's past contributions and in his or her wealth, yes, but also in other things such as fame.

One fact of life in many health care institutions is that "VIPs" are given specialty treatment. A *VIP (very important person)* may not only be given the best bed in the facility and royal treatment by staff but also jump to the head of the line for precious resources. VIPs sometimes are literally royalty but more often are popular public figures who are given high social status: government officials, rock or movie stars, CEOs of major corporations, major league athletes, etc. What is your feeling response to professionals who assign merit to famous or powerful people?

Even when one takes the VIP situation out of the picture, merit reasoning based on social criteria of worth poses a challenge. Who is the better investment in the following case?

Two men are brought into the emergency department of a community hospital in a small town after the crash of a small plane carrying 16 passengers. Both need emergency life-saving surgery immediately, but only one operating suite and team is available. Mr. A., a brilliant, 26-year-old PhD researcher is on the brink of making a major breakthrough in Alzheimer's disease research. His ability to pay for care is limited because of the burden of his large student loans. Mr. B., who is 75 years old, is a wealthy, world-renowned, retired concert pianist who is now showing the first stages of Alzheimer's disease and is the process of completing a bequest to endow a world-class Alzheimer's research unit at Mr. A's facility.

 Reflection

What qualifications do each have that might influence the type of thinking that an "investment" or merit approach to allocation would take? Do you agree with this approach? Why or why not?

_____

_____

In brief, three basic perspectives on the way to address ethical dilemmas of justice are presented here in somewhat "pure" form: rights, need, and merit being the governing criteria. However, they are presented as if they are completely distinct from each other. In fact, practices and policies often are based on many factors and may include components of each of them. For instance, a health care benefits package that takes shape from the basic premise that health care is a right may be founded primarily on assessments of relative need among different groups and also include a sliding scale of "copayments" according to difference in people's ability to pay for care.

 SUMMARY

In situations of moderate scarcity, justice decisions about the distribution of goods depend on assessments of rights, relative need, and relative merit.

As you can see, there is not always agreement about how justice best can be served. As you begin practice, you can help maintain your professional integrity by actively engaging the issues of justice that often become a part of your clinical reasoning and decisions.

Steps 4 and 5: Explore the Practical Alternatives and Complete the Action

In previous chapters, the application of Step 4 almost always placed you (or the clinicians in the story) solely in the moral role of advocate for an individual patient and acting in accordance to what a caring response entails. That is the role John Krescher and the ICU team have to maintain throughout their relationship with Mr. Lacey and Mr. Lacey's family. What additional alternatives to the one they are facing can be explored? Here are a few we have identified:

- The team can check further to discern whether the medical need of those waiting to be admitted to the unit is in fact as urgent as Christopher's need for continued ICU care.
- They can check to be sure there has been an attempt to wean Christopher from some of the life-supporting interventions in the ICU to see his response instead of abruptly transferring him.
- They can inquire whether there is a step-down unit between the ICU and the general medical unit to which he may be moved soon and if so, do it.

- The team can acknowledge that Christopher Lacey's sister is a clinically informed source as a nurse. She can be an important ally, but her concerns have to be attended to.

All of these alternatives to quickly moving the patient at least have the benefit of buying a little time to more fully assess what his status is and how he will tolerate the transfer.

At the same time, this chapter is designed to help you focus on the larger social context of which health professionals also are a part, so that moral agency considerations include participation in policy too. The alternative of passively letting others make policy decisions and then reacting to them distorts the role of the professional as a moral agent today. Some alternatives to the team members not being involved in policy include:

- Some members of the team should insist on being involved in developing ICU policies in their institution. This can help them minimize their justice dilemmas even if they cannot totally eliminate them.
- Allocation policy often is set by insurers, government bodies, and other extrainstitutional bodies. The ICU team members must be willing to participate in commissions, review committees, and other public forums, thereby taking advantage of their opportunity to contribute considered opinions and provide documentation and data regarding their experiences.

Thinking clearly about these alternatives allows you to bring the concerns of care and justice more fully into alignment. All the "Mr. Laceys" are the beneficiaries of your preparatory work, so that whatever the outcome in Mr. Lacey's immediate situation, you have done the best you can for him and created an awareness of the vicissitudes of limitations imposed by scarce resources. You will be able to add your insights into current debates about whether health care is a right, should be a resource to respond to basic need despite ability to pay, or is a commodity. In other words, in allocation decisions, your moral agency can be effective at both practice and policy levels.

Step 6: Evaluate the Process and Outcome

There is an expression, "The proof is in the pudding," which means that only if the pudding tastes as good as it looks or smells should one conclude that the chef has succeeded. The team should engage in a reflective review of what Mr. Lacey's situation has taught all of them for future dilemmas of justice. The proof of a caring response to Mr. Lacey is that he has received the best clinical care available within reasonable constraints on resources, resources that are being allocated according to a nonarbitrary (fair) process. At the level of policies, basic equity considerations have been taken into account and the amount of compromise of resources for an individual patient such as Mr. Lacey is strictly proportionate to the actual scarcity.

Rationing: Allocation and Dire Scarcity

Having given careful attention to the way the general principle of distributive justice works, consider the companion notion of *rationing*. Some use the term rationing to denote any intentional method of distributing a desired good when there are far too many qualified claimants for a good, or the good is much too costly for all to have it. As you can easily discern, this is the way we have been describing distributive justice as a general principle guiding allocation. Traditionally, rationing decisions were made when there was a *dire scarcity*, a severe shortage, of the good, and it is from this traditional stance that we address it. Currently, an active discussion about this type of rationing focuses on the sobering prospect of a desperately inadequate supply of lifesaving or basic quality of life interventions. For example, across the globe, there is increasing attention to plans for how to respond to a bioterrorist attack in a large urban area that would thrust an entire population into a sudden position of dire scarcity. Every major medical center knows that there is no way to stockpile sufficient supplies to effectively combat such a horrifying situation. Who should be admitted into the hospital and other medical facilities? Who should receive antidotes against the toxic agents used in biowarfare? Who should be admitted after the first wave of emergent care?[7]

Natural disasters also can create chaos in spite of the best thought-out approaches to justice. Many who witnessed the flood after Hurricane Katrina in New Orleans experienced this phenomenon as an entire city went under water. Common situations include natural disasters such as an earthquake, drought, or flooding. It can also include a smaller group of people trapped by circumstance, such as a plane wreck in a remote area, a boycott on goods coming into an area, or the movements of people into overcrowded refugee camps (Figure 15-1). Obviously not all health professionals find themselves providing services in such situations, but some volunteer to be available as first response teams or join organizations such as Doctors Beyond Borders or the International Red Cross. Others are pulled into it by unforeseen circumstance, such as being caught in the situation while on vacation.

Analyses that address basic health care needs and a dire scarcity of resources do not all do so in the context of a big blow-out like a dirty bomb or major flood. There are many who project a more gradual but persistent move into an unsustainable health care system as we know it today based on diminishing resources. Among the most prevalent themes are arguments that pit the well-being of younger generations against the demands of a currently aging one. In 2008, the United States spent more than four trillion dollars on health care. The estimates were that roughly a third of the total was spent on those over 65 years, although they constituted only about 10% of the population. Combining this with the advent of post–World War II baby boomers now coming into retirement age, the 2010 figure of 38 million "senior citizens" over 65 years will proliferate to more than 75 million just 15 years later (2025).[8]

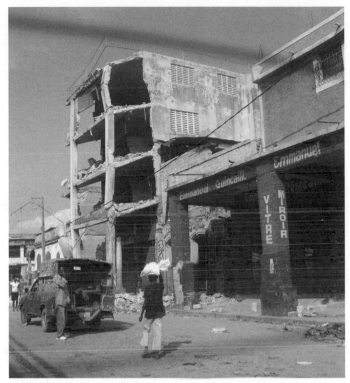

Figure 15-1. Natural or human made disasters create chaos that may require triage and rationing of resources. *(Courtesy of Angelina Rayno.)*

Soothsayers raise serious questions about how, if at all, justice can sustain us as we witness a rapidly exploding population of older people. Many others do not see such a clear-cut progression of an older population persistently taking with them their children's and grandchildren's health care resources.

Currently, another impetus to create ration-based approaches to health care resources is being occasioned by new technologies. As we briefly noted at the outset of this chapter, Callahan recently has argued that the need for rationing has become more painfully acute mainly because we are seeing the rapid proliferation of costly "last chance" therapies. A recent article in the New Yorker magazine convincingly showed that there are immense differences in what such technology costs from one region of the United States to another, suggesting that the price in a particular place cannot be accounted for by the true value of the equipment or skill. One can only imagine that as the technology becomes more available, the demand will continue to increase without assurance that the cost will decrease.[9]

Criteria for a Morally Acceptable Approach to Rationing

Several criteria have been developed to assist in the difficult, usually tragic, situation occasioned by the severe shortage of an essential life-sustaining good or service.

A Demonstrated Need

There must be proof that rationing is necessary. At times, politicians and others have declared that rationing of a particular good or service is necessary because of "dire scarcity." Any use of this powerful argument not based on well-documented data is just plain wrong. Rationing means that some groups who would benefit will not receive any of a desperately needed service or good. In contrast, the one who would benefit is the essential focus of clinical decisions. The widespread idea that health care responds to a basic human need requires that the burden of proof be placed on anyone declaring that it is necessary to ration some aspect of health care.

A Last Resort Move

It follows from the preceding criterion that every other approach must be exhausted before the decision is made to exclude from care individuals who would benefit. For example, one necessary approach is to place priority on research designed to discover less expensive but effective modes of treatment affordable to everyone who needs it. Health plans such as the one in which Mr. Lacey is enrolled take the tack of research using pooled data from many similar patients before him to determine what works best and then eliminate other interventions with the hopes of keeping costs within everyone's reach. But when rationing is required after such alternatives have been exhausted, the argument is that the whole society is at such a risk of total breakdown that priority must be given to those who are the most likely to be able to help the group or society get back on its feet, not necessarily those with the most need. As this book is being prepared, we are witnessing the aftermath of a terrible earthquake in Haiti that illustrates the deep quandary of health care providers in this kind of situation. For this reason, some have said that rationing in the face of dire scarcity turns usual understandings of justice upside down because it may be that the least needy are the ones to receive priority.

An Established Standard of Care

For some order to be brought into these desperate kinds of situations, an agreed-on standard of care must be established. Many groups have attempted to establish a baseline level to help ensure equity for everyone, even in these extreme circumstances. If the situation becomes so desperate, at least a standard was set. For example, the Ethical and Religious Directives for Catholic Health Care Services set a standard that poor people be a focal point of consideration. The reasoning is that if their basic needs are met, it is likely that others' needs will be too.[10] Philosopher John Rawls's proposal is that an unequal distribution of basic goods in a society must be acceptable from the standpoint of the least well off.[11] Many nations have used a set of basic benefits everyone must receive as a bottom line standard, no matter how minimal. Although applaudable in spirit, the practical downside of this criterion is that in some instances there is so little to go around that no one benefits.

An Inclusive Process

Representatives and advocates for all groups that will be affected should participate in the allocation process. An interesting experiment in rationing was conducted by the state of Oregon in regard to its Medicaid recipients. A random group of taxpayers was asked to rank many treatment interventions, the idea being that when the results were tabulated, the state dollars allocated annually to health services would be directed to people needing those treatment interventions determined by the citizens themselves to be the most important. Others would be left out. Much has been written about the pros and cons of this experimental approach. It goes beyond the purposes of this book to go into more detail, but if you have interest in learning more about this innovative experiment, you can do so by searching "The Oregon Health Plan."

Proportionality and Reversibility

The beneficial services that are withheld must be proportional to the actual scarcity. *Proportionality* means that just enough, but no more, constraint is adopted to meet the difficult demands of scarcity in a situation than absolutely is needed. Moreover, cuts or cutbacks are justifiable only as long as true and serious scarcity exists so that the constraints on care can be reversed as soon as the dire scarcity situation no longer exists.

Box 15-1 summarizes all five criteria for rationing.

Random Selection and Tragic Choices

In the unthinkable possibility of eliminating some people from receiving resources altogether, a *lottery approach*, or process of *random selection*, has been suggested by some as a procedure that can help to make a decision more just when the claim is for an essential life-saving treatment unavailable to everyone who needs it.

Box 15-1   Criteria for a Morally Acceptable Approach to Rationing of Health Care Resources

1. Rationing is necessary.
2. Rationing is a last resort move.
3. A high standard is the goal.
4. The process is inclusive.
5. The cuts are proportionate and reversible.

In random selection, a prior medical judgment of medical need and suitability has been made, and the patient's freedom to refuse possible treatment has been ascertained. In an attempt to be as unbiased as possible in selecting who is to receive treatment among those still found eligible, "rolling the dice" has been suggested as a model. In extreme circumstances, such as an earthquake, terrorist attack, or other horrendously tragic situations, the method has been upheld in the courts of the United States as a procedure that expresses an equal consideration of the equal right of each person to his or her life (United States v. Holmes).[12] The actual situation that led to this decision was around the tragic moment in which survivors of a shipwreck, while lost at sea, realized that all would die if one or more were not "sacrificed." They decided among themselves to draw lots, and those who lost were thrown overboard. Eventually, the remainder were rescued and had to stand trial regarding the death of their life raft mates. It was the court's conclusion that under extreme life-threatening circumstances, drawing lots was a just solution.

It also has been argued by proponents of this position that those unfortunate people who are excluded (in the lifeboat situation, from continued life; but in our context of discussion, from treatment) may find it easier to accept their fate because they have not been excluded on the basis of individual traits they have or do not have.

Nonetheless, not everyone agrees that random selection is the most humane way of proceeding. Some maintain that once patients have been selected as being similarly situated in terms of medical need, it makes sense to give weight to such merit-related social factors as the likelihood of future service to society, the extent of past services, or family responsibilities. These positions take seriously into account that people are seldom viewed in isolation but rather in context as members of their larger communities.

 SUMMARY

Random selection attempts to remove the opportunity for discrimination, but some criticize its deeply impersonal nature.

Summary

Discussion of the proper moral response to Christopher Lacey's situation, viewed from the lens of what distributive justice considerations would require, raises many questions regarding the most morally defensible way to proceed with his care. A caring response may counsel one course of action, but real limits may require a different course. Inherent in the judgment are considerations of fairness and equity and the appropriate criteria for a rationing approach if one is needed.

What Sidney McCally, John Krescher, and the other members of the health care team decide to do that is the most consistent with a caring response will be based on clinical *and* policy considerations. In the ethical dimensions of the decision, they are faced with the issues of fairness and equity. They need courage to act on their decision in addition to wisdom to decide well. They will also see the wisdom of participating in policy formation and review to try to minimize the harm that may result in situations of scarcity. Policymakers who take seriously what equity means in this type of situation help the health professionals do the morally correct thing.

Questions for Thought and Discussion

1. This exercise can be performed as an individual or group exercise.

You have an opportunity to advocate for services that you judge should be included or excluded in your state's health care rationing plan for Medicaid recipients (i.e., persons in the United States whose financial burdens qualify them for government-assisted health care). You take this task seriously for many reasons, but one is that the federal government has given your state the opportunity to develop a rationing plan for Medicaid recipients nationally.

On the basis of the Oregon plan, the first step was to poll a random group of citizens to set priorities among services. Your task force has gone one step further than the Oregon plan. Oregon polled only voting citizens. Your group has set a mechanism in place that also ensures input from a large contingency of Medicare recipients themselves. (One criticism leveled at Oregon policymakers was that their pool of voters did not include a proportionate number of Oregon Medicaid recipients.) Now the real crisis has come because several important services that the members of the task force hoped could be included are not. You now have to decide among yourselves how to make the final cuts but not tinker with the list created by the first part of the process that has received approval. The task force has before it six possible services that could be included for the state's 20,000 Medicaid recipients (all estimated costs are annual, and the task force has $46,136,000 to adjudicate).

   a. Preventive dental care for children ages 2 to 6 years. Includes a yearly check-up and teeth cleaning. Does not include fillings, orthodontics, or other acute dental or surgical services. Estimated cost: $3,760,000.

   b. Outpatient mental health services (initial evaluation and up to 12 visits) for children and adolescents (ages 4 to 19 years). Does not include medications or hospitalization. Estimated cost: $8,000,000.

   c. Smoking-related asthma treatments. Estimated cost: $8,860,000.

   d. Liver transplantation and follow up. Estimated cost: $12,200,000.

   e. Mammograms for women younger than 50 years. Estimated cost: $6,900,000.

   f. Coverage for pain management for patients with chronic back pain, including medications, rehabilitation, and pain centers, but not including surgery, which could be covered in another surgical category that ranked higher on the list of services. Estimated cost: $21,040,000.

   Rank order, with highest priority number 1 and lowest 6, and write your rationale below each one. When you have reached $46,136,000, you have exhausted the remaining available funds.

2. A friend of your mother has a rare progressive and eventually fatal disease. In the course of your work, you discover a highly experimental but potentially lifesaving medication that is being tested as a clinical trial at the institution where you are employed. You make a few inquiries and now have serious doubts about whether your mother's friend will be able to get into the study because the waiting list already is much longer than the experimental protocol allows. Still, you think the caring thing to do is to at least let her know that such an intervention is available. Knowing her, she will definitely want to go for it and will push you hard to try to influence your colleague to get her into the study. While you are thinking about these things, the clinician conducting the protocol calls you back to say that on the basis of your being a fellow employee, she may try to rearrange the queue to get your mother's friend into the study. No promises. Now you find yourself wondering if it is fair to those who already are in the queue if your influence does work and your mother's friend jumps ahead in the line.

   How do you go about deciding what to do in this situation that brings to your doorstep both your care for someone close to your mother with a medical need (although not a patient of yours) and your reflection about others eligible for inclusion in the study who may end up being ousted?

3. You are a clinical psychologist in private practice. Your receptionist asks if you can see an unscheduled new patient who is in such severe pain from a headache and is crying in the waiting room. You glance at the back-to-back appointments for the afternoon, sigh, and ask your assistant if he can get a better idea of what brings her here today with such an urgent need to see you.

   He interviews her, and after your next patient, you get this report: the patient, 35 years old, explained haltingly that her headaches began around the time she began suspecting her husband was having an affair. She then burst into tears saying, "It's the headaches that are driving him away." You know this woman needs help; her anxiety is overwhelming her and she may even be suicidal. She needs counseling preceded by a more thorough neurologic workup, neither of which you will be able to do for her and arrange today. You ask your assistant if he can handle this, and he says he thinks it would be better if you would just take a few minutes to talk with her because her sobbing and holding her head seems to be distressing the other patients in the waiting area. You suggest he try to schedule an appointment later in the week when you have more time to show her the care you are sure would be of some reassurance to her and perhaps get her headed in the right direction for a more thorough neurologic workup as well.

Your assistant comes back from this suggestion saying she is pleading persuasively, "Can't she [or he] at least see me for a few minutes now?" Her husband, a truck driver, has asked her to accompany him on a long distance trip, and she fears if she does not go with him, he will take someone else. She wants to know whether it is too dangerous for her to go with the headache such as it is. You are genuinely concerned about her but also conscious of the full waiting room outside your door.

What considerations of a caring response and the claims of distributive justice come into conflict in your deliberation about what to do? What will you do? Why?

REFERENCES

1. Sheehy, E., Conrad, S.I.., Brigham, L.E., et al., 2003. Estimating the number of potential organ donors in the United States. *N Engl J Med* 349 (7), 667–674.
2. Fleck, L.M., 2009. *Just caring: Health care rationing and democratic deliberation.* Oxford University Press, New York.
3. Callahan, D.T., 2009. *Taming the beloved beast: How medical technology costs are destroying our health care system.* Princeton University Press, Princeton, NJ, p. 2.
4. Hoffman, S., 2002. Actuarial fairness vs. moral fairness in health insurance. *Law Bioethics Rep* 1 (4), 2-4.
5. Powers, M., Faden, R., 2006. *Social justice: The moral foundations of public health and health policy.* Oxford University Press, New York.
6. Braveman, B., Bass-Haugen, J.D., 2009. Social justice and health disparities: An evolving discourse in occupational therapy research and interventions. *Am J Occupational Ther* 63, 7–12.
7. Ruben, E.R., Osterweis, M., Lindeman, L.M. (Eds.), 2002. *Emergency preparedness: Bioterrorism and beyond.* Association of Academic Health Centers, Washington, DC.
8. Fleck, L.M., 2002. Rationing: Don't give up. *Hastings Center Rep* 32 (2), 35–36.
9. Gawande, A., 2009. The cost conundrum: What a Texas town can teach us about health care. *The New Yorker,* June 1, 2009 Available from: <http://www.newyorker.com/reporting/2009/06/01/090601fa_fact_gawande>.
10. Committee on Doctrine of the National Conference of Catholic Bishops, 2001. *Ethical and religious directives for Catholic health care services.* United States Catholic Conference, Washington, DC.
11. Rawls, J., 1971. *A theory of justice.* Harvard University Press, Cambridge, MA, pp. 54–114.
12. *United States v. Holmes,* 1842. 26F Case 36 (No 15, 383) C.C.E.D. Pa.

16

Compensatory and Social Justice: Societal Sources of Claims for Health Care

Objectives

The reader should be able to:

- Distinguish some key differences and similarities in distributive justice, compensatory justice, and social justice perspectives.
- Identify a range of policy options that could be adopted in situations in which compensatory justice is being considered as an appropriate response to a group that has been harmed.
- Describe some cautions that should be taken into account when social justice approaches are applied toward the goal of a more equitable society.
- Discuss the "dilemma of difference" in regards to labeling and its affect on a just allocation of resources.
- Evaluate why stigma and social marginalization are barriers to creating just health care policies based on the ideals of social justice.
- Discuss how the goal of solidarity transforms current problems of justice.
- Identify and evaluate the role of personal responsibility for health maintenance from the standpoints of distributive justice, compensatory justice, and social justice perspectives.

New terms and ideas you will encounter in this chapter

compensatory justice	interdependence	vulnerability
stigma	altruism	social marginalization
workman's compensation	reciprocity ethic	solidarity
collective responsibility	social need	personal responsibility for health
communitarian approach	labeling	
	"the dilemma of difference"	

Topics in this chapter introduced in earlier chapters

Topic	Introduced in chapter
Beneficence	4
Nonmaleficence	4
Distributive justice	15
Social justice	15
Equity	15

Introduction

Justice issues often are difficult to grasp because they require professionals to move beyond their usual one-on-one interaction to consider the well-being of whole groups of people. As you learned in the previous chapter, distributive justice focuses on medical conditions as the basic approach to justly allocating resources. This chapter introduces two other related dimensions of justice that are pertinent in some of the situations you will face as a health professional. *Compensatory justice* and social justice (introduced in Chapter 15) both arise from the observation that not everyone has the same chance as others to benefit from basic societal services and goods. The similarity between the two types of justice is that each takes into account additional factors to medical conditions, those factors being related to the person's or group's relatively disadvantaged position in society. Compensatory justice has built into it an assumption that the person or group at least has a role (e.g., worker) that is valued by mainstream society. In contrast, social justice is a "no fault" position that says regardless of social role it is simply the societal disadvantage that matters. The assumption is that a well-working society has to respect everyone where they are and try to make adjustments regarding who needs what. At the core of the issue for our study here is the concern that some groups of people have health problems related to their disadvantaged position in the larger society. We devote most of the study in this chapter to compensatory justice but also demonstrate how it is one aspect of the broader concept of social justice, the latter of which focuses on serious disparities in health and health care allocations.

The story of the Maki brothers is an example designed to help you focus on how social contexts factor into compensatory justice considerations and how you, the health professional, are involved.

🐍 The Story of the Maki Brothers

Mr. Eino Maki is an asbestos miner who emigrated from Finland to the United States in 1975. He was born into a poor rural family that lived in a small remote village near the Russian border. Eino did not attend school in

Finland after the first grade because he was a "slow learner" and could not keep up with the other students. Although most students in his country received excellent educations, his family refused to send him to a special school in Tampere, some 300 miles away, saying they needed his help on the farm.

One dreadful morning in 1972, a fire destroyed the family's home and Eino's parents perished in the fire. Eino and his sister were sent to live with an aunt and uncle in Helsinki. At the age of 18 years, he could not find work in Helsinki, so he emigrated to the United States to live with his unmarried older brother in an area where there are many asbestos mines. The community where his brother lives is about 90% Finnish.

When Eino arrived in the United States, his brother John attempted unsuccessfully to find him a job in the railroad construction company where he was employed as a section worker. After several months, Eino did secure a job in a nearby asbestos mine.

He has been employed by this same mining company and has held essentially the same position for the last 36 years. Although at work he still suffers the ridicule at times associated with his being "slow" at grasping ideas, he is an excellent worker and participates in the social life of the community. Many evenings at the local bar, the men spend time reminiscing about the "good old days" in Finland, and everyone talks about going back. Privately, however, John and Eino agree that it is unlikely they will ever return.

In the last 2 or 3 months, Eino has had increasing difficulty breathing. Occasionally, he has coughed up blood-tinged sputum, and he often has pains in his chest when he awakens, but they disappear after he has been up and around for a couple of hours. At first, he does not say anything to John, but one November morning he realizes that he cannot make it to work. He asks John to take him to the company physician.

Eino has never liked doctors. In all of his years of employment, he has visited the company clinic only for the required routine annual physical examinations and once when he suffered a dislocated shoulder in a fall from a mine platform. He has always passed the physical examinations with a "clean bill of health."

After the examination, the physician assistant who conducted the initial tests tells Eino that some further tests are needed and for them he will have to be admitted to a hospital, which is about 120 miles away. Eino is angered at this news but realizes that he cannot go back to work feeling the way he does. He tells John he wants to rest at home until he feels better, but John, seeing the trouble his brother is having, insists he goes and drives him there.

Five days later in the hospital, Eino takes a sudden turn for the worse. John is called and drives back to the hospital. When he arrives, he is met by Dr. Kai Nielson, a young physician who looks to John as if he cannot be a day older than 16 years. Dr. Nielson invites John into a little room next to the nurse's desk and closes the door. "Mr. Maki, I'm afraid I have some bad news," he says. "Your brother has not been told yet, but he has cancer and has had it for quite a long time. Ideally, we should start a type of treatment immediately that his company's health plan does not totally cover."

So far, John has barely been hearing what the young doctor is saying. His mind is racing wildly. He vaguely recalls Eino's report of a discussion at a union meeting a year or so ago regarding a rumor that work in the asbestos mines causes cancer and that their union was looking into it. This concerned John greatly, but Eino brushed it aside and said it was "a bunch of hogwash" and he was "healthy as a horse," refusing to discuss it further. Later he told a friend, "you know that Eino is not only healthy as a horse but stubborn as a mule. What could I do? I let the matter drop."

Finally, John realizes that Dr. Nielson has been talking to him. "We could do the treatment, but unless Eino has additional insurance coverage, the treatment is going to cost him a lot of money."

John tells the physician that they own a small cottage together, with about two acres of unfarmed land around it. They have no savings, only the pension that their respective companies provide, but that benefit cannot be realized until Eino is 65 years old. Dr. Nielson replies sympathetically, "Well, there is a chance your brother will be eligible for federal assistance, but unfortunately it may mean you will have to sell your house to become eligible for it once you've expended the earnings you'd realize from that. I don't know exactly how it works, but I'll have the social worker talk to you. Of course, we can't guarantee that the treatment will beat the disease, but we feel reasonably sure that it would at least slow down the rate of growth of the cells."

There is a pause. Then he adds, "It is, of course, a big decision. It is entirely up to you and your brother what you decide to do. We haven't talked to him or, rather, been able to talk to him. He doesn't like doctors much. Why don't you two talk it over with the social worker here or the physician assistant he saw back at his company clinic? Remember, it's your decision and your brother's. But don't take too long in deciding. . . .I think every day counts. Do you have any questions?" John shakes his head "no." "Well," Dr. Nielson concludes, "if you do after talking with the others I've recommended, have them set up an appointment for you to see me again."

As John stands, Dr. Nielson extends his hand and John shakes it warmly. John glances up into the doctor's face and sees genuine compassion in the young man's eyes. John blurts out, "Was the cancer caused by the mines?" The young doctor drops John's hand and studies his own hands as he answers, "Mr. Maki, the cause of cancer is often complex. It can be the result of a combination of factors. But the type of cancer that your brother has is the same type that asbestos miners get at a higher rate than the general population. Primarily it attacks the lungs."

John thanks Dr. Nielson. Outside the doctor's office, he wanders over to a window and stares outside into the snowy darkness for a long time, his hands in the pockets of his overalls. He has not cried since their brother Matt was killed in a tractor accident many years before, but he feels a lump rising in his throat now. He feels totally unable to move, as if he is glued to the floor. He struggles to think clearly, but his mind remains a blank.

The story of John and Eino Maki raises numerous ethical questions. For instance, some people reading this story have questions about confidentiality. Why is Kai Nielson sharing all of this potent information with John when Eino, a competent adult, is the patient? What about Eino's informed consent? Is it appropriate for the physician to put the burden of sharing the bad news with Eino on John's shoulders? What should the role of the physician assistant and social worker be? These are certainly important ethical questions. However, we beam our lens in this chapter on the justice issues that patients in similar situations to Eino's raise. Their basic similarity is that they are among the members of society who are dismissed or even disdained by members of mainstream society even though they contribute in ways that society needs for its overall well-being.[1]

The Goal: A Caring Response

Eino Maki, a seemingly healthy, hard-working man, becomes a victim of circumstances that leave his health compromised. A caring response by health professionals requires that they do whatever is "best" or, in the language of ethics, is beneficent for this patient. In the story, the physician assistant and Kai Nielson have been doing exactly that in their attempt to get at the clinical root of Eino's symptoms, and they each make strong recommendations about what he needs to do. At the same time, they know that matters are fast slipping out of their hands. There is an environmental source of his cancer, a death-dealing cancer we presume, triggered by his employment in a company where he likely has been exposed to toxic levels of asbestos over a prolonged period of time. Mr. Maki's decision about what to do for his cancer treatment will depend in part on the availability of funds from his employing company or a government source to help pay for them. If the professionals think this through to its logical conclusion, they will realize that a caring response requires that they try to help build and strengthen institutions and societal arrangements that support individuals in such predicaments. Involvement at this level is aimed at policies that reflect justice for groups of people who are societally disadvantaged. The "Eino Makis" do not have the same opportunity to choose among desirable job options to the extent that persons who are better situated financially and socially do. Such policies are not designed only for one person (e.g., Mr. Maki) the way a treatment plan is created for a specific patient but outline a program that covers him and others like him. There is a subgroup of institutional and social arrangements that address legal mechanisms to compensate persons for harms incurred in the larger environment whether workplace, home, or publicly shared spaces. Compensatory justice deals with this reality from an ethical and legal standpoint, and it is the ethical considerations we consider here.

The Six-Step Process in Compensatory Justice Decisions

In Chapter 15, you studied about allocation dilemmas when whole groups of individuals become eligible for goods or services because of their medical need.

Now the lens of justice turns to include an additional question. What ethical difference does it make when a patient's medical need is caused by injury or illness but this person's condition is also caused by his societal position and the lifestyle people in that position have? Eino Maki is one excellent example. He is carrying out a type of work that is dangerous to his health but remains in a job available to him and others who have similar low social and economic status in society. You might respond that others who are at more financially secure levels of society have an opportunity for this kind of work too. True, but this reasoning is akin to the French political philosopher during the French Revolution who observed that "both the rich and the poor have an equal right to sleep under the bridges of Paris at night." Eino's autonomy to select a safer or more pleasant work environment is greatly diminished or absent.

Thoughtful individuals have pondered the role that such societally determined differences among patients should play. To help elucidate some of their thinking, let us first consider the relevant information in the story of the Maki brothers.

Step 1: Gather Relevant Information

We are making an assumption that Eino's situation is caused by his work environment. We can do that for the purpose of encouraging you to think about compensatory justice situations, but of course, in an actual clinical evaluation, your gathering of relevant information first requires clarifying further his stage of lung cancer and whether tests substantiate the source being the asbestos to which he has been exposed as a mining company employee.

Another relevant piece of information that is a question we would have to explore is how much responsibility the company took to help prevent undue exposure. The way risks were presented and action taken to minimize them could make a difference in how we view this situation.

We do know that Eino, and people like him, carry out labor tasks and other societal functions that are needed for the society to function well but often are not valued in other ways and may carry high risks to the workers. Of course, some "high-risk" situations are respected, and individuals who carry out the tasks are given extra financial benefits, and a high status. Examples are firefighters, members of a police force, or U.S. Navy Seals. Others, like Eino, are relegated to greater risk and "less desirable" jobs because of their overall lower social status, often accompanied by poverty or other characteristics that carry a stigma with them. *Stigma* in this social sense is a term first used by Goffman,[2] a sociologist, to depict persons held in low regard because of qualities they have. Status comes into being when mainstream society members, those in control and authority, make arbitrary judgments about the value of different kinds of lives and assign low priority to some whom they devalue. The most explicit negative effect on stigmatized groups comes through their disproportionately small allotment of the society's goods and services. It can be argued that even if Eino did have the full cognitive capacity to comprehend the danger he was in, he would have been able to do little to change his situation.

Step 2: Identify the Type of Ethical Problem

The idea of "compensation" at the root of compensatory justice issues arises out of society's consciousness that it is the morally right thing to be fair. But not everyone has the same chance at basic lifesaving or life-enhancing benefits from the get-go. Some people are born into situations that, through no fault of their own, force them into a disadvantageous societal position. You are probably familiar with the idea of a "handicap" among competitors in the sports arena. In that environment, good sportsmanship dictates that the handicapped player be given additional "points" to try to make up for the disadvantage. There is an intuitive correctness about this attempt to "even the playing field." But this compensation activity is not always the case in the larger society, so it is not surprising that the problem it raises is characterized as a dilemma of justice.

Compensatory justice acknowledges due regard for groups of individuals by offering them compensations for harms occasioned by their basic societal disadvantage. The compensation is not necessarily to make up for a consciously perpetrated wrong by another person or society, though one application is criminal justice situations where the perpetrator is required to pay for his or her injury to another. But more generally conceived, it is enough to make it a morally relevant issue that a person or group is vulnerable from the standpoint of having limited access to that society's available valued goods and services. As for Eino, we have reason to believe that his work in the mines led to a life-threatening, industry-related condition. If the company knowingly placed workers in harm's way to benefit the company's bottom line, moral responsibility to redress this wrong squarely can be placed on management. If they, too, are surprised by this bad news, society's understanding of the wisdom of compensating individuals in such a situation has led to certain mechanisms for spreading the cost of the compensation across the larger society with taxes and other common resources. (In the United States, *"workman's compensation"* grew out of this idea originally, but since has come to be considered a protection for anyone injured on a job, no matter their social status, economic security, or other variables.) Sometimes the wisdom of providing compensation has come from pressure by interest groups such as unions or other organizations (e.g., nonprofits run by various religious groups) who try to provide a voice for those who are not in a position to speak effectively against such wrongs themselves. Recently, concern has been expressed in the press and literature that labor unions' effective voice may be suffering from divided loyalties within the unions themselves.[3]

However voiced, the idea that a moral claim for compensation should influence how resources are allocated makes this problem a justice dilemma.

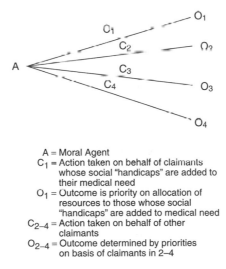

A = Moral Agent
C_1 = Action taken on behalf of claimants whose social "handicaps" are added to their medical need
O_1 = Outcome is priority on allocation of resources to those whose social "handicaps" are added to medical need
C_{2-4} = Action taken on behalf of other claimants
O_{2-4} = Outcome determined by priorities on basis of claimants in 2–4

Compensatory Justice Problems.

Similar reasoning has been applied to priority setting for shelter, food, or other basic goods of society, the underlying assumption being that not everyone comes equally supported by society to adequately take part in life's basic benefits.

  SUMMARY

Compensatory justice assumes that the allocation of resources should be made to address health care problems of an individual or group on the basis of more than medical need alone. Their position in society also is a relevant factor.

Step 3: Use Ethics Theories or Approaches to Analyze the Problem

In Chapter 15, you were introduced to several ethical theories and principles for analyzing the morally appropriate allocation of resources according to distributive justice reasoning. We present two key ones that clearly also apply to the analysis of compensatory justice reasoning: equity and the principle of nonmaleficence.

Equity

To review, equity means that every effort must be made to treat each person in a similarly situated circumstance alike, allowing for departures from that baseline of equality on the condition that differences are derived from ethically acceptable criteria.

For example, Mr. Maki works in a dangerous environment that is not highly regarded as a career line for mainstream members of society. Other miners are "similarly situated." They are in a class all their own, equal with each other but not with mainstream society. A compensatory justice approach takes into account that mainstream society has more opportunities and resources to deal with crises such as Eino faces. So "similarly situated" means that all like him fall within the same general category of claimants on health care resources. The compensation in the idea of compensatory justice is that there is a moral pull on a just society to respond to the disadvantages that Eino faces as one who is lower on the rung of the social and economic ladder of society through no fault of his own. It may take priority standing or more societal resources to be sure he receives quality care equal to his mainstream counterparts with similar clinical need. The fact that he is contributing an important service that others usually do not choose adds to the argument that those with more resources have a moral responsibility to help the larger society stay intact through compensations to those like Eino who are less well off.

Where does health care as a right fit into the compensatory justice framework? It certainly helps support the idea of compensatory justice if health care is viewed as a right that everyone should have access to in contrast to the opposite idea that health care is a commodity like all other products to be bought by those who can afford to do so. In some cases, the right may require that those who are better off as members of mainstream society are required to do whatever is needed to support access for all.

The Principle of Nonmaleficence

In Mr. Maki's case, a compelling argument in favor of supporting his medical treatments financially is not only that he has a terrible medical condition (which, indeed, he has) but that he has the condition because he is in a job that carries with it the albatross of a carcinogenic agent that is well established scientifically and can be tested for before damage to a person's health. Many people examining Eino Maki's plight have an intuitively sympathetic response in favor of compensating him for his job-related cancer. It seems wrong, from a moral point of view, that he should have to suffer the ravages of a debilitating, painful, and incurable disease because he has been working in a setting that economically disadvantaged individuals are more apt to accept because it is one of the only options open to them and that carries a life-threatening hazard with it (Figure 16-1).

The principle of nonmaleficence, "do no harm," includes the idea that there should be a commitment to prevent harm and remove harm when possible. Thus, compensation is a positive response to Eino's harm. For many, this case for compensation is strengthened by the possibility that the company might have known about the risk to the miners and failed to take humane measures and strong precautions on their behalf.

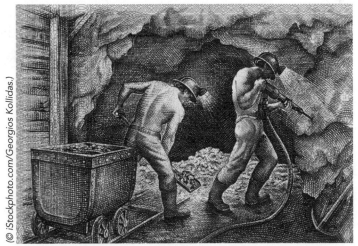

(© iStockphoto.com/Georgios Kollidas.)

Figure 16-1. Mine workers are one example of people whose jobs carry significant dangers to health and safety.

SUMMARY

Compensatory justice holds that some persons are at a societal disadvantage in ways that require the larger community or some aspect of it to respond to harms that occur because of the person's or group's societal position.

The key point for you to remember is that in compensatory justice approaches medical need is a fact that requires attention, just as it does in distributive justice deliberations. The additional factor that requires attention in compensatory justice deliberations is the societal disadvantage that some persons and groups have. We do know that societal disadvantage today creates disparities in health status and a disproportionally small allocation of health care resources goes to the disadvantaged groups. [4]

Step 4: Explore the Practical Alternatives

The compensatory justice issue can be highlighted by comparing several policies that might be adopted by companies, governments, or other policy-making bodies. All but one of them suggest that there is a *collective responsibility* by a company or government agency to respond to harm. You have an opportunity to explore six major alternatives we have outlined. As you do, try to think about which ones you could support from an ethical standpoint and why. In each case, you can choose whether you support or do not support the policy and provide reasons to help you defend your decision.

1. The company should offer Eino (and all similarly situated employees) a sum of money equal to that which would pay for their treatment and provide early retirement with all retirement privileges if the person is unable to return to work. It is up to the affected employee to decide whether to spend the money on treatment or something else.
   Support _____ Do not support _____
   Consider:
   • the most caring response to all similarly situated employees;
   • Eino's rights, autonomy, and moral responsibility;
   • the company's moral responsibility and rights and needs; and
   • the larger society's involvement.
2. The company should pay for the employee's treatment with the understanding that he or she will return to work if medically able and, if unable, will be retired with full privileges of retirement that would have accrued if he had worked until regular retirement age.
   Support _____ Do not support _____

(Continued)

Consider:

- the most caring response;
- Eino's autonomy and moral responsibility;
- the company's moral responsibility and rights and needs; and
- the larger society's involvement.

3. The company should pay for the employee's treatment with the understanding that he or she will return to work if medically able. If unable, the person will be terminated with whatever retirement has accumulated up to the time of termination.
Support _____ Do not support _____
Consider:

- the most caring response;
- Eino's rights, autonomy, and moral responsibility;
- the company's rights and moral responsibility; and
- the larger society's possible involvement of supplementing Eino's income if he has little or no retirement income (society as a "safety net").

4. Federal or state funds from tax dollars or other public sources should provide Eino (and all similarly situated people) a sum of money equal to that which would pay for treatment and arrange to supplement his current retirement earnings up to his company's full retirement level if he is unable to return to work. It is up to the affected person to decide whether to spend the money on treatment or on something else.
Support _____ Do not support _____
Consider:

- the most caring response;
- Eino's rights, autonomy, and moral responsibility;
- the company's lack of involvement for compensation beyond what Eino has already earned; and
- the larger public's collective contributions and assurance of being able to be supported in Eino's situation.

5. Federal or state funds from tax dollars or other public sources should pay for full medical coverage for people like Eino but not offer them a cash equivalent. That is, the compensatory considerations are limited to medical treatment directly related to the "injury." The understanding is that the person will return to the former employment if medically able. If unable, he or she will be retired by the company with full privileges, and the company will receive a subsidy from the government.
Support _____ Do not support _____
Consider:

- the most caring response;
- Eino's rights, autonomy, and moral responsibility; and
- the shared moral responsibility of company and the larger public

and how it is divided (society as provider of medical compensation, "safety net" of the company).
6. No company or public compensation should be provided for Eino or
similarly situated people.
Support _____ Do not support _____
Consider:
• the most caring response;
• Eino's rights, autonomy, and moral responsibility;
• the company's rights, autonomy, and moral responsibility; and
• the public's rights, autonomy, and moral responsibility.

As you can see, each of these six alternative courses of response provides a variety of possible conflicts of interest or opportunities for com-
munity-wide solidarity efforts. The conflicts may be seen as competing
interests of similarly situated harmed individuals, the private sector of
society, and the larger public sector of society. Questions of the most caring
approach (all things considered), rights, autonomy, and the sphere of
moral responsibility of each should be taken into account in the analysis of
any of them. Options 1 through 5 support the compensatory justice position that compensation should be provided for the harm suffered by people
such as Eino Maki, although the form, amount, and source of compensatory funds differ according to the political and social context in which the
compensatory mechanisms are situated. Many ethicists who address health
care issues support the position that at least a basic safety net of health care
benefits should be provided by federal, state, or local governments (the
public sector). The position that the whole community of society should
work together to find common solutions because it will, in fact, more likely
benefit all is called a *communitarian approach*.[5] Although there are several
varieties of communitarian thinking, they reflect a basic theme of *interdependence*. We are fundamentally not autonomous after all, and at some
time, each of us depends heavily on others to help sustain us. The first five
options all have elements of such thinking. Each provides some compensation for Eino and other people made vulnerable by circumstance. The tradition of the United States has carried some communitarian themes in it
but is largely based on the individual autonomy of individuals living
within structures and institutions where markets drive what each individual or group will rightly enjoy.[6] Canada and almost all European countries take a more communitarian approach. Eino and John Maki are good
examples of people who want to "earn their own way," the hallmark of this
type of thinking. There also are several varieties of this liberal approach
within modern society. The sixth option most fully conveys the extreme of

the liberal society free market approach, treating health care as a commodity as we discussed in Chapter 15. In this reasoning, Eino, like anyone else, should not be provided for by public funds. He does have a job and like anyone else may have to spend what he and his brother believe is a disproportionate level of income on these goods and services. Proponents of this argument feel that Eino chose to work in the mines, perhaps even knowing the risks involved. As you can see, this latter approach in its bare form leaves no room for the idea of compensatory justice in health care.

 SUMMARY

Compensatory justice approaches require an assumption of deep interdependence of people in society.

The previous discussion illustrates that compensatory justice cannot be discussed apart from determination of who in the population should bear the burden of costs incurred as a result of policies based on compensatory reasoning. For example, the first three options suggest that the cost should be borne privately, in this case, by the company. Options 4 and 5 remove the responsibility from the private sector. Taxes to pay for compensation plans come from those people who, under the U.S. doctrine of personal liberty, have been able to become and remain self-sufficient. As taxes increase for the purpose of supporting groups or individuals with situations such as that of Eino Maki, compensatory justice may be viewed as impinging on the personal autonomy of people who currently are not ill or in need of medical services. This hits deep in the North American psyche. As one U.S. colleague reflected recently, autonomy has a monopoly on our moral attention. Resistance grows out of anger that having earned the means of paying for health care, it is unfair that such persons then may be required to forego being financially able to send their children to colleges they otherwise would choose, put additions on their homes, buy sports and exercise equipment to keep fit, or, for some, even heat their homes properly because of a societal mandate to help support basic needs of strangers. This debate around the question of the conditions by which each of us must become our brothers' [and sisters'] keeper currently is raging as yet another round of national health care reform measures are placed before the U.S. public and legislature.

Step 5: Complete the Action

To arrive at a policy that supports public financing in whole or part for Mr. Maki, policymakers must decide how much personal liberty the more societally advantaged members of society are willing to contribute towards mechanisms that allow compensatory justice to be upheld. Those in favor of the community-oriented spirit of compensatory justice argue that it is a "contribution" instead of a "sacrifice" or loss. One example is that such a contribution yields the rewards of altruism. *Altruism* is the act of doing something on another's behalf with no thought or expectation of return, a concept that is found in almost every major religious tradition.[7] Another is the idea of a *reciprocity ethic*. In the latter, a contribution to someone else's well-being creates a societal environment in which others are willing to contribute to one's own well-being when the need arises. Those who have written the most extensively from this orientation as an ethical approach emphasize its similarity to the Golden Rule of the Christian Bible: "Do to others what you want them to do to you." Other writers show analogues in most other religious and many philosophic theories.

Reflection

Having considered all the ramifications, suppose that you are a member of a policymaking body that must vote on the six policy options discussed. You have already made your personal selection by completing the exercise. Now you are confronted with people who may hold different views from your own. Of the arguments opposing your choice, what do you think will be the most powerful?

_____

_____

_____

_____

Although you have been a responsible committee member, what (if any) lingering reservations do you have regarding your own choice?

_____

_____

_____

_____

In participating in this type of policy decision process, you have exercised your ethical reasoning in a manner similar to that which you will be asked to use in the policy-related aspects of the practice of your profession: in your process of coming to a decision, you have had an opportunity to engage in the step-by-step process of decision making. You have brought to consciousness the expressions of caring, considered the relevant facts, dealt with the ethical dilemma of justice in the situation with which you are faced, and, through that, arrived at the selection of your option.

Step 6: Evaluate the Process and Outcome

Although much can be said in support of compensatory justice, the determination of groups in society to be singled out for preferential treatment requires that they be designated as a special class. This raises at least two important caveats: one emerges from the double edge of labeling, and the other is from the specific label of "vulnerability." We take you through these considerations one by one, but to do so, we shift your attention from compensatory justice situations alone to the larger context of social justice. The topics we cover now show the ways in which compensatory justice and social justice approaches are related.

Social Justice, Social Need and Respect for All

By focusing on Eino Maki's situation and the type of contribution he is making as a worker, we can begin to see how a person's societal position impacts a deeper understanding of what justice requires. However, there are some important shortcomings in relying solely on the fact that a person is contributing to the workforce as the means of triggering the wheels of justice. To be sure, it does illustrate one example of social justice introduced in Chapter 15 insofar as it illustrates that medical need alone does not explain fully how health care must be allocated to meet the criteria of a just society. Social justice embraces situations like Eino's but goes further to tackle the issue of serious and pervasive disparities in health that persist amongst millions of less well-off people in the United States and global society (Figure 16-2).

Some argue the folly of allowing these disparities from a utilitarian approach. Nobel-winning economist Amartya Sen[8] submits that we cannot realize the benefits of a healthful society overall until we uncover the *de*valuation of stigmatized groups who simply by virtue of skin color, ethnicity, physical or mental condition, age, or gender bear the brunt of discrimination. He shows convincingly that our fate is intertwined and that without respecting the capacities that every single member of society brings to the society, all eventually lose.[8] By disentangling "capacity" from the Western ideal of societal worth measured by "contribution," he honors the life situation of all, whatever the societal interpretation of their economic worth. As you can see, the principle of interdependence is embedded in this utilitarian conception of society. In short, the disproportionately small allotment of the society's goods and services to devalued members of society arise from prejudices that threaten to trade the idea of equality and respect for all at the price of well-being for everyone.

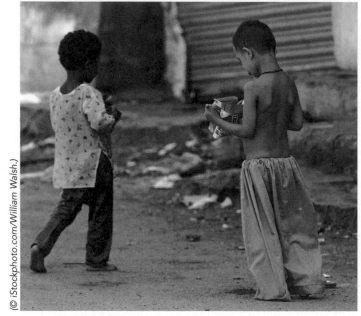

(© iStockphoto.com/William Walsh.)

Figure 16-2. Economic impoverishment touches all areas of a person's life.

Others argue, similarly to the reasoning in compensatory justice, that disparities are just plain wrong from the standpoint of the ethical standards of equity and the principle of nonmaleficence. To counter the negative effects of inequality, the concept of social need is a useful tool.

Social need means that a person is in a societal environment that is not friendly to basic needs being met to the same degree that mainstream society enjoys. How social need is established then becomes a key consideration. Two societal tools to do so are presented for your consideration: labeling and vulnerability.

Labeling: A Double Edge

Labeling is an important mechanism used to help identify significant similarities among members of a group. Labeling was designed to help ensure that by grouping such persons their needs better could be met and often has been helpful in identifying great need. However, Martha Minow[9] points out that "Difference . . . is a comparative term . . . different from whom? I am no more different from you than you are from me . . . The point of comparison is often unstated . . . " She says that at the root of this issue is *"the dilemma of difference."*[9] Labels can succeed in identifying differences among groups and thereby assist in seeing that justice is done, but they can also be a barrier: "When does treating people differently . . . emphasize their differences and stigmatize or hinder them on that basis? And when does treating people the same become insensitive to their differences and likely to stigmatize them or hinder them on that basis?"[9] As you read in Chapter 13, persons whose chronic conditions receive a genetic label often find themselves disadvantaged with insurers and others because of the label. Labeled groups are not always given the positive treatment promised them and may be even further discriminated against.

A case in point is an extensive screening program for sickle cell disease that was initiated in the United States in the latter quarter of the 20th century. The important point from a social justice perspective is that sickle cell disease affects primarily African Americans, a group that traditionally has suffered stigma and the resulting discrimination on many fronts. It is a painful condition that manifests itself in infancy and continues throughout a shortened life span. Symptoms associated with it include infarction of the soft tissue and bone, which causes acute pain. It also affects the spleen, liver, and kidneys.[10] The screening designed to identify affected individuals and therefore identify them as a group deserving of special attention was conducted. However, once labeled, these individuals did not realize the benefits of large-scale treatment programs. Instead, in many instances, African Americans identified through the screening process found that insurance, employment, and other records carried stigmatizing information regarding their status as carriers of the sickle cell trait.[11]

 SUMMARY

Labels are designed to identify special needs or characteristics. However, populations who have been societally disadvantaged and experienced previous social wrongs do not necessarily benefit from placement in a labeled group.

The "Vulnerability" Criterion

Vulnerability or "vulnerable populations" are general labels applied to establish a stigmatized group's disadvantageous societal circumstances. Again, the intent is to provide a way to determine special needs that befall some members of the group and to respond positively. Some at-risk groups include women, elderly individuals, people with disabilities, poor people, groups of people in racial and ethnic minorities, and other people who are consigned to relatively low societal status within mainstream society.[12]

But in fact, traditionally some of these socially stigmatized groups labeled as vulnerable have been viewed as the *cause* of the "unfortunate" situation they are in because of a personal, genetic, or cultural "defect" or sin.[13] As recently as the beginning of the AIDS epidemic in the United States, one commonly heard the opinion that men who had sexual encounters with other men deserved their fate because of their sin. There was a similar backlash to "feminists" who sought equity in the work environment, the reasoning being that they belonged in the home. Whether or not specific vulnerable groups are seen as the cause of their societal position today, the fact is they are *socially marginalized* when compared with mainstream society and collectively are excluded at disproportionately high rates from desired opportunities and the goods and services of society.[14] Legal mechanisms to help minimize the discrimination against them are helping to provide some opportunities for fuller participation.

The idea of social need gets at the heart of the issue because it focuses priority on the societal situation of the relatively less well off and detaches it from the idea that some deserve to have less than others. It goes beyond the compensatory justice reasoning based in part on Eino's contribution to the workforce. The idea of vulnerable groups goes deeper into a kind of "no fault of their own" assumption that takes people where they are no matter what the reason is for their landing in this place. Their need is medical need for health care services, but the additive factor of societal disadvantage is best captured in the idea of social need. If the demands of social justice are to be met, there is an urgent onus on society to be more inclusive.[15]

 SUMMARY

Mainstream society plays a major role in social marginalization with resulting serious health disparities. The appropriate moral response must be found in paying attention to how labels and the criterion of vulnerability do not necessarily result in allocations that address social need or bring about social justice. A commitment to more inclusive societal arrangements is essential.

Justice and Solidarity

Anderson[16] in her article "What Is the Point of Equality?" critiques some of the thinking that has supported social justice policies. Her major point is what we just shared, namely, that at the root of the problem is our lack of inclusiveness. She says that in some ways we have moved out of "blaming" people for their place in society and recognized that "the fundamental aim of equality is to compensate people for undeserved bad luck—being born with poor native endowments, bad parents, and disagreeable personalities, suffering from accidents and illness, and so forth."[16] The compensatory and larger social justice goal for such individuals having drawn a so-called short straw in the natural lottery of life is to mitigate or eliminate the negative impact of their predicament. But ultimately, Anderson rejects this concept of the goal of compensatory and social justice because, she argues, there is no way around an assumption embedded in it that the disadvantaged group has inferior basic worth, is "sadly inferior."[16]

In contrast, she proposes (with other thinkers today) that a more considered understanding of justice would work toward the aim of creating "a community in which people stand in relations of equality to others"[16] based on true and deep respect (Figure 16-3).

Silvers[17] emphasizes that this can be achieved by giving priority to societal arrangements that allow everybody to optimize their freedom at all times, no matter their capacity. The basic conceptual underpinning is captured in the sociopolitical notion of *solidarity*. Groups who make claims on another could do so through virtue of their socially recognized equality with mainstream groups.

With this perspective beginning to emerge, the construction of an inclusive social environment may be viewed by some as utopian, but substantive changes that already have been made show it to be a practical alternative. From a cost-sensitive approach alone, the costs to society in lost productivity and need for caregivers (professional and otherwise) makes the neglect and exclusion of whole groups of people a bad idea. Health professionals are in a good position to be one important voice advocating for such changes.

Individual Responsibility for Health Maintenance

Now we come to a potential snag in the evolving compensatory and social justice reasoning and a more solidarity-oriented approach to allocation. As we noted previously, there is an idea that vulnerable populations who are

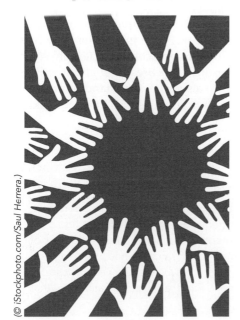

Figure 16-3. True respect for all strengthens everyone in society.

(© iStockphoto.com/Saul Herrera.)

socially marginalized when it comes to the allocation of goods and services may be disadvantaged through no fault of their own. We never fully addressed the question of Eino's responsibility, if any, of preventing his current ill health. Eino was a hard-working miner in a dangerous environment, and at least some people who read his story probably are sympathetic toward him. However, we also know that he may have refused to admit earlier that he was having symptoms that warranted medical attention. And some would ask whether he had really had no other choice but to work in the mines.

A similar kind of question has been raised in regards to social justice-based policies that work to give all persons a more equal chance of health. For instance, we presented a sympathetic picture of African Americans who were diagnosed as having the debilitating effects of sickle cell disease and felt that they had been identified without receiving the promised interventions. A part of their feeling of betrayal came from their recognition that they are in a group whose forbearers arrived as slaves and that overall dark-skinned people have never been given the same advantages as light-skinned ones. Some critics are not sympathetic, maintaining that once identified, they had a responsibility to take matters into their own hands to avoid further debilitation as much as medical care could provide it.

Today, there is a lively discussion about how the social responsibility of society to allocate resources justly must be balanced against each individual's *personal responsibility for health*. As you read earlier in the chapter, there is a strong ethos of autonomy in the United States and other Western societies that supports the idea that each of us has the freedom to be responsible for maintaining our own health.

The subsequent example illustrates some of the complexities that arise in the process of trying to exercise justice for everyone in a society. We have chosen the story of Jane who has a life-threatening condition (emphysema) in part because, like Eino, she is having difficulty breathing and it will get worse without intervention. Viewed from a social justice standpoint, she is vulnerable. But her situation is different from Eino Maki's in some striking ways too.

The Story of Jane Tyler and Sam Puryo

Jane Tyler, a 32-year-old single woman and mother of three children (5, 8, and 12 years old), has been living on public assistance since her first child was born. Jane lives in a small apartment above her mother's in a part of town most people never go. Her mother helps with light housekeeping and child care. Now that all three children will be in school, Jane has successfully applied for a grant from the local Woman's Fund, a private organization, that will allow her to train to become a business information technology assistant so that she can make a living for herself and her family. Receiving this award was a tremendous boost to her self-esteem, and she sees it as a bright doorway out of her "no exit" life situation. The one nagging anxiety she is experiencing is a severe shortness of breath at times and unusual fatigue. Before taking on this additional load of schooling, she decides to have a checkup at her neighborhood clinic.

It comes as a devastating blow to her to learn that she has emphysema. She has been threatening to stop smoking for a long time, but her two pack-a-day habit has had a strong grip on her. It is an even greater shock to learn that although the emphysema is only in the beginning stages, she may not be eligible for state-of-the-art curative treatment because she is on public assistance. The state legislature presented to the voting public the opportunity to decide priorities for high-cost interventions provided through public funds by sending a questionnaire to a sample group. (Some readers will recognize this general approach as the innovative tactic passed by the Oregon state government in 1989 that became known as "The Oregon Experiment.") Three physicians concur that Jane's smoking is a direct cause of her emphysema. One of them believes there may be cofactors that lead some people to actually manifest the symptoms of emphysema, whereas others do not. The other two are completely convinced her smoking directly has created her serious health problem. Because two of the physicians of the three are needed for this policy to take effect, she is able to receive only cursory treatment. Her only opportunity for an adequate treatment regimen is for her to find some way to pay for it.

Sam Puryo is a caseworker in the public assistance office. Jane has been one of his clients for several years. He is upset at what he judges to be the apparent injustice of the laws that have put her in her current dilemma. He tries to call his state senator to see whether there are any loopholes in the law that could help her or whether an exception can be made for this woman who Sam sees as exceptional. The senator is not encouraging; she is sympathetic but knows of no loopholes and is pessimistic about an exception being made.

During a coffee break, Sam gets into a discussion of the new rulings with his colleagues at the welfare office. His fellow social worker is strongly in favor of the approach taken by the legislature. All the people at lunch agree that it is important to be willing to consider the arguments.

 Reflection

Now is your opportunity to join Sam and the others in their discussion. Consider the following questions. What is morally due Jane Tyler and other people in similar situations? More importantly, how should her situation be approached to ascertain what she should receive, if anything?

_____

_____

_____

_____

Viewed from a justice perspective, at least three variables are relevant in trying to sort out what, if any support, for her treatment is due Jane Tyler. One is her medical need, a second is her personal habit that apparently has contributed significantly to her health condition, and the third is her low economic status.

Medical Need and Individual Responsibility

The first variable, her medical need, is relevant from the perspective of distributive justice. Therefore, if we view Jane's predicament solely as a distributive justice question based on her symptoms, we have to conclude that optimal medical care is due her on the basis of her medical need. The state legislature obviously has not made their judgments strictly on the basis of medical need, which means Jane's situation is not only a distributive justice allocation decision.

Personal Habits and Individual Responsibility

Now comes the complication of her smoking-induced condition. From a social justice standpoint, this does not factor in as a strike against her. However, you can see compensatory justice reasoning working against Jane Tyler. Most of us believe—in theory, if not in practice—that responsible citizens should positively contribute something to society and attempt to refrain from destructive behaviors. Now she is viewed tacitly, if not explicitly, as doing harm through her smoking habit. The harm is not only the destruction of her lungs; she may also be viewed as causing harm to others by using societal resources and contributing to a drain on tax money that might be needed for her care and that of her small children as her condition deteriorates. Finally, some would argue that given mounting evidence of the harm of secondhand smoke, she is putting her children at risk for ill health.

One defining factor is the extent to which Jane is in a position to be held accountable for her tobacco addiction now and the ensuing difficulties it has brought on her. Distinguishing between disadvantages that a person brings on himself or herself and those that result from external forces over which he or she has no or little control is not easy to do. Most readers know that a person's conduct is determined in early childhood and is reinforced by one's cultural, ethnic, and socioeconomic group (to name some influences on adult behavior). However, many join society's individualism-based judgment that all she would have had to do to break her habit was "just say no." Moreover, there are many aids to stop smoking on the market.

Reflection

Do you think that she is voluntarily harming herself and others, or is this an example of blaming the victim? What reasons support your judgment about her conduct?

_____

_____

_____

_____

Economic Disadvantage and Individual Responsibility

Finally, her low socioeconomic situation and being a single mother with three children ensures that she is vulnerable. Her stigmatized status tends to exclude her from beneficial societal supports, a factor that is relevant from a social justice perspective. At the same time, she is not totally excluded because she has been receiving publicly funded assistance to help sustain her and her three children. But even this support is against a backdrop of her poverty. Her economic status may become another decisive variable because of the following lines of observation:

- Poor people are at a financial disadvantage in their opportunities to acquire an education, and through that means, increase their range of choices regarding careers, where they work, and how much money they make.
- Women in poverty are more economically disadvantaged than men.
- Finding an avenue to a skilled worker position through education could be an important turning point in her life and in her children's welfare. She has found funds for bettering herself, but now her health needs may be the barrier.

You can see how social justice reasoning adds these economic considerations that go well beyond medical concerns taken alone.

Reflection

Do you think that these social factors should influence your decision about her eligibility for the optimal health care for her medical condition? Why or why not?

_____

_____

_____

_____

You now have three perspectives on individual responsibility all tied up in this one case, leaving you to make the final decision about whether or not she should be eligible for the optimal care for her worsening emphysema. This discussion and your responses are germane because you are entering the health professions at a time when there is much debate about how much responsibility individuals must take for their own health.[18]

Individual Responsibility and a Caring Response

Although you cannot help but have opinions and personal feelings about issues related to others' destructive habits and behaviors, it is important to remember that in policy the relevant arguments are usually general, not specific. Therefore, a caring response to a group in deciding what role their behaviors should play in the allocation of publicly generated resources for health care (or other basic goods) must begin with humility toward the complexity of "what makes people tick." Although it cannot be reasonably expected that the larger society will support any and all types of self abuse and self neglect, the prior moral responsibility is to get to the root causes of a group's behavior. This cannot be accomplished without sound research data combined with skills that allow for culturally competent approaches to the variety of situations we find ourselves in at anytime allocation decisions are being made.

SUMMARY

Currently, there is much debate about the role each individual must play in assuming responsibility for his or her own health. Such assessments must be made within the larger societal context in which individuals reside to ensure that inequities are not placed on them.

Summary

The compensatory and larger social justice issues raised in this chapter admit of no easy answers, theoretically or in their practical application. In your professional practice, you will have ample opportunity to reflect further on the implications of how distributive justice, compensatory justice, and social justice approaches foster the larger societal goals of a caring response in the face of limited resources. The underlying concerns presented by social marginalization and the complementary roles that individuals, their institutions, and the larger public should play in upholding the tenets of a flourishing society all are relevant considerations in implementing just policies. Only when just policies are in place can individual health professionals and others be confident that just practices will be possible.

Questions for Thought and Discussion

1. Some have argued that because the extent to which people value health in relation to other goods (such as food, shelter, clothing, a car, living where there is fresh air, and so on) varies from person to person, the most just health care resource distribution would be to give the same amount of money to each citizen (a "voucher" or "savings account") and let him or her spend it however he or she chooses over a lifetime. Discuss the strengths and weaknesses of this arrangement. At what age should this allocation be made? Why?
2. A group project:
   Discuss the pros and cons of the following proposed legislative bills from the point of view of distributive, compensatory, and social justice considerations. Vote for the one you support based on your reasoning.
   Condition A is a progressive disease of the central nervous system. It first affects the spinal cord and in its later stages infiltrates the brain, resulting in progressive spasticity and later in multiple movement and thought disorders. It occurs primarily in white, middle-class men 40 to 55 years of age and leads to certain death within 15 to 20 years. The cause and course of the disease is well understood. It is an autoimmune condition. Recently, a medication has been discovered that can help to slow the progress of Condition A dramatically. Currently, however, the cost of the medication needed for treatment is estimated to be about $10,000 per year for each patient. About 7500 people in the United States have been diagnosed with the disease, and the incidence rate seems to be increasing. It is believed that many more cases will surface if the medication becomes available for any who need it.

Legislation has been introduced into the U.S. Congress to make possible the processing and administration of the drug to all patients "in
the name of humanity." A conservative estimate is that the cost to U.S.
taxpayers will be about $17.5 million per year.

When the bill is being debated, a counterproposal is introduced.
Proponents propose that the funds be allocated to provide full annual
physical examinations, free of charge, to any refugee child in the
United States up to 12 years of age whose parents fall under the poverty
line economically. This free medical insurance will be compartmental-
ized from other federal or state funding for medical care because some
of those plans do not cover annual exams and some do not cover the
children of undocumented (i.e., illegal) immigrants. The estimated total
cost is close to that in the competing bill but "will serve 10 times as
many, each of whom is equally deserving of services as the people in
the competing bill." The core of the argument is that in general the latter
individuals are discriminated against in the United States, that only the
poorest among even that group has been targeted for public support,
and that legislators and policymakers must take this factor into account
in determining health care priorities.

3. James is a 29-year-old man who incurred a spinal cord injury at C3 in a
diving accident while on his company outing in Aruba. After several
days in a coma from hitting his head on a rock, he woke up to the
shock of having no movement from his neck down.

James worked as an investment banker before his injury and saved
a substantial amount given his 80-hour work week and single status.
Most of these funds he placed in 401k retirement accounts. James has
medical insurance; however, his medical bills are mounting, and the
social worker recommends that he apply for state disability to receive
additional coverage for long-term services that he will need but are not
covered by his private insurer. James decides to do so and then realizes
that to become eligible he must spend down his present dollar assets,
including his 401k accounts. He is furious and yells at the social worker,
"You've got to be kidding me. Do you think just because I'm crippled I
don't want to retire comfortably? This is grossly unfair."

Given what you have studied in this chapter, what sources of support,
and at what cost to his personal savings, do you think would meet the
demands of a just allocation of resources for him and others like him?

REFERENCES

1. Purtilo, R., 2004. Social marginalization of persons with disability: Justice considerations for Alzheimer disease. In: Purtilo, R., ten Have, H. (Eds.), *Ethical
foundations of palliative care for Alzheimer disease*. Johns Hopkins University
Press, Baltimore, MD, pp. 290–304.

2. Goffman, E., 1963. Information control and personal identity. In: Goffman, E., *Stigma: Management of spoiled identity.* Simon and Schuster, New York, pp. 41–105.

3. Fletcher, B., Gapasin, F., 2008. *Solidarity divided: The crisis in organized labor and a new path toward social justice.* University of California Press, Berkeley, CA.

4. Berkman, L., Epstein, A., 2008. Beyond health care-socioeconomic status and health [editorial]. *N Engl J Med* 358 (23), 2509–2010.

5. Bell, D., 2009. Communitarianism. In: Zalta, E.N. (Ed.), *Stanford encyclopedia of philosophy,* Spring 2009 edition. Available from: <http://plato.stanford.edu/archives/spr2009/entries/communitarianism> (acessed 25.01.10).

6. Appiah, A., 2001. Liberalism, individualism and identity. *Crit Inquiry* 27, 305–332.

7. Green, W.S., 2005. Introduction. In: Neusner, J., Chilton, B., (Eds.), *Altruism in world religions.* Georgetown University Press, Washington, DC, pp. x–xiv.

8. Sen, A., 2004. *Inequality reexamined.* Belknap Press of Harvard, University Cambridge, MA.

9. Minow, M., 1990. *Making all the difference: Inclusion, exclusion and the American law.* Cornell University Press, New York, pp. 20–21.

10. Centers for Disease Control and Prevention, 2010. *CDC features: Sickle cell disease: 10 things you need to know.* CDC National Center for Birth Defects and Developmental Disabilities, Division of Blood Disorders, Washington, DC. Available from: <www.cdc.gov/features/sickle cell> (accessed 24.01.10).

11. Anionwu, E., Atkin, K., 2001. *The politics of sickle cell and thalassaemia.* Open University Press, Philadelphia, PA.

12. Luna, F., 2009. Elucidating the concept of vulnerability: Layers not labels. *Int J Feminist Approaches Bioethics* 2 (1), 121–139.

13. Carlson, E.A., 2001. *The unfit: A history of a bad idea.* Cold Spring Harbor Press, Cold Spring Harbor, NY.

14. Purtilo, R., 2004. Social marginalization of persons with disability: Justice considerations for Alzheimer disease. In: Purtilo, R., ten Have, H. (Eds.), *Ethical foundations of palliative care for Alzheimer disease.* Johns Hopkins University Press, Baltimore, MD, pp. 290–304.

15. Miller, F.A., Katz, J.H., 2002. Part 1: The need for an inclusion breakthrough. *The inclusion breakthrough: Unleashing the real power of diversity.* Barrett-Koehler, San Francisco, CA, pp. 1–40.

16. Anderson, E.S., 1999. What is the point of equality? *Ethics* 109, 287–337.

17. Silvers, A., 2000. The unprotected: Constructing disability in the context of antidiscrimination law for individuals and institutions. In: Francis, L.P., Silvers, A. (Eds.), *Americans with disabilities: Exploring implications of the law for individuals and institutions.* Routledge, New York, pp. 126–145.

18. Steinbrook, R., 2006. Perspectives: Imposing personal responsibility for health. *N Engl J Med* 355 (8), 7533–7756.

17

Professionals as Good Citizens: Responsibility and Opportunity

---

Objectives

The reader should be able to:

- Describe how the concepts of moral agency and professional responsibility apply to the health professional's role in addressing civic issues.
- Identify three spheres of moral agency that constitute a health professional's scope of professional responsibility and how they differ from each other.
- Discuss what a caring response entails when the "patient" is the public at large.
- Compare the focus of shared fate and self-realization careers in relation to your role as a professional involved in civic issues.
- Identify two ethical principles that apply to a health professional's participation in trying to resolve threats to health in the larger society.
- Describe the relevance of virtue theory in preparing professionals for participation in civic issues.
- Describe four criteria of moral courage expressed by people who act courageously.
- Describe how the idea of a civic self becomes an orienting notion when acting on behalf of the common good.
- Reflect on how a basic respect for people may mean that the health professional will become involved in pressing social issues outside of health care.
- Discuss the reasons why health professionals are global citizens and what that means for their professional involvement in larger societal problems.

New terms and ideas you will encounter in this chapter

good citizenship	self-realization	moral courage
civic responsibility	service ethic	civic self
spheres of moral agency	public interest versus common good	global citizen
shared fate orientation	contributions	

Topics in this chapter introduced in earlier chapters

Topic	Introduced in chapter
Professional role	1
A caring response	2
Professional responsibility	2
Agency	3
Moral agency	3
Moral distress	3
Utilitarian theory	4
Ethical reasoning	4
Deontology theory	4
Duties and principles	4
Nonmaleficence	4
Beneficence	4
Ethics of care	4
Virtue theory	4
Solidarity	16

Introduction

Finally we come to the last chapter in this study of ethics, and it is fitting that its focus is back on you: you the health professional, but also you the citizen. *Good citizenship* is of course everyone's responsibility, and the activities that express good citizenship are captured in the idea of *civic responsibility*. Both "citizen" and "professional" are labels that carry assumptions about a person's role in society. Being a good citizen and being a good professional do have much in common. For example, each requires a measure of conscientiousness, engagement with societal needs, communication skills, and a willingness and ability to work with and on behalf of others.

Many interesting questions surround this dual role. For example, does your professional training provide you with any special opportunities and imply any special duties and responsibilities as a citizen? What is your special role, if any, that makes you the most appropriate person to take leadership on a civic issue that affects your community? Do you owe anything to society because it has bestowed on you the privileges of being a "professional," a status that has always been held in high esteem in Western cultures? If asked, are you morally obligated to respond to a pressing civic need, or can you just say no? There are certainly civic situations from which you are not exempt because you are a professional, such as paying taxes and jury duty. Are you a professional person 24-7, or can you blend into society as an ordinary citizen, leaving any special tugs on your moral conscience at your professional workplace? We attempt to address all these questions in this chapter.

To help focus our discussion, consider the following story.

The Story of Michael Merrick and ExRad Corporation

Two years ago, the residents of Peetstown, a small town in the Northeastern United States, welcomed the arrival of ExRad Corporation. The town had suffered terribly when Cal Mode Textiles Corporation closed, leaving in its wake more than 400 unemployed individuals. A major recruitment by town officials and its residents resulted in ExRad's choice of Peetstown for its new location.

Michael Merrick is a pharmacist working in Peetstown. He grew up in the beautiful hills 10 miles from where he now works, although for several years, he went to school and worked in New York City. He, his wife, and their three children moved back to Peetstown 2 years ago.

Recently, Michael and his family went on a walk along a path by the stream that flows through the small town. The stream provides recreation for children and adults alike along its banks, and fishing and swimming. All of the family simultaneously smelled a strong, sweet odor. Michael's 10-year-old son, John, ran upstream and discovered a small pipe just under the surface of the water. The odor was distinctly stronger in the pool that had formed there, and the water was a purple-tinged color.

Michael suggested that they not go too near the water. They continued their walk. But that night, he took a small jar and went back to collect a sample of the water. The next day, he drove 40 miles to visit a chemist friend who works in the chemistry department at the community college. The friend agreed to analyze the water and a week later called to say it contained large amounts of trichloroethylene, a toxic chemical that Michael remembered had poisoned the water supply in a town in Pennsylvania not long ago. Alarmed, Michael told a physician colleague who makes biweekly visits to the local clinic in Peetstown about his findings. The two decided to go to a county health official, who then promised to take care of the problem. "Let me know what happens," he said to the official as they left his office. "Sure will," said the man.

A month went by, and Michael heard nothing. He called the county official's office with no success. Finally, he saw the man at the monthly Rotary Club meeting and asked him what was happening. The man took him aside and said, "Don't worry about it. It was nothing. The injection well belongs to ExRad Corporation, and they are looking into it." Then he added, "You know we need that corporation. You can just let the matter drop."

The next day, Michael returned to the stream again. The odor was stronger than ever. When he got back to the clinic, he called the physician and related his story. She said, "I guess we had better pursue this ourselves, Mike." That night after dinner, Michael discussed the matter with his wife. Both of them were worried about what lay ahead if they took on what now appeared to be a very unpopular issue with the town officials. Michael called the physician and told her he felt he had to pursue the matter as best he could on his own because he was concerned about the effect of this toxin. She said, "It's the right thing to do. Count me in. I couldn't live with myself if I knew you were out there tackling this problem alone. We'll make a plan next week when I'm back in Peetstown."

Reflection

Does the action that Michael and his physician colleague have taken so far demonstrate any special character traits that a good citizen would not also have (so that you would have to attribute it to their being health professionals)?

_____

_____

_____

_____

As you reflect on it further, is anything required of them as a duty because they are health professionals that would not also be required of any ordinary citizen?

_____

_____

_____

_____

Anyone reading about the situation probably feels that Michael and his physician colleague are responsible, caring citizens. He did not just ignore the worrisome thing he encountered, leaving a question about whether his children or other members in the community were at risk. But this does not distinguish him from any caring citizen. Nor does it answer the question as to whether there is anything in his and her roles as health professionals that made them uniquely responsible to decide to pursue the matter over the responsibility of, say, a housewife, or CEO of a company or a plumber who stumbled on to the same situation. We personally believe that the professional role per se seldom sets professionals uniquely apart from other caring citizens, although there may be some exceptions to this general rule of thumb. Some good thinking about this very issue has been done, and we welcome sharing key aspects of it with you here. We will examine the now familiar idea of seeking a caring response to gain insight into how and why your civic responsibilities will sometimes emerge from or combine with the fact that you are a professional. We will also explore how in some situations your opportunities to contribute to society's well-being will be enhanced because you are one.

The Goal: A Caring Response

Two basic ethics notions presented early in this book help to provide a paradigm of understanding for what constitutes a professional's caring response to civic issues. The first is the idea of moral agency, accenting situations in which you can be expected to take charge. The second is the concept of professional responsibility.

Spheres of Moral Agency

As you recall, the important concepts of agency and moral agency were introduced in Chapter 3 and have been reinforced time and again throughout the book. To review briefly, agency means that you have an authoritative voice in a matter and are in a position to legitimately exercise that authority. You are in charge, and for a reason that you and society affirm. Approaching your role as a moral agent as having *spheres of moral agency* provides a way to distinguish different kinds of circumstances where you might become involved in civic issues (Figure 17-1).[1*]

As a professional, direct patient care decisions that fall within your area of professional expertise represent the major focus of your agency. Because there is a moral dimension to direct health care service, in Sphere One, your professional actions clearly are as a moral agent.

A second sphere of authority exists when you encounter a situation that is not direct patient care but you have important knowledge, insight, or skills that can help to effectively address the issue. In Sphere Two, the more

---

*We acknowledge with gratitude the authors of this excellent article and their graphic representation that helped to refine our own thinking on the health professionals' role in public life. Their article addresses the situation of physicians specifically, proposing a definition and conceptual model for physician advocacy. It also frames a public agenda for individual physicians' and physician organizations' involvement in larger health-related issues. Their goal, as ours in this chapter, is to promote health professionals' involvement beyond traditional health care and health policy boundaries. The difference between their and our emphases is that we broaden the scope to include the roles of health professionals more generally and take the discussion beyond health issues to others in the public arena.

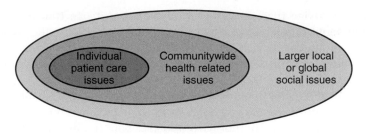

Spheres of Moral Agency

Figure 17-1. Health professional responsibility and good citizenship. (Adapted from Gruen, R.L., Pearson, S.D., Brennan, T.A., 2004. Physician-citizens—Public roles and professional obligations. *JAMA* 29 (1), 94–98.

your role as a professional prepares you better than any other group in society to address it, the more you will be looked to as an authority. For example, the more education a dietician has on the effects of snack food on childhood obesity, the more other parents on the school PTA board will look to her for advice regarding the proposed debate to institute a public mandate regulating the vending machines contents. When there are deep values involved, you are viewed as a moral agent by fellow citizens in this second sphere of your activity. A current trend in some Western nations reported in the International Social Work[2] journal is the movement from professional organization-based to citizenship-based regulation of traditional professions, one effect of it being the decreased distinction between the professions and citizens. This trend relies on the idea of traditional professional expertise to help enrich the understanding of what a professional really contributes but in other ways decreases the difference between professional and citizen characteristics. If this trend increases, the second sphere of moral agency may rely heavily on the expertise of professionally prepared citizens such as you are preparing to be, but your authority will be around your area of knowledge and skills only. Over time, agency could spread to rely less on the difference between professional and citizen.

The outermost Sphere Three shifts the emphasis from your knowledge and skills base to the fact that professionals are held in high regard in society. Health professionals, lawyers, religious leaders, and others often have a high status, even though they become the brunt of deep criticism when they do not stand up to society's realistic (or even unrealistic) expectations. Often, the gravity or urgency of a situation is expressed more forcefully when professionals get behind the cause and provide leadership in endorsing it. This is seen in everything from television ads to appeals for financial contributions for societal issues. Your voice can influence the outcome by virtue of being a professional, although you may have little significant or unique knowledge that situates you as an authority. In this sphere, you represent someone who is worthy of being taken seriously; therefore, you become an authority by virtue of your societal status. Again, when the issue involves societal values, which it almost always does, you are seen as a moral agent.

These three spheres provide general guidelines for the relationship of your role as a professional to your role as a citizen. As you can probably quickly conclude, there are not hard and fast boundaries separating these three spheres. Your clinical expertise may be operative in any of them to some degree, and your position of high regard in society supports activity at the very core of your decision-making authority.

A second conceptual notion that you were introduced to in Chapter 2 is essential in helping you to further fine-tune your civic priorities.

Professional Responsibility: Accountability and Responsiveness

Your responsibility as a professional must be calibrated according to a combination of accountability and responsiveness to a situation. All too often responsibility is viewed solely in terms of accountability, reducing responsibility to a duty that is inherent in the idea of professionalism and suggesting that when an opportunity to act arises you are obliged to do so. The standards of accountability by which you are measured range from the dictates of your professional codes, to patient care standards established by your profession and other licensing bodies, to institutional policies. You can see that in the center Sphere One of moral agency (concerned with direct patient care) they are appropriate and, in fact, designed for that purpose.

As you consider becoming involved in the other two spheres, the companion idea of responsiveness also is critical to understanding your actual responsibility. Being responsive means being relational at a deeper level that requires sensitivity to and understanding of the other or others who will be impacted by your action. The urge to act must be balanced with detailed attention to the narrative or human story you are encountering and with it, a genuine humility reminding you that your professional expertise does not prepare you to be an expert in every societal problem that falls into your path. As you continue outward towards Spheres Two and Three, your experience as a citizen and as a professional coincide more fully. In the second, you may quickly discern whether or not the type of health-related problem you encountered as a societal issue draws quite closely on what you know from your professional training. If yes, you can more closely identify with the details of the situation and what should be done.

As you move into Sphere Three, you are increasingly acting as a citizen who is a health professional. Yet, others may view you primarily as a health professional because most people think of professionals as being a doctor, or lawyer, or pharmacist or other professional 24-7. For example, if you have not already been prodded for your professional advice when someone recognizes you at a supermarket check-out counter, at a party, or elsewhere on the street, we can guarantee you will be. However, your professional identity is at work in Sphere Three only as a member of a citizenry who is granted moral authority on the basis of your societal position. You are not drawing on the content of your professional training and you will be acting more fully on what you know and can learn in the same way as any other citizen who becomes involved in societal issues.

 SUMMARY

By combining three spheres of moral agency with your professional accountability and ability to give serious attention to the relevant human implications of a situation, you have a general framework from which to discern a caring response. This response is consistent with a level of ethical duty you are in a position to exercise competently as a professional when becoming involved in various societal issues.

The Six-Step Process in Public Life

Michael and his physician colleague are not faced with a clinical or health policy situation in the same regard that we have invited you to explore the professional's involvement in them in other parts of this book. They may have no thoughts at this point about whether their decision to try to get at the root of a problem they believe is potentially causing harm to their community is related to their professional roles. Their lack of imagination or reflection on this issue is understandable because the health professional's idea of "care" usually is thought of as being contained to situations between individuals. Yet they feel as if they should do something as citizens, and we can assume that they are being driven in part by a motivation that they should be of service whenever they can. There is a lot of writing about this motivation among professionals, one aspect of which we present briefly here through the lens of different kinds of careers.

We touched on the career choice issue in Chapter 16 when a part of Eino Maki's situation was analyzed from the point of view that he was in a job open to him as a worker with some societal strikes against him, and you met Jane Tyler who was trying to increase her life options through the financial aid she had been granted to realize a career. All professionals fall within the category of having had an opportunity to choose a career, an option not open to most of the world's population. Having a career choice means that you are able to pursue your specific tastes, framing a life plan to suit your own character. Norman Care's[3] classic article on the nature of careers suggests that people choose between two basic types of careers: those with a *shared fate orientation* and those oriented to *self-realization*. The former focuses on service to society, the latter solely on self-satisfaction.[3] Health (and other) professionals fall within both categories to some extent but primarily are in the shared fate category, with its straightforward *service ethic*, or inclination to be of service. This inclination again has been revisited recently from a sociological analysis of the utility of the professions in the 21st century workforce that you are entering.[4] In short, both from a personal leaning towards helping others and from a pragmatic consideration of our usefulness, the idea of service is deeply engrained in many professionals.

Now that you have been introduced to the three spheres of moral agency, each involving a caring response, and reminded of the idea of professional responsibility, you have an expanded framework to think from as we walk with Michael and his colleague through the six-step process of ethical decision making regarding this opportunity to be of service.

Step 1: Gather Relevant Information

What information do we have?

Michael knows there is a deadly toxin in the stream near his home and other homes in their neighborhood. Every action he has taken so far suggests that he knows this is not a benign situation; rather, it is a problem that should arrest the attention of others. He surmises, though does not have certainty, that something more is going on, perhaps an attempt by other leaders in the community to cover up any wrongdoing by the ExRad corporation that has brought needed jobs. His suspicion is shared by his physician friend who has offered to link arms with him in pursuing the issue. They are concerned just as any other good members of the community would be concerned.

However, we know that these two individuals also are not like many other citizens in the community. It stands to reason that they have been exposed in their professional training to some understanding of how various environment pollutants affect health. As a pharmacist, Michael may have quite specific information about the toxic effects of trichloroethylene. At the very least, they have ready access to literature that will inform them in technical language they can more readily comprehend than many ordinary citizens. Whether or not they have direct knowledge of how polluted water supplies are damaging the health of whole communities, we do not know for sure. But we do know that starting about a decade ago, the World Health Organization made waterborne sources of ill health one major focus worldwide[5] and that this type of information is broadly being researched and the findings disseminated to medical and other health professions who provide direct patient care.[6] From just these perspectives alone, we can assume that Michael and his colleague's moral agency would fall more fully within the second sphere of professional responsibility to become involved in this civic issue than if the issue involved a heavily used bridge whose construction may be called into doubt by some members of the community.

We can also safely assume that this doctor and pharmacist are in a position to be heard if they speak up. The fact that the official took Michael aside and quietly implied that he not pursue the issue further suggests that he knew Michael and the physician could call attention to ExRad's conduct. They work in a relatively small town, a type of closely knit community usually loyal to their professionals. Michael belongs to the Rotary Club, a social and service organization to which leaders in a community must be invited by other leaders. Their roles carry a certain amount of status and weight in relation to most citizens. So, all things being equal, they can be viewed as moral agents in this situation in the third sphere by virtue of their status and role.

However, there is another human dimension that informs Michael's situation. It depends on his having grown up with these people. In discerning his professional responsibility, accountability is one thing, but then there is responsiveness at a more detailed level. He can be sensitive to nuances of this community that others would not be able to detect. For one thing, he knows how much the livelihood of this community does depend on jobs and the fragile line between abject poverty and at least minimal needs being met. ExRad is meeting an essential economic need. Michael knows that while he is "one of them," he also jumped ship and went to live in, of all places, New York City. Having come back, he is welcomed on the one hand as "a hometown boy who made good" but also may still be viewed with suspicion as an "outsider" who can be dismissed (and discriminated against) as a troublemaker. He and his family may become ostracized, even if his concern about ExRad is proven to be correct. So, he is hesitant about what to do next, not because he is ignorant of his or his colleague's power but because they understand that getting into this issue may be a messy business.

Finally, he and his colleague are faced with uncertainty about the outcome of their endeavor. They know they may be able to prove nothing.

Reflection

Are there other types of information you would consider relevant but that we have not touched on? If so, what are they?

_____

_____

_____

_____

Step 2: Identify the Type of Ethical Problem

Michael and his colleague are facing an ethical problem in the form of moral distress. There is some uncertainty about the morally correct course of action, but for the most part, their distress is focused on the barriers, consistent with moral distress Type A. They feel compelled to be sure this community has at least been warned that their water is being polluted with a toxin and would like to be sure someone is taking care of the problem to prevent harm that may be befalling the townspeople.

 Reflection
With the diagram here, sketch out some details of the barriers causing their distress. Recall that Michael and his colleague are moral agents (A) who want to take a course of action (C), but the course hits up against barriers that must be overcome to arrive at what they believe is the correct outcome (O). Fill in the key barriers you imagine they are facing in this civic action they want to take.

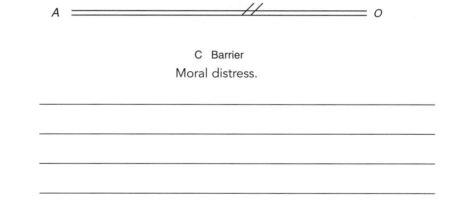

A ═══════════════ // ═══════════ O

C   Barrier

Moral distress.

_____

_____

_____

_____

    This situation highlights that the basic ethical problem termed moral distress is as helpful a tool for ethical decision making when the problem calls for action in one's professional role involving civic decisions as those decisions pertaining to direct patient care or health policy ones presented earlier in this book.

    Also, recall that emotions are one of the clues that you are encountering an ethical problem. Think of emotions and the specific response of fear or reticence it is generating in these two professionals as an interior barrier in themselves that combines with the external barrier of resistance from at least one powerful sector of the community to keep them from doing what they believe is right.

Step 3: Use Ethics Theories or Approaches to Analyze the Problem

Having identified their problem as one of moral distress, let us look more closely at these two moral agents in a predicament they do not welcome. We have already addressed the ethical idea of professional responsibility as a resource in these types of situations. It is a combined activity of discerning one's professional duty (being accountable to a standard) and getting the details of the narrative clear in one's mind (being responsive) before deciding one's actual course of action.

Utilitarian Reasoning as a Resource

An approach based on utilitarian theory would require these moral agents to weigh all the consequences of their proposed action as far as they can determine them. What are they? Not to be underestimated is their feeling that their integrity depends on what they do or not do. Other important factors have been discussed, among the most obvious the potential harm of the pollutant to the community if nothing is done, and if the issue is raised, the risk of ExRad's retaliation either to the agents or by moving to another community and leaving hundreds of people unemployed. Benefits of their going ahead with their plan to pursue the truth of the matter include, of course, preventing harm (or further harm) from the toxic pollutant and being sure that those in positions of power in this community are held accountable for their conduct. There are other less obvious but important benefits, too, one being that the community can count on its knowledgeable professionals to try to help maintain a safe and flourishing environment.

 Reflection

Approaching this moral distress problem as a utilitarian, what other factors would you want to add if you were balancing the benefits and risks of the professionals' pursuing a course of action designed to expose the presence of this toxin, its source, and a demand for corporate accountability?

_____

_____

_____

_____

Does your reasoning factor in the idea that their involvement is not around a Sphere One direct care issue but instead a Sphere Two issue (i.e., their professional role probably gives them insight into the clinical effects of the toxin) and a Sphere Three issue (i.e., they believe they can lend their authoritative voices as leaders in the community to help resolve the problem)? How, if at all, does this affect your reasoning?

_____

_____

_____

_____

Duties and Principles Approaches as Resources

The traditional oaths and codes of professional ethics depend heavily on deontology theory. They delineate the health professional's duties but say little about the professional's duties to society at large, except that patient care can be viewed as having a positive impact on the health of the larger society. The focus was on Sphere One duties and, to a lesser extent, on Sphere Two, an understanding of your role that persists in these documents with few exceptions today.

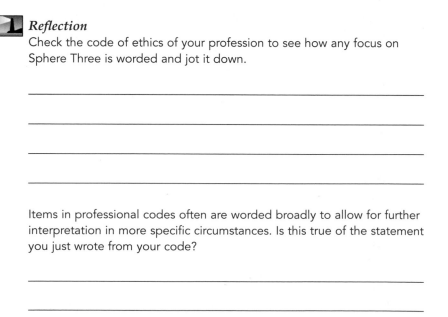 *Reflection*

Check the code of ethics of your profession to see how any focus on Sphere Three is worded and jot it down.

_____

_____

_____

_____

Items in professional codes often are worded broadly to allow for further interpretation in more specific circumstances. Is this true of the statement you just wrote from your code?

_____

_____

If they were using the statement as their guide, would Michael and his colleague receive any guidance about how to proceed in their situation of moral distress?

You should now be aware that to discern your behavior in today's complex health care environment you need to do more than rely solely on even the best code of ethics. You must engage in ethical reasoning using the various concepts, theories, and approaches of ethics. We have just walked with you through an ethical reasoning process from a utilitarian standpoint. Some of the ethical principles you learned earlier in this text now come to your aid when thinking about your moral agency and the extent of your professional responsibility in civic matters.

Nonmaleficence and beneficence are at the core of this approach. Now your focus is society in general, not just an identified patient or client. Jennings, Callahan, and Wolf[7] distinguish two types of societal involvement of professionals, each of which meets the criteria of nonmaleficence and beneficence. The first is service that seeks to promote the public interest, and the second is that which promotes the common good.[7] We submit that both are instrumental in preventing harm in civic life and in promoting types of good that honor the dignity of all.

Uses of your legitimate moral agency for Sphere One and Two involvements are what Jennings, Callahan, and Wolf identify as *public interest* activities. Public service that promotes the public interest includes the profession's contribution of technical expertise to public policy analysis and community problems. It also provides indirect service to civic society as a byproduct of direct health care provided to its individual members. In other words, the spheres of influence and the value of your civic contribution are governed by your technical and professional expertise.

The use of your legitimate moral agency for some Sphere Two and all Sphere Three involvements promotes *the common good*. This includes the distinctive and critical perspective the various professions have to offer on basic human values and on facets of the human good and the good life. It also includes the profession's contribution to what may be called civic discourse—that ongoing conversation in a democratic society about our shared goals, our common purposes, and the nature of the good life in a just social order. Your influence is determined in large part by your relatively high social standing in the community as a professional.

As Jennings, Callahan, and Wolf conclude, there is a duty to contribute to "the well-being of the community: its safety, the integrity of its basic institutions and practices, the preservation of its core values."[7]

Reflection

What important civic values could be served by Michael's involvement in this problem that would count as contributing to the prevention of harm to the community and to promoting the common well-being of all?

_____

_____

_____

_____

Michael's and his physician colleague's concern is with unclean water, but they are tapping into a deeper sensitivity about health and human flourishing. We are learning that among the most important values today is the safety of all living beings as a planet-wide, interdependent ecosystem: people, animals, and plants; and the air and water and soil working together or being destroyed together. In Chapter 16, we discussed the ethical principle of solidarity and how it transforms our understanding of relationship. Here the notion of solidarity is expanded to include more than solely human life as a civic value. The development of a worldwide document titled The Earth Charter,[8] signed off on by leaders across the globe, highlights that we must become acutely aware of the fragility of ecosystems and of the deleterious effects of their imbalances on human and nature's healthfulness and survival. Viewed from this insight, Michael's and his colleague's decision to enter the public arena to prevent or to remove harm to the whole community have more far-reaching health consequences than their direct patient care interventions. Their involvement provides an opportunity for us to think out of the box about what a caring response entails for today's health professionals, a theme heralded by Leonard Boff[9] in his piece The Ethics of Care: "Among so many other fine things, the Earth Charter proposes a new way of seeing that gives rise to a new ethic . . . " including its emphasis on respect and care for the [whole] community of life, ecological integrity, and social and economic justice (Figure 17-2).

"This sustainable way of life is equivalent to happiness in traditional versions of ethics deriving from the Greek, medieval and modern traditions. The supreme value now, that which must save the system of life . . . comes under the sign of care. It represents the new collective dream of humankind."[9]

Virtue Theory and Civic Involvement: Moral Courage as a Model

A caring response directed to involvement in civic issues provides an opportunity for us to assess the role of moral character and the virtues that support positive professional action. There are many that may apply in the case under discussion: compassion, a commitment to professional competence, integrity, honesty, and trustworthiness. All of these can come into play to help motivate action in any of the three spheres of moral agency.

However, recall that one of the barriers to action facing Michael and his physician colleague is their fear of what might happen if they go forward with what they believe is the morally appropriate thing to do. Their fear gives us an opportunity to explore the sometimes neglected resource of moral courage in health professionals' ethical decision making.

Moral courage is a readiness for voluntary, purposive action in situations that engender realistic fear and anxiety to uphold something of great moral value.[10] It is not surprising that Michael and his colleague are afraid. One way to view their reticence is that they are doing their homework by assessing the full picture of what they are up against. If they had no fear, they may

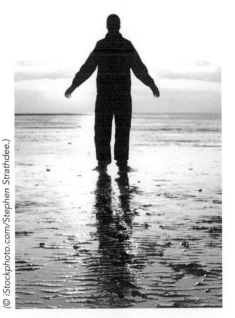

Figure 17-2. A vision of care that includes each other and nature sustains human flourishing.

bumble into the civic fray without thinking of the important byproducts of their good intentions.

Courage can be built up by preparation for such moments as Michael and the physician are facing now. In 1999, one of the authors had the privilege of learning this through a series of interviews with exemplars of courageous action by professionals and others who fought the injustices of the apartheid system in South Africa. Several common themes emerged, among them the following ways in which courageous resisters identified the step-by-step process that allowed them to act courageously:

1. Name the seriousness of the situation. Do not pretend that what is happening, or not happening, is acceptable and that it will go away. It is not, and it will not. Michael and the physician seem convinced of that.
2. Believe that good will prevail over wrongdoing. (One might call this the optimism of courage, or "hoping courage.")
3. Take the opportunity to nurture and be nurtured by essential sources of support. Everyone emphasized this, no matter their individual circumstances in other regards. In this chapter, we see Michael, the physician, and Michael's family as one "support coalition" that already is in place, and others will surely follow as the word gets out.
4. Become fully invested in the outcome. As one interviewee said, "The cause I started out to embrace eventually embraced me."[11]

There were other themes, but these four seem to fit the situation facing Michael and the physician as they begin to stake out their strategies. Even if they find that their inquiries and probing reveal no wrongdoing, they will have prepared well and will benefit from the experience of having done so. In fact, in a report on their studies of moral development and moral agency in professionals, Bebeau, Rest, and Narvaez[12] attribute to Rest the idea of defining moral character as "having the strength of your convictions, *having courage*, persisting, overcoming distractions and obstacles, having implementing skills, [and] having ego strength." [emphasis added] He singles out moral courage as the attribute needed to turn disposition into moral action.[12]

 SUMMARY

Moral courage is a virtue that, when cultivated, prods one to the right action, even in the face of fear or other difficulties.

Step 4: Explore the Practical Alternatives

With all of the information we have provided in this chapter about their situation, these two professional moral agents are still faced with the very personal decision about whether and how much to get involved. We have evidence from their story that they are motivated in part by a sense that their professional commitments should involve them in doing what they can in the larger society to make the world a better place.

They can of course, reverse direction and do nothing. Or Michael could decide to move his family out of town.

We see some other alternatives that fall more fully into what appears to be consistent with their motivation to address the issue.

The health professionals can bypass (or first inform) the county official and go directly to the leadership of ExRad to be sure the corporation is aware that the polluting source has been identified with them and report that the county official claims they know of the hazard. If there is a convincing positive response that this issue is being swiftly and adequately addressed, the professionals can link arms with the corporation to plan a strategy to correct the situation. They can also help ensure that the plan includes an effective mechanism for compensating anyone with health threats that already may have resulted from the polluted water supply and have a plan in effect to address longer term negative effects of the poisoning.

The professionals can call local print and other media to avail them of the situation with the hope that they will provide leadership in exposing the health hazard.

Michael can share his concern during the next Rotary Club meeting, hoping that others of the town's leadership will take up the cause with him.

They can also build a coalition of professionals and other citizens who will work with them on a plan to address this issue before taking the issue to the broader public. As you saw of the interviewees who exercised moral courage, all of them emphasized the essential feature of having a support system in place. Western cultures often believe that because we want to act responsibly, we must carry the moral weight of an issue on our individual shoulders. William May[13] points out that this is just one of the burdens we assume mistakenly. He reminds us that to cultivate strong, nurturing societies we must cultivate our civic self:

> *"The civic self, as opposed to the imperial self, understands and accepts itself as limited and amplified by others. The civic self recognizes that it enjoys an expansion of its life in and through its participation in community."*[13]

Finally, we believe they can take some steps to further enhance their judgment about how much difference their involvement is likely to make. This may not govern their decision about how and whether to proceed. It will, however, fully prepare them for their task by affirming that their act is about who they, as professionals and citizens, want to be in spite of what they may or may not be able to do about resolving this serious societal situation. This preparation helps ensure they will go forward with integrity and the inner strength they need, whatever the outcome.

Reflection

What questions do you still want answered before deciding which of several practical alternatives that Michael and his physician colleague might follow will be the best one?

_____

_____

_____

_____

Steps 5 and 6: Complete the Action and Evaluate the Process and Outcome

Reflection

Which option would you take to best achieve a caring response? Why?

_____

_____

_____

_____

For purposes of our discussion, we will assume that Michael and the physician decide they will continue to pursue the issue.

Whichever of the alternatives they choose, they will have had the opportunity before taking action to consider their roles not only as traditional members of the health professions but also as citizens in one civic issue. After the fact, they will have an opportunity to use the three spheres of moral agency that they have as professionals combined with the idea of professional responsibility to help them reflect on the experience. What they learn will help them navigate through the many civic issues they will be asked to participate in. They will also have the opportunity to share what they have learned with their professional colleagues. Sharing their knowledge and reflections will widen the knowledge of others and may inspire moral courage.

When they are engaged in their reflection, they would benefit by taking time to look outside of their own immediate situation to be reminded of other models of courage that have allowed common ordinary people to do remarkable things benefiting the society, We share one such account with you from a great American novel, John Steinbeck's[14] The Grapes of Wrath. It is a powerful literary statement about our interdependence and the will to try to help fulfill high ethical goals. In this excerpt from the novel, Tom, who sees the victimization of migrant workers during the great dust bowl years in the United States, has already begun to speak out against the perpetrators. Now we feel that the cause he embraced is embracing him. He is becoming a person of courage, deciding to join the ranks of people struggling against the injustices, and goes to let his mother know he will be leaving:

> They sat silent in the coal-black cave of vines. Ma said, "How'm I gonna know 'bout you? They might kill ya an' I wouldn' know. They might hurt ya. How'm I gonna know?"
>
> Tom laughed uneasily. "Well, maybe like Casy says, a fella ain't got a soul of his own, but on'y a piece of a big one: an' then:"
>
> "Then what, Tom?"
>
> "Then it don' matter. Then I'll be all aroun' in the dark. I'll be ever'where: wherever you look. Wherever they's a fight so hungry people can eat, I'll be there. Wherever they's a cop beatin' up a guy, I'll be there. I'll be in the way kids laugh when they're hungry an' they know supper's ready. An' when our folks eat the stuff they raise an' live in the houses they build: why, I'll be there. See?"[14]

Tom has made the decision to be where he sees an opportunity to exert his moral agency and where he believes he is situated to make a difference.

Before we leave this exploration into the coherence between your professional role and opportunity to participate effectively as a good citizen in society, we turn the lens to the question of local versus global environments where your moral agency can be effective.

Good Citizenship: Local or Global?

There is a popular adage designed to liberate caring citizens from trying to be all things to all people, namely, "Think Global, Act Local." The wisdom of this phrase seems self evident insofar as it suggests correctly that having a "global" awareness of how a local need connects to the larger human condition is a valuable resource. It also reflects that because many health professionals are by nature adventurers, wanting to save the world (while seeing the world), they can ignore their professional responsibility to be effective moral agents in their local environment where they may actually be of much more service. Their responsibility is limited to accountability to the larger world that beckons them. The idea that professional responsibility requires responsiveness to the deeper human needs of a community finds support in the idea of acting locally. Generally speaking, professionals usually can more fully comprehend the needs of a familiar community and assess what they can do to help in any of the three spheres of moral agency than if working in a geographic and social environment that is foreign. For instance, we assumed that Michael, the hometown boy who returned, had an advantage insofar as he knew these townspeople and how they might respond.

That being said, we believe your generation of health professionals will be *global citizens,* requiring new paradigms in education and practice that replace current ones based primarily on the idea of local versus global preparation and service. Some of you have come from areas that were homogenous ethnically, religiously, and in other ways, only to see the population mix dramatically shift in your lifetime. The globe is at your doorstep and, to some degree, at everyone's doorstep, everywhere. Some trends that point to an increasingly globalized world that will require our deep interdependence with others worldwide and make all health professionals global citizens include:

- An increase in the number of community-based disease prevention and health maintenance programs in all parts of the globe that can more efficiently be administered as international initiatives and that require knowledge of deeply diverse health-related issues.
- Convincing evidence of the relationship of the spread of poverty worldwide and the power of even simple on-the-ground solutions involving basic health care and clean drinking water to help minimize or reverse this fundamental source of human suffering. Such solutions already are inspiring many health professionals to seek service in poverty-immersed areas locally and globally, although almost none of them come from such environments themselves.[15]
- The health professions' response to the need for global preparedness to combat new viral strains, drug-resistant infections, and the health effects of bioterrorism, none of which are confined to national boundaries.
- Increased reliance worldwide on information technology for sharing effective diagnostic and clinical interventions.
- The ability to reach people living in the most remote areas along with more and more clinical and basic science research opportunities in their local environment.[16]
- More movement across nations and continents by unprecedented numbers of immigrants and refugees along with millions of global tourists and business people annually.
- More than ever before, opportunities for long-term or short-term professional service "abroad."
- Increasing numbers of people entering the professions with a background of international travel and living, providing them with language and other skills that increase their vision as to where their "place" in the workforce is.

Given these realities, the idea of "citizen" is comprehensible only in the context of being a global citizen. Understanding our mutual interdependence as "global civic selves" allows us not only to call on our colleagues and others worldwide to resolve problems they are more suited to handle but also to count on their support for addressing our challenges. The paradigm we offer that combines the three spheres of moral agency along with awareness of the dual aspects of responsibility is useful for determining in a general way where and around what issues you should become involved in. Your moral agency potentially can be exercised in your hometown, at the national level, or literally anywhere else in the world, depending on where you feel at home professionally.

Reflection

Of the many places you may find yourself employing your professional expertise, do you imagine them being exercised locally, or also nationally or internationally?

_____

_____

_____

_____

Summary

In this final chapter, you have had an opportunity to see yourself as a moral agent in regard to important social issues that face the larger human community. You will find a niche where your expertise, skills, standing in the community, interests, and the urgency of the needs will help you set priorities. Attentiveness to how and when to become involved depends in part on understanding the characteristics of moral agency in the three spheres of moral agency where you can express your professional responsibility. Your readiness to be a positive force in civic society whatever the circumstances is a resource well worth cultivating as a part of the larger role you have a splendid opportunity to play!

Questions for Thought and Discussion

1. Because you cannot become involved in every social issue that comes along, it is a good idea to choose the issues that hold some interest for you. If you were to become involved in trying to solve three social problems today, what would they be? Do they fall within Spheres One, Two, or Three of your moral agency?

2. Your place of employment has been designated a first response site in case of the unthinkable—a bioterrorist attack. The administration has decided to identify key personnel on a volunteer basis, hoping to create a core group that will become the chief managers and caregivers in such an exigency. Each professional employee is asked to indicate his or her willingness to be a member of the core group, and each is asked also to discuss the matter with loved ones before arriving at this decision. Some issues you are asked to consider are the heightened danger (in respect to the general population) you will be in either because the facility is hit directly or because exposed victims may quickly contaminate the facility, the likelihood that all communication will be cut off with the world outside your workplace, the likelihood that a triage network will be set up to include—and exclude—some victims for desperately needed attention, and the likelihood that you will be "locked in" and not free to leave the site until such time as you are deemed not to be a biohazard to others. Will you volunteer? On what factors do you base your decision?
3. You have been invited to become a member of a state commission that will examine how to best use public space (parks, gardens, beaches, parking areas, and so on) for the welfare of the citizens. They have asked you because they think "your expertise as a health professional is needed." What, if anything, do you think you can you bring to such a commission from the point of view of your professionalal training and expertise?
4. Homelessness has reached momentous proportions. What can your profession do about meeting the health-related needs of people for whom the street is their "home," those who do not have so much as a roof over their heads? What can you personally do? What resources do your profession and you personally have to attend to their larger social, spiritual, and psychological needs? What benefits will such involvement offer you and your profession?

REFERENCES

1. Gruen, R.L., Pearson, S.D., Brennan, T.A., 2004. Physician-citizens—Public roles and professional obligations. *JAMA* 29 (1), 94–98.
2. van Ewijk, H., 2009. Citizenship-based social work. *Int Social Work* 52 (2), 167–179.
3. Care, N., 1984. Career choice. *Ethics* 94 (2), 283–302.
4. Sullivan, W.M., 2004. *Work and integrity: The crisis and promise of professionalism in America.* Jossey-Bass Publishing Company, New York.
5. World Health Organization, 1999. *World Health report 1999.* World Health Organization, Geneva, Switzerland.

6. Blakeney, A.B., Marshall, A., 2009. Water quality, health and human occupations. *Am J Occupational Ther* 63 (1), 46–57.

7. Jennings, B., Callahan, D., Wolf, S., 1987. The professions: Public interest and the common good. *Hastings Center Report* (Suppl), 3–11.

8. United Nations Commission on Environment and Development, 1994. (Approved 2000. *The earth charter.* UNESCO Headquarters, Paris, France. Available from: <www.earthcharter.org> (accessed 02.02.10).

9. Boff, L., 2008. The ethics of care (P. Berryman, Trans.). In: Corcoran, P.B., Wohlpart, A.J. (Eds.), *A voice for Earth: American writers respond to the Earth Charter.* University of Georgia Press, Athens, GA, pp. 129–145. Quote, 149.

10. Purtilo, R., 2000. Moral courage in times of change: Visions for the future. *J Physical Ther Educ* 14 (3), 4–7.

11. Purtilo, R., 1999. Step up, speak out, stand firm! Moral courage: Lessons from South Africa. *Creighton Magazine* Fall, 20–25.

12. Bebeau, M., Rest, T., Narvaez, D., 1999. Beyond the promise: A perspective on moral education. *Educ Res* 28 (4), 22.

13. May, W.F., 2001. *Beleaguered rulers: The public obligation of the professional.* Westminster John Knox Press, Louisville, KY, pp. 188–189.

14. Steinbeck, J., 1939. *The grapes of wrath.* Penguin Books, New York, p. 535.

15. Sachs, J.D., 2006. *The end of poverty: Economic possibilities for our time.* Penguin Books, New York, pp. 233–234.

16. Millum, J., 2010. How should the benefits of bioprospecting be shared? *Hastings Center Report* 40 (1), 24–33.

Index

Page numbers followed by *b* refer to boxes; page numbers followed by *f* refer to figures; and page numbers followed by *t* refer to tables.